A PSYCHIATRIST'S GUIDE TO ADVOCACY

A PSYCHIATRIST'S GUIDE TO ADVOCACY

Edited by

Mary C. Vance, M.D., M.Sc.

Katherine G. Kennedy, M.D.

Ilse R. Wiechers, M.D., M.P.P., M.H.S.

Saul M. Levin, M.D., M.P.A., FRCP-E, FRCPsych

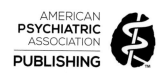

AMERICAN
PSYCHIATRIC
ASSOCIATION
PUBLISHING

If you wish to buy 50 or more copies of the same title, please go to www.appi.org/specialdiscounts for more information.

Copyright © 2020 American Psychiatric Association Publishing

ALL RIGHTS RESERVED

First Edition

Manufactured in the United States of America on acid-free paper

24   23   22   21   20   5   4   3   2   1

American Psychiatric Association Publishing
800 Maine Avenue SW
Suite 900
Washington, DC 20024-2812
www.appi.org

Library of Congress Cataloging-in-Publication Data
Names: Vance, Mary C., editor. | Kennedy, Katherine G., editor. | Wiechers, Ilse R., editor. | Levin, Saul M., editor. | American Psychiatric Association, issuing body.
Title: A psychiatrist's guide to advocacy / edited by Mary C. Vance, Katherine G. Kennedy, Ilse R. Wiechers, Saul M. Levin.
Description: First edition. | Washington, D.C. : American Psychiatric Association Publishing, [2020] | Includes bibliographical references and index.
Identifiers: LCCN 2020000545 (print) | LCCN 2020000546 (ebook) | ISBN 9781615372331 (paperback ; alk. paper) | ISBN 9781615373116 (ebook)
Subjects: MESH: Community Psychiatry | Patient Advocacy | Patient Rights
Classification: LCC RC454 (print) | LCC RC454 (ebook) | NLM WM 30.6 | DDC 616.89—dc23
LC record available at https://lccn.loc.gov/2020000545
LC ebook record available at https://lccn.loc.gov/2020000546

British Library Cataloguing in Publication Data
A CIP record is available from the British Library.

Contents

Part I
Understanding Advocacy

Part II
Practicing Advocacy

Part III
Advocacy for Special Populations

Contributors

Steven J. Ackerman, Ph.D.
Staff Psychologist, Austen Riggs Center, Stockbridge, Massachusetts

Rohul Amin, M.D., FAPA, FACP
Major, Medical Corps, United States Army; Staff Psychiatrist and Internist and Assistant Professor, USUHS-SOM; Program Director, NCC Military Psychiatry Residency Program, Bethesda, Maryland

Bachaar Arnaout, M.D.
Assistant Professor, Department of Psychiatry, Yale University, New Haven, Connecticut

Daniel S. Barron, M.D., Ph.D.
Resident Physician, Department of Psychiatry, Yale University, New Haven, Connecticut

Jessica S. Bayner, M.D.
Child and Adolescent/Adult Forensic Psychiatry Fellow, University of Pennsylvania, Philadelphia, Pennsylvania

Rebecca Weintraub Brendel, M.D., J.D.
Director, Master of Bioethics Degree Program; Associate Director, Center for Bioethics; Assistant Professor of Psychiatry, Harvard Medical School, Boston, Massachusetts

Kristin S. Budde, M.D., M.P.H.
Assistant Professor of Psychiatry, Yale University, New Haven, Connecticut

R. Dakota Carter, M.D., Ed.D.
Medical Director, Rock Prairie Behavioral Health; Medical Director, Brazos Valley Psychiatry; Adjunct Faculty, Texas A&M University Department of Psychiatry, College Station, Texas

John Chaves, M.D.
Captain, Medical Corps, United States Army; Staff Psychiatrist, Blanchfield Army Community Hospital, Fort Campbell, Kentucky

Joan M. Cook, Ph.D.
Associate Professor, Department of Psychiatry, Yale University, New Haven, Connecticut

Gary Epstein-Lubow, M.D.
Associate Professor of Psychiatry and Human Behavior and Associate Professor of Medical Science, Warren Alpert Medical School of Brown University; Associate Professor of Health Services, Policy and Practice, Brown University School of Public Health, Providence, Rhode Island

Thomas N. Franklin, M.D.
Service Chief, The Retreat at Sheppard Pratt, Baltimore, Maryland

Andrew J. Gerber, M.D., Ph.D.
President and Medical Director, Silver Hill Hospital, New Canaan, Connecticut; Associate Clinical Professor of Psychiatry, Columbia University Medical Center, New York, New York

Falisha Gilman, M.D.
General Psychiatry Resident, Department of Psychiatry, Yale University School of Medicine, New Haven, Connecticut

Jessica A. Gold, M.D., M.S.
Assistant Professor, Department of Psychiatry, Washington University in St. Louis School of Medicine, St. Louis, Missouri

Stephanie V. Hall, M.P.H.
Ph.D. student, Department of Learning Health Sciences, University of Michigan, Ann Arbor; Research Health Science Specialist, VA Ann Arbor Healthcare System, Ann Arbor, Michigan

Ayana Jordan, M.D., Ph.D.
Assistant Professor, Yale Department of Psychiatry, New Haven, Connecticut

Katherine G. Kennedy, M.D.
Assistant Clinical Professor, Department of Psychiatry, Yale University School of Medicine, New Haven, Connecticut

Jennifer Kononowech, L.M.S.W.
Project Manager, Center for Clinical Management Research, VA Ann Arbor Healthcare System, Ann Arbor, Michigan

Debra Koss, M.D., FAACAP, DFAPA
Clinical Assistant Professor, Department of Psychiatry, Rutgers-Robert Wood Johnson Medical School, Piscataway, New Jersey

Harold Kudler, M.D.
Adjunct Associate Professor, Psychiatry and Behavioral Sciences, Duke University School of Medicine, Durham, North Carolina

Saul M. Levin, M.D., M.P.A., FRCP-E, FRCPsych
Chief Executive Officer and Medical Director, American Psychiatric Association; Chair, Board of Directors, APA Foundation; Clinical Professor, George Washington University School of Medicine and Health Sciences, Washington, D.C.

Luming Li, M.D.
Assistant Professor, Department of Psychiatry, Yale School of Medicine, New Haven, Connecticut

Myra Mathis, M.D.
Addiction Psychiatry Fellow, Yale Department of Psychiatry, New Haven, Connecticut

Danna E. Mauch, Ph.D.
President and CEO, Massachusetts Association for Mental Health, Boston, Massachusetts

Eric Plakun, M.D.
Medical Director/CEO, Austen Riggs Center, Stockbridge, Massachusetts

Debra A. Pinals, M.D.
Clinical Professor of Psychiatry, University of Michigan Medical School; Clinical Adjunct Professor, University of Michigan Law School; Director, Program in Psychiatry, Law, and Ethics; Medical Director of Behavioral Health and Forensic Programs, Michigan Department of Health and Human Services, Ann Arbor, Michigan

Allison Ponce, Ph.D.
Associate Professor of Psychiatry, Yale School of Medicine, New Haven, Connecticut

Michelle B. Riba, M.D., M.S.
Professor, Department of Psychiatry, University of Michigan; Associate Director, University of Michigan Depression Center, Ann Arbor, Michigan

Michael Rowe, Ph.D.
Professor of Psychiatry, Yale School of Medicine, New Haven, Connecticut

Kaila Rudolph, M.D., M.P.H.
Attending Consultation-Liaison Psychiatrist, Boston Medical Center; Instructor of Psychiatry, Boston University School of Medicine, Boston, Massachusetts

Adam J. Sagot, D.O., FAPA
Child and Adolescent Psychiatry Fellow, Thomas Jefferson University
Hospital, Philadelphia, Pennsylvania

Melanie Scharrer, M.D.
Geriatric Psychiatry Fellow, Department of Psychiatry, University of
Wisconsin School of Medicine and Public Health, Madison, Wisconsin

Jennifer Severe, M.D.
Assistant Clinical Assistant Professor, Department of Psychiatry, University of Michigan, Ann Arbor, Michigan

Jeanne Steiner, D.O.
Professor of Psychiatry, Yale School of Medicine, New Haven, Connecticut

Allan Tasman, M.D., DFAPA, FRCP
Emeritus Professor, Chairman, and Schwab Endowed Chair in Community and Social Psychiatry, Department of Psychiatry and Behavioral Sciences, University of Louisville School of Medicine, Louisville, Kentucky

Kenneth Thompson, M.D.
Medical Director, Pennsylvania Psychiatric Leadership Council, Philadelphia, Pennsylvania

Onyi Ugorji, M.D., M.B.A.
Board-certified psychiatrist, Miami, Florida

Mary C. Vance, M.D., M.Sc.
Assistant Professor of Psychiatry and Scientist, Center for the Study of
Traumatic Stress, Uniformed Services University of the Health Sciences,
Bethesda, Maryland

Ilse R. Wiechers, M.D., M.P.P., M.H.S.
Associate Professor of Clinical Psychiatry, University of California San
Francisco, San Francisco, California; Assistant Clinical Professor of
Psychiatry, Yale University School of Medicine, New Haven, Connecticut; Associate Director, Northeast Program Evaluation Center, Office of
Mental Health and Suicide Prevention, Department of Veterans Affairs,
New Haven, Connecticut

J. Corey Williams, M.D.
Child and Adolescent Psychiatry Fellow, Children's Hospital of Philadelphia, Philadelphia, Pennsylvania

Eric Yarbrough, M.D.
Past president of AGLP: The Association of LGBTQ Psychiatrists; Chair,
Council on Minority Mental Health and Health Disparities, American
Psychiatric Association, New York, New York

Kimberly Yonkers, M.D.
Associate Professor, Department of Psychiatry, Yale University, New Haven, Connecticut

Kara Zivin, Ph.D., M.S., M.A.
Research Scientist, VA Ann Arbor Healthcare System; Professor, Department of Psychiatry, University of Michigan, Ann Arbor, Michigan

Disclosures

The following contributors to this book have indicated a financial interest in or other affiliation with a commercial supporter, a manufacturer of a commercial product, a provider of a commercial service, a nongovernmental organization, and/or a government agency, as listed below:

John Chaves, M.D. *Funding:* APA Public Psychiatry Fellowship

Gary Epstein-Lubow, M.D. Member: Advisory Council on Alzheimer's Research, Care, and Services, Certification Group, Division of Nursing Homes, CMS Center for Clinical Standards and Quality; National Committee for Quality Assurance Exclusions Expert Work Group

Adam J. Sagot, D.O., FAPA *Member:* Advisory Committee, American Academy of Child and Adolescent Psychiatry; Regional Council of Child and Adolescent Psychiatry Eastern PA/Southern NJ; Advocacy Committee, New Jersey Psychiatric Association; Graduate Medical Education Committee, Rowan University School of Osteopathic Medicine

Mary C. Vance, M.D., M.Sc. *Funding:* APA Public Psychiatry Fellowship

The following contributors have indicated that they have no financial interests or other affiliations that represent or could appear to represent a competing interest with the contributions to this book:

Steven J. Ackerman, Ph.D.; Rohul Amin, M.D., FAPA, FACP; Bachaar Arnaout, M.D.; Rebecca Brendel, M.D., J.D.; Kristin S. Budde, M.D., M.P.H.; Thomas N. Franklin, M.D.; Andrew J. Gerber, M.D., Ph.D.; Falisha Gilman, M.D.; Stephanie Hall, M.P.H.; Katherine G. Kennedy, M.D.; Jennifer Kononowech, L.M.S.W.; Debra Koss, M.D., FAACAP, DFAPA; Harold Kudler, M.D.; Saul Levin, M.D., M.P.H.; Luming Li, M.D.; Debra A. Pinals, M.D.; Michelle B. Riba, M.D., M.S.; Kaila Rudolph, M.D., M.P.H.; Jennifer Severe, M.D.; Ilse R. Wiechers, M.D., M.P.P., M.H.S.; Kara Zivin, Ph.D., M.S., M.A.

Foreword

As psychiatrists, we are some of the greatest advocates that our patients have. We work on our patients' behalf every day, convincing insurance companies that a patient needs the mental health care we are recommending, writing letters supporting a patient's request for workplace accommodations, and educating family members about the patient's illness and what the patient needs from them to get the most out of psychiatric care.

Advocacy beyond the level of the individual patient, such as before state or federal governments, takes place on a broader scale but is not very different. Rather than promote the interest of an individual patient, we focus on what the community of mental health patients, their psychiatrists, and the overall health care system needs to make quality mental health care accessible and affordable.

As a resident fellow, I was introduced to advocacy when I became a member of the American Psychiatric Association's (APA's) Joint Commission on Government Relations, now called the Council on Advocacy and Government Relations. Advocacy giants taught me the importance of having practitioners and patients speak regularly to their legislators on the national and state levels about the difficulties they are facing and how these problems can be solved. It became clear to me that if we as psychiatrists did not advocate for our patients and the profession, we would never achieve parity between mental health care (including for substance use disorders) and all other medical care. And, in fact, that is what we did.

Collectively, the tens of thousands of psychiatrists who belong to the APA combined forces with other advocates for mental health and worked tirelessly for years to convince Congress that mental health was not less significant than cancer or diabetes to the health of our nation. As a result, we saw the passage of the Mental Health Parity and Addiction Equity Act in 2008. This act was a significant step toward equality for mental health care, payment parity for psychiatry, and equity in the treatment of the serious diseases with which our patients struggle.

Through actively educating decision makers, building relationships with them and their staff, and repeatedly making personal contact, we can effect meaningful change.

Supporting advocacy in the political context is also extremely important. Through APA's Political Action Committee, psychiatrists are able to support candidates who are willing to listen to our patients' stories, promote a mental health agenda that includes better access to care, advocate research funding, and allocate the funds necessary for psychiatric residency programs to meet the growing demand for mental health care.

I quickly learned that we do not need to be professional lobbyists to effectively advocate for our patients and our profession. Indeed, it is often the personal stories of constituent patients, family members, and psychiatrists that are the most persuasive and motivating in conversations with our elected representatives. Our knowledge, experience, professional affiliation, ability to share experiences, and right to vote all give us tremendous power. Psychiatrists are in a position to impact where and how patients receive their care, the quality of care they receive, and the future of our profession.

I encourage all of my colleagues to embrace this opportunity to improve lives and to ensure continued progress in the diagnosis and treatment of mental illness, including substance use disorders. I acknowledge that the beautiful iconic buildings of Washington, D.C., such as the U.S. Capitol, and similarly beautiful state capitol buildings can be very intimidating. However, we need to remember that legislators are influential people and are in a unique position to help or produce challenges for our profession and our patients.

This book helps you build the skills and confidence that make advocacy less intimidating and mysterious in those grand settings of legislators. In addition to discussing the critical work of legislative advocacy, the book also explores multiple other forms of advocacy that can create meaningful change and addresses the specific advocacy needs of several special populations. I am impressed with the expertise and experience of the contributors to this book. Their insights make for a good educational read that provides illuminating facts and case studies that will enable you to engage families, patients, and other physicians to become advocates for improving mental health access and the quality of mental health care in this country.

Enjoy, learn, and *act* on that knowledge. APA and its advocacy and policy experts are standing by ready to assist you!

Saul M. Levin, M.D., M.P.A., FRCPhysicians-E, FRCPsych

Acknowledgments

The editors would like to thank the following individuals for their generous contributions of time, expertise, and assistance with the process of bringing this book to fruition: James Batterson, Tanya Bradsher, Colleen Coyle, Yoshie Davison, Jon Fanning, Kristin Kroeger, Katie Ling, John McDuffie, Craig Obey, Ranna Parekh, Erika Parker, Debra Pinals, Mary Raucci, Laura Roberts, Patrick Runnels, and Daphna Stroumsa.

In addition, we would like to express our deep gratitude to our families and friends, who helped us with all aspects of our lives, from housework to homework to health issues, while we labored over language and struggled with sentence structures. A special shout-out goes to Marcus and Izzy; Ted, Kiley, and Teddy; and Mike and Maggie.

PART I
Understanding Advocacy

What Is Advocacy, and Why Is It Important?

Mary C. Vance, M.D., M.Sc.
Ilse R. Wiechers, M.D., M.P.P., M.H.S.
Katherine G. Kennedy, M.D.

Learning Objectives

By the end of this chapter, readers will be able to:

- Define the role of the physician-advocate
- Provide historical and recent examples of advocacy by physicians
- Describe why psychiatrists are needed as advocates in this era of rapidly changing mental health care systems

Physicians as Advocates: Defining Advocacy in Medicine

All physicians can be advocates.

In recent years, advocacy as a professional responsibility has begun to gain widespread recognition in the "house of medicine." In 2001, the American Medical Association adopted the "Declaration of Professional Responsibility: Medicine's Social Contract With Humanity," which states that physicians should "advocate for social, economic, educational, and political changes that ameliorate suffering and contribute to human well-being" (American Medical Association 2001, p. 195). Advocacy is generically defined as "the act or process of supporting a cause or proposal" (Merriam-Webster 2019). Applied specifically to health care, advocacy can be defined as *the public voicing of support for causes, policies, or opinions that advance patient and population health.*

When we consider this health care–specific definition and terminology, we can understand *advocacy* as a broad term that encompasses a wide variety of actions physicians can take to improve the health of patients and the health care systems that serve them—or fail to serve them. We can define *physician-advocates* as physicians who strive to enact changes that will be beneficial to patients and crucial to the continued improvement and even survival of our health care systems. Furthermore, physician-advocates consistently strive to act in the best interests and according to the values of the patients, communities, and populations served. Although such advocacy may require that we take stances on political or legislative issues, it does not provide an opportunity for us to express our personal political beliefs (which is more appropriately accomplished by advocating as private citizens). Any stances we take as physicians should reflect our informed medical opinions on how best to advance the health care that our patients receive and the health of the communities in which they live, in accordance with their values and best interests.

Advocacy may not be formally taught during medical training, but it is a ubiquitous part of physicians' daily work. (New efforts to teach advocacy in psychiatry residency training programs are described in Chapter 8, "Education as Advocacy.") For example, a physician may advocate by calling an insurer repeatedly for authorization of health care coverage that has been unfairly denied to a patient or by pointing out discriminatory practices in medical settings against individuals who have mental illness and/or who are members of other historically marginalized groups (Chapter 5, "Patient-Level Advocacy"). An organizational physician-advocate may join a hospital task force that is aimed at improving care for chronic conditions by assisting with logistical barriers to attending appointments (Chapter 6, "Organizational Advocacy"). Advocacy at the population level, such as with local, state, and federal governments (Chapter 7, "Legislative Advocacy"), can spur critical changes to the system of health care. Writing op-eds and posting on social media our professional opinions about health care topics are forms of advocacy (Chapter 10, "Engaging the Popular Media"), as are educating medical trainees to be attuned to inequities in the health care system (Chapter 8, "Education as Advocacy") and producing high-quality research that helps to shape more informed and humane public policies (Chapter 9, "Research as Advocacy").

Although we began this chapter with the statement that all physicians can be advocates, as you can see, most of us already *are* physician-advocates—perhaps without even realizing it.

Psychiatrists as Advocates: A Call to Action

The field of psychiatry is in need of physician-advocates. Mental health disorders, including substance use disorders, affect a large proportion of the U.S. population: an estimated 1 in 5 adults, or 46.6 million people, suffer from mental illness in a given year (National Alliance on Mental Illness 2019). Among youth, approximately 1 in 5 American adolescents ages 13–18 have experienced mental health problems during their lives (National Alliance on Mental Illness 2019). In fact, the World Health Organization (2011) attributes a full 30.9% of the global burden of disease in the United States to psychiatric disorders. Mental health disorders are well known to contribute to decreased quality of life and premature death, including from suicide but also from treatable medical conditions such as cardiovascular disease (Brown et al. 2010). In addition, the economic cost of mental illness is enormous; the World Economic Forum (2011) estimates that mental illness accounts for the largest share of global economic burden among noncommunicable diseases.

Despite the prevalence and individual and societal toll of mental illness, less than half of individuals with mental illness received any treatment during the past year (National Alliance on Mental Illness 2019). Access to care is a pressing issue, especially given the shortage of psychiatrists nationwide and the lack of enforcement of mental health parity laws in many jurisdictions (Douglas et al. 2018). Stigma against mental illness, including substance use disorders, also looms large and prevents many individuals from seeking necessary treatment.

Moreover, patients with mental illness may be less able to effectively advocate for themselves than are patients with nonpsychiatric diagnoses. This is in part because their psychiatric symptoms may interfere. For example, they may be too disorganized or too depressed to be able to effectively advocate for themselves. Even when they are able to advocate, societal stigma, bias, and discrimination against individuals with mental illness may still limit the extent to which their voices are heard. For example, other people may not believe legitimate concerns voiced by an individual with mental illness, on the assumption that the illness is affecting the person's judgment. These factors mean that individuals with mental illness are less likely to have social and political capital, and their needs and wishes are more likely to be ignored or unknown.

Psychiatrists are uniquely equipped to provide medical leadership beyond clinical issues toward larger societal issues pertaining to mental health. As physicians, we receive extensive training in the biology of the body and mind during medical school and then during residency gain deep expertise in the diagnosis of the full range of mental illnesses as well as their treatments, both psychopharmacological and psychothera-peutic. Some of us undertake even more subspecialty training during fellowships prior to entering practice. We are critical to the functioning of the mental health care system and have a broad view of its workings. As physicians, our job title and medical expertise also give us a place of respect within society. For these reasons, we are ideally positioned to lead the way in advocacy for mental health.

Psychiatry is also arguably the most controversial specialty in the house of medicine, which only increases the need for advocacy in this field. Because the illnesses we treat are often "invisible" (both physically and in terms of diagnostic testing) and because they can profoundly alter the way individuals experience and are experienced by the world, they are imbued with a mystique that can quickly escalate to fear and judgment, especially during times of political turmoil. Across nations and across time, psychiatric labels and treatments have been particularly vulnerable to being used as tools of social control. Among medical diagnoses, mental illness diagnoses are especially prone to being influenced by changing societal attitudes about what is behaviorally "normal" or "abnormal."

These factors contribute to a variable and at times hostile perception of psychiatry in modern popular culture. There is no "anti-pediatrics" or "anti-nephrology" movement, but there is an active and vocal anti-psychiatry movement. Chemotherapy, which has both lifesaving properties and potentially severe side effects, is not generally considered to be a barbaric and unnecessary treatment, but electroconvulsive therapy, which also has lifesaving properties and potentially severe side effects, sometimes is. Given the historical background and the current atmosphere surrounding psychiatry, our field urgently needs ethical, effective, and humanitarian advocates at its helm, both to promote the fair and equal treatment of individuals with mental illness and to guard against potential future injustices against our patients and our profession.

In addition, before the advent of the medical-industrial complex and today's complicated health care systems, the quality of care that a patient experienced depended primarily on factors within the provider-

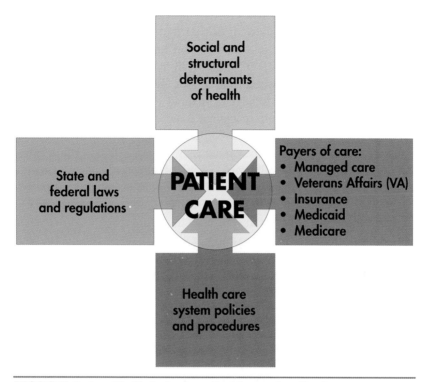

FIGURE 1–1.   **Multiple factors that impact patient care.**

patient dyad. Today, however, the provider and patient are no longer truly autonomous when they make mental health care decisions, and multiple factors now impact the type and quality of care that a patient receives. These include the payers who finance the care, the health care systems where the care is received, and the state and federal regulations that govern the care. Also, we now understand the powerful role that social and structural determinants of health play in contributing to health care outcomes, including mental health outcomes, and these must also be considered whenever we as physicians engage in advocacy. Given this complex interplay of factors influencing mental health care in the modern era (Figure 1–1), psychiatrist-advocates are needed now more than ever to ensure high-quality, equitable care for our patients.

Finally, our mental health care system is in the process of undergoing enormous transformation. The decisions made in the next few years will impact the way health care is organized and delivered for generations to come. Understanding how to advocate for a better mental health care delivery system is critical to ensuring that patients have access to quality mental health care services.

All of these various considerations boil down to one point: we, as psychiatrists, must advocate for our patients. In some cases, such as when patients are incapacitated by symptomatic mental illness, we must advocate *on behalf of* our patients, by acting in their best interests when they have a diminished capacity for effective advocacy. In other cases, such as when they do have the agency to advocate for themselves but need a physician's help to navigate the complexities of the health care system, we must advocate *in support of* our patients and lend our voices and our expertise to the causes they believe will have the greatest positive impact on their well-being. In still other cases, such as when patients and psychiatrists are both stakeholders who would be impacted by proposed legislative changes, our role is to advocate *alongside* our patients, joining with them in solidarity to ensure a health care system that will benefit both their care and our ability to deliver it. Our clinical work as psychiatrists already improves the mental health of patients— and our advocacy work as psychiatrists will improve the mental health of patients, populations, and nations.

Health Advocacy: Historical Context and Recent Trends

There is no single, unified history of health advocacy, in part because what we consider advocacy in this book and in these times has been, and still is, known by various names. That being said, the field of social medicine offers a useful example of an academic medical discipline that contains components of advocacy at its core (Geiger 2017). German physician Rudolph Virchow (1821–1902), a foundational figure in social medicine, wrote, "Medicine is a social science, and politics nothing but medicine at a larger scale" (Mackenbach 2009, p. 181). It has been argued that this oft-quoted statement is a summary of "public health's biggest idea: human health and disease are the embodiment of the successes and failures of society as a whole, and the only way to improve health and reduce disease is by changing society by, therefore, political action" (Mackenbach 2009, p. 181). In this spirit, social medicine looks beyond the health of individuals to the health of populations and holds that physician involvement in shaping what are known today as the social and structural determinants of health is necessary for healthy individuals, populations, and societies. This involvement can take place through public health efforts and, of course, through political and other forms of advocacy.

The history of medicine contains many examples of advocacy, at both the individual and the collective levels, by both physicians and nonphysicians. In the area of mental health, perhaps one of the best-known historical examples of advocacy is that of Dorothea Dix (1802–1887), whose vigorous and steadfast advocacy efforts on behalf of impoverished individuals with mental illness led to the opening of the first mental asylums in the United States. Florence Nightingale (1820–1910), the founder of modern nursing, also led multiple advocacy efforts that resulted in social reform, including for improved hospital sanitation and for increased acceptance of women in the workforce, especially as nurses. Dr. Ignaz Semmelweis (1818–1865), a Hungarian physician, advocated for the practice of handwashing prior to contact with obstetric patients in order to reduce infection; although he was ridiculed for this advice and died years before his practice was validated, we remember him today as a pioneer of germ theory who saved the lives of numerous mothers. Examples of more recent advocacy efforts in medicine, including by physicians, are the promotion of seat belt use in vehicles, the placement of health warning labels on cigarette packs, the removal of homosexuality as a DSM diagnosis, and health education campaigns about the human papillomavirus (HPV) vaccine. Many more examples of recent and current advocacy efforts by physicians, especially psychiatrists, ranging from the everyday advocacy associated with individual patient care to collective advocacy efforts for sweeping changes in health care, can be found throughout the pages of this book.

As these examples show, health advocacy can take many forms and span many health concerns. Furthermore, physician health advocates need not limit themselves to speaking out only about issues directly related to health care (e.g., cigarette smoking, seat belt use); there are precedents in which physicians have sought to, and succeeded in, advocating on larger societal issues that are likely to impact health (e.g., nuclear warfare, climate change). Finally, not all of the examples we discuss in this book feature what are universally considered to be forms of advocacy, but we argue here, and throughout this book, that they really *are* forms of advocacy. We believe that this more inclusive approach democratizes the idea of advocacy, encourages more engagement in advocacy, and allows previously unacknowledged ways of impacting meaningful change to be named and appreciated as the acts of courage and vision that they are.

Traditional medical training is not known for producing advocates. In fact, if we consider advocacy to be an act of enlarging our view beyond the problems of individual patients to the problems of populations and societies, traditional medical training does the exact opposite: it finely hones our ability to understand health and disease in individual patients, while largely ignoring how societal contributions influence those states of health and disease. One factor underlying this educational omission can be attributed to the need to prioritize basic competency in the care of individual patients, which, of course, is required in order to be a physician. Another factor may have to do with prevailing attitudes about the physician's proper role in society.

There are those who assert that advocacy beyond the level of the individual patient falls outside of a physician's professional concerns because "political advocacy is detached from the doctor-patient relationship" (Huddle 2011, p. 380). However, this assertion is based on the underlying belief that there is such a thing as "pure" medicine untouched by the "toxins" of the social and political contexts in which that medicine is practiced—a belief we argue is both erroneous and detrimental to our patients and our profession because it allows sociopolitical interest groups, often financially motivated, to capitalize on our inaction. As the saying goes, "If you're not at the table, you're on the menu." If we as psychiatrists, the physician leaders in mental health care, do not advocate for our patients, then who will? Silence on our part would mean putting our patients at risk for even greater disenfranchisement and discrimination. Psychiatrists must advocate to block actions, programs, and legislation that could potentially harm patients or worsen the systems in which patient care is embedded, as well as to advance those that serve our patients' best interests and improve their health and well-being.

Fortunately, over the past several decades, the medical profession has come a long way in confronting the reality of the social and political factors that influence our patients' health and the health care system. Interest in health advocacy among physicians and other health care professionals has increased substantially, in concert with rising concerns about the sustainability of the current health care environment and the efficiency, quality, and value of the health care that is currently delivered. As a rough demonstration of this burgeoning interest, entering the term "health advocacy" into Google Ngram Viewer (a search engine that charts the frequencies of words and phrases found in printed sources over time) shows a dramatic and continuing increase in the use of the term since the late 1960s (Figure 1–2).

Advocacy as Professional Responsibility

Both professional societies and medical training organizations have increasingly acknowledged advocacy as a core professional responsibility among physicians. As mentioned at the beginning of this chapter, in 2001, the AMA listed advocacy as a fundamental responsibility of phy-

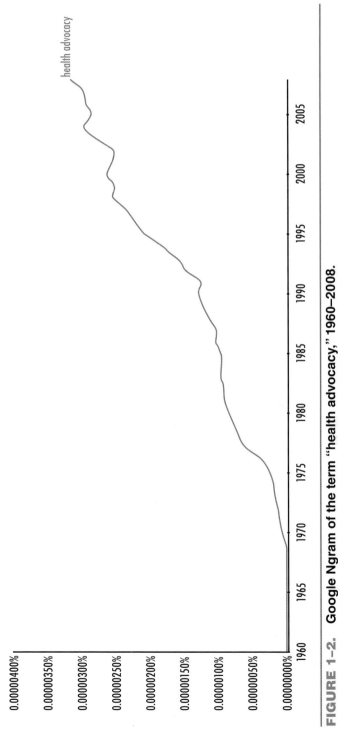

FIGURE 1–2. **Google Ngram of the term "health advocacy," 1960–2008.**

Source. Google Books: Ngram viewer. Available at: https://books.google.com/ngrams/graph?content=health+advocacy&year_start=1960 &year_end=2008&corpus=15&smoothing=3&share=&direct_url=t1%3B%2Chealth%20advocacy%3B%2Cco. Accessed August 19, 2019.

sicians in its Declaration of Professional Responsibility (American Medical Association 2001). Similarly, the medical training framework of the Royal College of Physicians and Surgeons of Canada includes the "health advocate" role as one of seven essential competencies to be addressed in medical education (Frank et al. 2015).

Psychiatry has followed suit in this trend toward increased recognition and teaching of advocacy. In 2002, the American Psychiatric Association's (APA's) Board of Trustees officially endorsed the AMA's Declaration of Professional Responsibility, including its clause on advocacy (American Psychiatric Association 2002). In terms of advocacy teaching, the Accreditation Council for Graduate Medical Education (ACGME) in psychiatry now considers "advocating for quality patient care and optimal patient care systems" to be a competency under the domain of "systems-based practice" (Accreditation Council for Graduate Medical Education 2019). The Psychiatry Milestone Project, a joint effort of the ACGME and the American Board of Psychiatry and Neurology (ABPN), also mentions advocacy as a competency under multiple domains, including those of medical knowledge, systems-based practice, and professionalism (Accreditation Council for Graduate Medical Education and American Board of Psychiatry and Neurology 2015).

Still, compared with some other medical specialties, psychiatry has a less robust tradition of advocacy teaching and lags behind in terms of advocacy engagement and effectiveness (for more information, see Chapter 8, "Education as Advocacy," and Chapter 11, "Advocacy for Children and Families"). Because psychiatry is a specialty with a high need for advocacy, encouraging a greater culture of advocacy among our fellow psychiatrists is of paramount importance if we are to effect broad and lasting changes for our patients and our profession. This attention to advocacy as one of our core professional responsibilities should begin in medical school, continue throughout residency and fellowship, and last over the entire course of a psychiatrist's career. However, that is easier said than done because advocacy remains a "frontier" in medical education and practice. Achieving a strong and sustained culture of advocacy in the field of psychiatry will require a mass paradigm shift in the way we think about our professional responsibilities to our patients, our profession, and our society as a whole—which begins by clearly conceptualizing what advocacy is and defining its boundaries, norms, and best practices.

About This Book

It is our hope that this book will lay the foundation for how we can all embrace our role as psychiatrist-advocates, by providing both a theoretical understanding and a practical toolkit for mental health advocacy in its myriad forms. We firmly believe that there are many ways to advocate, and therefore we have devoted chapters to multiple types and levels of advocacy and to the specific advocacy concerns of particular populations. We further firmly believe that at all stages of our careers, we as psychiatrists can be effective advocates and that each generation of psychiatrists contributes its own unique and critical advocacy voice and vision. To reflect our conviction, we have invited psychiatrists from a wide variety of career stages to author chapters in this book, and the book contains guidance that is relevant to new and seasoned advocates alike, from medical students to late-career psychiatrists.

To this point in the chapter, we have defined *advocacy* as it applies to health care; argued for the importance of advocacy, especially in psychiatry; and given historical and recent examples of health-related advocacy. In the rest of Part I, "Understanding Advocacy," we address how to think about advocacy conceptually and outline general ethical principles to consider when engaging in advocacy (Chapter 2); describe several seminal advocacy issues within psychiatry that impact both our patients and our profession, as well as ways we might tackle them (Chapter 3); and provide an overview of the skills and knowledge needed to become an advocate (Chapter 4).

We then shift from discussing the theoretical aspects of advocacy in psychiatry to discussing its practical aspects—that is, how to actually do the work of advocacy in multiple contexts. In Part II, "Practicing Advocacy," we consider advocacy engagement at several of the different levels of advocacy (Chapters 5–7) as well as within several of the different types of advocacy (Chapters 8–10). Although we cannot exhaustively cover all of the possible levels and types of advocacy, we believe that the chapters in this part of the book provide a foundational introduction to some of the most common ones.

In Part III, "Advocacy for Special Populations," we home in on the unique advocacy needs of certain special populations (Chapters 11–20). Again, this part of the book is not an exhaustive catalogue of all the patient populations that may have unique advocacy needs. However, it aims to be a starting point for conversations about how we can best advocate for these and other patients whose specific concerns and social and structural determinants of health must be taken into account both in clinical care and in advocacy.

Finally, Chapters 3, 4, 6, and 10 include short interviews with *advocacy role models*. These are real psychiatrist-advocates at different stages of their careers who come from a variety of backgrounds and have dedicated themselves to addressing different advocacy issues through various methods of advocacy. We hope that the advocacy success stories of these psychiatrists will inspire and motivate you and other current or budding psychiatrist-advocates who are reading this book to keep sharpening your advocacy skills and to stay confident that our efforts *do* make a difference.

All psychiatrists can be advocates, and more psychiatrists are becoming advocates every day. By sharing our experiences, encouraging each other, and fostering a culture of advocacy within our profession, we will become an organized, impassioned, and effective group of psychiatrist-advocates at the front lines of shaping the future of mental health care.

References

Accreditation Council for Graduate Medical Education: ACGME program requirements for graduate medical education in psychiatry. Chicago, IL, Accreditation Council for Graduate Medical Education, 2019. Available at: www.acgme.org/Portals/0/PFAssets/ProgramRequirements/400_Psychiatry_2019.pdf?ver=2019-08-26-134127-827. Accessed December 14, 2019.

Accreditation Council for Graduate Medical Education, American Board of Psychiatry and Neurology: The Psychiatry Milestone Project. Chicago, IL, Accreditation Council for Graduate Medical Education, July 2015. Available at: www.acgme.org/Portals/0/PDFs/Milestones/PsychiatryMilestones.pdf. Accessed August 19, 2019.

American Medical Association: Declaration of professional responsibility: medicine's social contract with humanity. Mo Med 99(5):195, 2001 12025762

American Psychiatric Association: Declaration of professional responsibility. Psychiatric News, July 19, 2002. Available at: https://psychnews.psychiatryonline.org/doi/full/10.1176/pn.37.14.0004a. Accessed August 19, 2019.

Brown S, Kim M, Mitchell C, et al: Twenty-five year mortality of a community cohort with schizophrenia. Br J Psychiatry 196(2):116–121, 2010 20118455

Douglas M, Wrenn G, Bent-Weber S, et al: Evaluating state mental health and addiction parity laws: a technical report. The Kennedy Forum, 2018. Available at: https://pdfs.semanticscholar.org/22e4/c65c3c24a407a7d764d76f847c0a56462abe.pdf. Accessed August 19, 2019.

Frank JR, Snell L, Sherbino J (eds): CanMEDS 2015 Physician Competency Framework. Ottawa, ON, Canada, Royal College of Physicians and Surgeons of Canada, 2015

Geiger HJ: The political future of social medicine: reflections on physicians as activists. Acad Med 92(3):282–284, 2017 28030421

Huddle TS: Perspective: Medical professionalism and medical education should not involve commitments to political advocacy. Acad Med 86(3):378–383, 2011 21248605

Mackenbach JP: Politics is nothing but medicine at a larger scale: reflections on public health's biggest idea. J Epidemiol Community Health 63(3):181–184, 2009 19052033

Merriam-Webster: Advocacy. Merriam-Webster Dictionary, 2019. Available at: www.merriam-webster.com/dictionary/advocacy. Accessed August 19, 2019.

National Alliance on Mental Illness: Mental health by the numbers. Arlington, VA, National Alliance on Mental Illness, 2019. Available at: www.nami.org/Learn-More/Mental-Health-By-the-Numbers. Accessed August 19, 2019.

World Economic Forum: The global economic burden of non-communicable diseases. Cologny, Switzerland, World Economic Forum, September 2011. Available at: www3.weforum.org/docs/WEF_Harvard_HE_GlobalEconomic BurdenNonCommunicableDiseases_2011.pdf. Accessed on August 19, 2019.

World Health Organization: Mental health atlas 2011. Geneva, Switzerland, World Health Organization, 2011. Available at: www.who.int/mental_health/evidence/atlas/profiles/usa_mh_profile.pdf?ua=1andua=1. Accessed on August 19, 2019.

2

Conceptualizing Advocacy

Ilse R. Wiechers, M.D., M.P.P., M.H.S.
Debra A. Pinals, M.D.
Danna E. Mauch, Ph.D.
Kaila Rudolph, M.D., M.P.H., M.B.E.
Katherine G. Kennedy, M.D.
Mary C. Vance, M.D., M.Sc.

Learning Objectives

By the end of this chapter, readers will be able to:

- Understand the levels of advocacy
- Describe several usable theories for advocacy and policy change
- Discuss factors in effective advocacy
- Identify ethical considerations to keep in mind when engaging in advocacy
- Promote the idea of an advocacy specialization

To better develop the concept of a physician-advocate, in this chapter we discuss the different levels of advocacy, some usable theories for advocacy and policy change, factors in effective advocacy, ethical considerations in advocacy, and the idea of an advocacy "specialization." We hope that this conceptual discussion will provide a framework to guide your thinking about advocacy. This chapter provides a broad overview, and many of the concepts covered here will be explored in more detail in later chapters.

Levels of Advocacy

As depicted in Figure 2–1, advocacy can take place at various levels, ranging in scale from advocacy for an individual patient to advocacy for issues of national or even global impact. Establishing a clear understanding of the level at which an advocacy effort takes place helps to frame the scope of the work as well as to identify the stakeholders who need to be engaged.

Patient-Level Advocacy

Patient-level advocacy aims to improve the health and well-being of individual patients by attending to the societal forces that shape their life and health. Not uncommonly, advocating for individual patients means advocating for their families or caregivers as well because the same forces that impact patients often impact their families (for more information, see Chapter 11, "Advocacy for Children and Families"; Chapter 12, "Advocacy for Older Adults"; and Chapter 18, "Advocacy for Patients in Medical Settings"). Patient-level advocacy also includes advocacy on behalf of the patient within the medical team or among different teams or services providing care for the patient (see Chapter 18). This level of advocacy lies at the heart of health advocacy because it goes one step beyond the medical care we routinely provide and because it is the most accessible form of advocacy even when time pressures may make larger-scale advocacy goals seem more aspirational.

Organizational-Level Advocacy

Advocacy within an organization (e.g., hospital, health system, insurance company) can be highly impactful for patient care and is sometimes a more feasible way to create change for a population than directly addressing local, state, or federal legislation (see Chapter 6, "Organizational Advocacy"). This kind of advocacy often focuses on changing organizational policies, processes, or allocation of resources.

Stakeholders at the health system level may include hospital senior management such as the chief executive officer, clinical department heads, patient advocacy department members, physician and allied health care providers, and health care consumers (Pandi-Perumal et al. 2015). Health system–level advocacy working groups may comprise physicians, allied health personnel, hospital unit administrators, and research team members. The products and process of advocacy at the health system level may be disseminated though hospital-wide education campaigns, lecture series, the hospital website, the electronic medical record system, and academic publication.

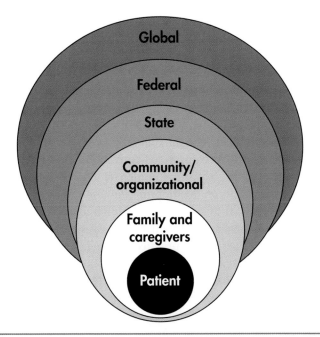

FIGURE 2-1. Primary advocacy levels.

Barriers to interventions at the health system level include prioritization of competing clinical duties, clinician lack of knowledge of the stakeholder engagement process, limited hospital mentorships and partnerships to support clinician completion of large-scale hospital-wide initiatives, and absence of hospital administrative support to coordinate stakeholder and team meetings. Despite these barriers, training, creativity, and persistence can go a long way toward building effective organizational advocacy efforts.

Population-Level Advocacy

Local, state, federal, and even global health reforms can be achieved by collaborating with key stakeholders to improve health laws, policies, funding, and social programming models to enhance population health. Key principles for legislative advocacy are discussed in detail in Chapter 7, "Legislative Advocacy."

Engaging community partners in advocacy at the local level—and often state and even federal levels—is essential for successful advocacy efforts. In accordance with the unique project goals, community partners may act as decision makers, provide guidance and feedback, or deliver health care services (World Health Organization 2003). A community organization may be selected for partnerships on the basis of such criteria as preexisting relationships with the health institution or history of successful partnerships, shared interests, target population, location, and skilled workforce.

The leader or leaders of a community and/or community organization should be contacted and a meeting arranged to discuss potential collaboration (Israel et al. 1998). Preparation for this meeting relies on principles reviewed earlier regarding stakeholder partnerships (see section "Organizational Level Advocacy"). With the support of a community leader, a joint meeting between the remaining members of the health institution and community organization teams should be arranged to solidify commitment to partnership development (Israel et al. 1998). Because power differentials between health professionals and community members may be present, it is critical to establish a safe environment in which group norms such as active listening, respectful disagreement, honesty, and acceptance will be practiced (Israel et al. 1998).

The community organization and health care professionals must then establish a set of shared goals and objectives to guide the partnership and specific tasks to be completed by each organization (Israel et al. 1998). It is important to determine in advance how decisions will be made, to have a plan for funding sources and resource allocation, and to decide on meeting frequency (Israel et al. 1998). Successful partnerships will generate a collaborative advocacy proposal for implementation, consistent with the shared organizational goals.

Usable Theories for Advocacy and Policy Change

When undertaking advocacy at a patient level, an organizational level, or a population level, new advocates might consider what is known in both theory and practice about impactful intervention. Knowledge of advocacy theory and practice can support physician-advocates in choosing a strategy that best fits the advocacy challenge and level of intervention in assessing advocacy capacity and achieving desired outcomes. A brief review of global and tactical theories of advocacy follows (for deeper detail on these topics, see Stachowiak 2013).

Brief Review of Global Theories of Advocacy

Global theories of advocacy include the following: policy windows or agenda-setting model, power politics or power elites theory/regime theory, coalition theory and advocacy coalition framework, and large leaps theory (Stachowiak 2013). In this subsection, we summarize two global theories commonly employed in health and social welfare advocacy initiatives.

Policy Windows or Agenda-Setting Model

Kingdon (1984) theorized that policy change advocacy is best undertaken during a "window of opportunity" when advocates can connect multiple components of the public policy process for larger impact. This linkage of components may involve some combination of 1) problem definition, 2) proposed policy solution, and 3) ripe policy climate. This window may arise as an opportunity to link a change in the making with your policy agenda to shape the result in a way that addresses your policy concern. Windows of opportunity often arise after media reports, following a high-profile incident, or with transitions in leadership.

For example, emergency department (ED) boarding is a system-level problem with patient-level consequences that disproportionately impacts psychiatric patients who wait hours, days, and in some cases weeks longer in emergency rooms than do other medical patients following screening for admission to hospital beds. ED boarding is a result of many factors, including poor staffing for psychiatric evaluation in EDs, higher thresholds for admission to psychiatric beds, problems of geographic accessibility of psychiatric beds, limited numbers of psychiatric beds serving certain age or diagnostic groups, prior authorization requirements of insurers, and inflexible inpatient staffing levels that dissuade units from admitting high-acuity patients. In some cases, ED boarding has been associated with increased use of law enforcement interventions, such as when a patient becomes angry about waiting, has a behavioral disruption, and is arrested out of the ED.

Case Example: ED Boarding

Dr. N, a psychiatrist who was serving as the chief medical officer for behavioral health of a large health insurer and health plan, was instrumental in changing prior approval and supplemental staffing policies, resulting in significantly reduced time in ED boarding for the plan's patients. As a physician leader who was recognized as a clinical expert and policy thought leader, Dr. N was able to leverage a high-profile series of press reports, legislative hearings, and research studies (problem definition) with the public-private sector effort to address ED boarding that followed (creating a ripe policy climate and window of opportunity). His long experience working in public and private systems lent credibility to and ensured feasibility of several defined policy solutions that would mitigate factors of ED boarding and provide relief to the health plan's members.

Case Example: ED Boarding *(continued)*

Dr. N used the data produced in the research studies, which revealed how many hours patients were delayed in EDs while the prior authorization process was under way, along with data detailing the number of patients denied admission at hospitals because they were considered "too acute" to admit given the current patient mix and staffing levels. These patients who were deemed "too acute" were often described as having behavioral challenges that in other cases might have been criminalized or have resulted in an arrest. Dr. N determined that lifting his health plan's prior authorization requirement for inpatient admission would save hours or even as long as a full day that his plan members languished in EDs. Similarly, he determined that establishing a protocol for selective approval of additional payments for authorized use of one-to-one staffing would clear the way for admission of certain patients who waited days in EDs for admission. Using his long-established credibility, his access to health plan executives, his command of the data, and his solutions that benefited patients and lowered costs, he was able to advocate for changed policy and solved ED boarding for a significant number of his health plan's patients.

Power Politics or Power Elites Theory

Mills (1956) wrote about policy change forged by working directly with individuals in positions of executive, judicial, or legislative power. Tasks might include forming alliances with those wielding power on issues of concern, focusing on policy decisions in support of program and practice change, focusing on legal and regulatory requirements to drive and cement change, and/or focusing on budget and reimbursement decisions to implement and sustain change.

Psychiatrists serving in leadership roles in state government agencies are in a unique position to advocate at a system level and to employ power politics or power elites theory. Those who serve as state mental health or behavioral health directors, medical directors, Medicaid directors, or mental health commissioners operate in the corridors of executive and judicial power on a daily basis and have opportunities to form working alliances with their colleagues across government. Examples of the power of their influence date to the 1970s and 1980s, when they deployed their advocacy to end long-term institutionalization of persons with psychiatric and developmental disabilities. The following are more recent examples:

- Psychiatrists in leadership roles are attempting to examine strategies to manage populations of individuals with mental illness who require expanded reentry services from jails and prisons.
- At New York City's Rikers Island jail complex, an inside psychiatric leader and others are helping to improve the conditions of confinement.
- In Massachusetts, inside advocates within mental health systems have partnered actively with judges and other stakeholders to expand and develop specialty courts.

Brief Review of Tactical Theories of Advocacy

Tactical theories of advocacy include messaging and frameworks or prospect theory, media influence or agenda setting theory, grassroots and community organizing theory, group formation or self-categorization theory, and diffusion theory or diffusion of innovations theory (Stachowiak 2013). Two tactical theories commonly employed in health and social welfare advocacy initiatives are summarized as follows.

Group Formation

As described by Tajfel and Turner (1986), the group formation approach represents policy change achieved through collective action with other members of an affinity group directly affected by a particular issue or set of related issues. Advocates encourage those identifying with the group to act in ways that align with group interests, policy, or change agendas. Theorists note that cohesion among an organization's members is a prerequisite for change, which speaks to a strategy of using groups with a history of working together for change.

Diffusion Theory

Rogers (1995) developed diffusion theory to represent change that happens when a new program model or policy idea is communicated to a critical mass of people or decision makers who view the innovation as superior or inevitable and agree to adopt the policy or practice. Change happens when positive program outcomes, proofs of concept, and/or return on investment analyses catch the attention of decision makers and policy leaders.

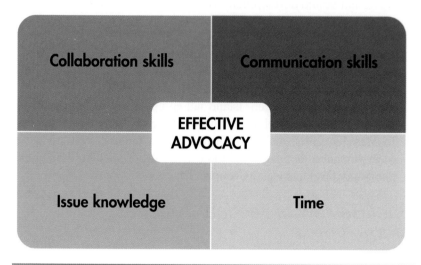

FIGURE 2–2. Factors in effective advocacy.

Factors in Effective Advocacy

Effective advocacy requires access to four key factors (Figure 2–2) either by the advocate or within an advocacy team. Depending on the population for which one is advocating (e.g., children, older adults, incarcerated individuals) and the level of advocacy (e.g., patient, population), various combinations of these key factors will be needed to attain a given advocacy goal. It is rare for effective advocacy to be achieved in the absence of one of these factors. The four factors are as follows:

- *Collaboration skills:* Advocates need to be prepared to work in concert with a variety of stakeholders and within a diverse array of cultures and systems. Methods that work in one system or culture may fail in others. For example, in one culture, a highly involved and hands-on approach may be necessary, whereas in a different culture, this same intensity of engagement may be perceived as intrusive or controlling. Advocates and their teams should strive to maintain flexibility, self-awareness, and openness to a range of possible ways that stakeholders may use to engage and collaborate. In addition, psychiatrists should be aware that their identity as psychiatrists may evoke distorted beliefs and misperceptions, which may color collaborative efforts.
- *Communication skills:* Advocates need to acquire the communication skills necessary to get the attention of their audience and to

clearly communicate the core message of their advocacy issue. These skills include effective messaging and oral and written communications skills across a range of platforms. (For further discussion about communication skills and methods, see Chapter 7, "Legislative Advocacy," Chapter 8, "Education as Advocacy," and Chapter 10, "Engaging the Popular Media.")

- *Knowledge of the issue:* Advocates should strive to be thoroughly briefed on whatever issue they are working on. Having only a basic or cursory understanding of an issue will leave advocates ill prepared to anticipate opponents' arguments or to counter critiques. To be fully prepared to advance an issue with strategies and policy solutions, advocates need to research and understand all substantive aspects of that issue.

- *Time:* Advocacy takes a considerable investment of time. Unfortunately, for many psychiatrists, advocacy is an unpaid activity that requires, but does not receive, protected time. Advocates should be aware that they will need to add time for advocacy to their schedules, and they should also plan for additional unexpected advocacy time requirements.

Ethical Considerations in Advocacy

There are several important ethical considerations to keep in mind when engaging in advocacy. First and foremost, when we advocate as physicians, we must always strive to do so in a way that puts our patients' best interests first and minimizes harm. The same ethical principles that govern our clinical care for patients should also extend to our advocacy for patients. These principles include not advocating for changes that could harm patients, advocating for changes that would protect patients from harm, advocating for changes that positively impact patients' health and well-being, advocating for just resource allocation and equitable health care access, and advocating from our position of expertise on the basis of the best available scientific knowledge and professional wisdom to date. As occurs in practice, ethical obligations in patient advocacy may come into conflict. Weighing competing obligations to patients, communities, and health care and political systems is complex and may require support from medical colleagues, as well as involvement of health care administrators and clinical ethicists. In some roles, psychiatrist-advocates may be called on to advocate for a whole population rather than an individual patient (a utilitarian perspective) or to advocate for one patient over another as prioritization principles come up. Policy options pursued through advocacy may be curtailed in order to open up other options or to deal with budgetary realities. At all times, advocates should avoid abandonment of individual patients, and respect for persons should remain central.

First, as a foundational principle, advocacy by physicians is distinct from one's personal values, beliefs, and political leanings and should be focused on enhancing patient care rather than being a self-serving endeavor. Although many topics in health care are politicized today and the line between a political party's agenda and what is best for patients is often blurred, we must practice continual self-awareness when taking on the role of physician-advocate. This will ensure that our advocacy efforts remain patient-centered and abide by our profession's ethical standards.

Second, it is important to understand and disclose the position from which we are advocating. We need to clarify whether we are speaking as private citizens or as representatives for a group and whether we have conflicts of interest regarding the topic about which we are advocating. When engaging in advocacy as physicians, we are speaking for our profession or on behalf of an organization or group with which we are affiliated. When we advocate as private citizens, we speak on the basis of our personal knowledge and experiences. Although we may be advocating on behalf of the field of psychiatry or a particular patient population, our voices are our own, unless we have been explicitly granted the authority to speak on behalf of a particular group (e.g., university, agency, employer). It is a critical ethical obligation to acknowledge any conflicts of interest up front (e.g., employer, major investments). These actions will help to instill trust and goodwill among the stakeholders with whom we engage.

Certain psychiatrists, especially those employed by the federal government (e.g., active duty military personnel or employees of the U.S. Department of Veterans Affairs), have particular restrictions placed on their political activities. The Hatch Act of 1939, a U.S. federal law, in general prohibits employees of the federal government from engaging in political activities while on duty or in the workplace (U.S. Office of Special Counsel 2016). Additionally, certain types of federal employees (e.g., career Senior Executive Service employees) have even further restrictions. The Hatch Act, however, usually in no way limits the opportunities for these individuals to engage in legislative advocacy during their personal time as private citizens, or to engage in other types of advocacy (e.g., patient-level advocacy, organizational advocacy, voicing support for policies that improve patient care).

Third, whenever we engage in advocacy alongside patients, such as when we provide testimony at a legislative hearing, we must pay especially close attention to the ethical concerns that may arise. Firsthand patient stories are a powerful form of advocacy, but consideration of ethical guidelines (e.g., American Academy of Child and Adolescent Psychiatry 2014; American Medical Association 2016, 2019; American Psychiatric Association 2013) is needed prior to our engaging in advocacy activities in concert with any patient or family member. Because of the power imbalance between ourselves and patients in general, it is critical to avoid any tone, language, or actions that could be construed as overly persuasive or coercive when approaching patients and families about joint advocacy efforts. In addition, power differentials, boundary crossings, and potential violations are magnified when we ask our own patients to advocate with us. Therefore, as a rule, we as psychiatrists should not invite our own patients to engage in joint advocacy efforts. Instead, we should find advocates through connections with patient and family advocacy organizations such as the National Alliance on Mental Illness. Asking the patients and families directly under our care to be advocates should be the exception and should be done only after careful consideration and discussion with colleagues about the ethical and clinical implications.

A final ethical consideration concerns the maintenance of patient confidentiality when providing examples of patient experiences in advocacy work. Psychiatrist advocates are encouraged to illustrate advocacy needs with patient stories, which is a routine occurrence during a range of advocacy activities. However, unless explicit written permission has been obtained from a patient, the psychiatrist advocate should conceal all identifiers to such a degree that the patient and family are unable to recognize themselves within the example. If the patient or family can identify themselves, then the duty of confidentiality has been breached.

Should Advocacy Be Promoted as a Specialization Within Medicine?

By definition, *to specialize* means to become an expert in a particular subject matter or skill set. In this sense, a physician who has deep expertise in the theoretical and practical aspects of advocacy and who regularly engages in the work of advocacy could certainly be considered an advocacy specialist. Given the considerable time, energy, and dedication needed to be an advocate, as well as the critical role that advocacy plays in advancing patient and population health, we argue here that advocacy deserves consideration as a distinct specialization or career track within the house of medicine.

Developing the specialty of advocacy would have important implications for the future of advocacy by physicians. Consider this: The establishment of clinician-educator tracks at medical schools was not uniformly a straightforward or noncontroversial process, but it was necessary to retain talented clinicians who also shouldered a large teaching load and to recognize them for their contributions (Bickel 1991). Furthermore, the push to link talent in teaching to recognition and promotion across many academic medical centers also likely encouraged more teaching innovations by giving clinician-educators the time and headspace to pursue new ideas and created more interest in medical education as a professional goal by institutionalizing support for this specialization as part of a viable career trajectory.

In the same way, we can imagine a future where physicians who participate in health advocacy receive some formalized acknowledgment for their efforts, such as the creation of clinician-advocate tracks at medical schools. Such an acknowledgment could very well shift the way we think about advocacy and turn it from an action that we pursue only in our spare time to a scholarly as well as practical endeavor that is taken seriously by our peers and our institutions.

Advocacy portfolios have been proposed as a framework for operationalizing completion and recording of high-quality advocacy work to enhance patient well-being and scholarship opportunities. Nerlinger et al. (2018) have developed a six-step framework to guide advocacy initiatives. This approach highlights the need for goal-setting, completion of preparatory tasks, strategy and methodology development, evaluation of results, effective dissemination, and critical reflection on the process and outcomes of advocacy. Advocacy portfolio tasks can then be categorized and presented within five core domains: clinical practice enhancement, establishing collaborative partnerships, teaching and mentorship, leadership and administration, and knowledge dissemination (Nerlinger et al. 2018). It is hoped that development and widespread implementation of frameworks for advocacy by physicians will facilitate a standardized approach to advocacy engagement and academic recognition of advocacy endeavors.

To encourage more physicians to specialize in advocacy, institutions can also consider requiring trainees to have some degree of advocacy education, be it in medical school, residency, and/or fellowship. This type of requirement would introduce physicians to advocacy early in their careers, reinforce the standing of advocacy as a core competency alongside other core competencies they are learning, and ultimately enable more physicians to become and remain active physician-advocates (for more information, see Chapter 8, "Education as Advocacy," and Chapter 11, "Advocacy for Children and Families"). Training in advocacy should be broadly available, regardless of the establishment of advocacy tracks or specialization, in order to expose and inspire as many physicians as possible.

Conclusion

We in medicine are just beginning to define what advocacy is and how it applies to our professional role as physicians. Although there are many ways to understand advocacy, and no consensus definitions, guidelines, or best practices are yet available, we have aimed in this chapter to outline some basic frameworks to consider when thinking about advocacy by physicians. In the rest of Part I, "Understanding Advocacy," we will further explore many of these concepts to help you gain a clearer understanding of what advocacy means.

References

American Academy of Child and Adolescent Psychiatry: Code of ethics. Washington, DC, American Academy of Child and Adolescent Psychiatry, September 6, 2014. Available at: www.aacap.org/app_themes/aacap/docs/about_us/transparency_portal/aacap_code_of_ethics_2012.pdf. Accessed August 19, 2019.

American Medical Association: AMA code of medical ethics. Chicago, IL, American Medical Association, 2016. Available at: www.ama-assn.org/sites/ama-assn.org/files/corp/media-browser/principles-of-medical-ethics.pdf. Accessed August 19, 2019.

American Medical Association: Ethics: political communications. Chicago, IL, American Medical Association, 2019. Available at: www.ama-assn.org/delivering-care/ethics/political-communications. Accessed August 19, 2019.

American Psychiatric Association: The principles of medical ethics with annotations especially applicable to psychiatry, 2013 edition. Arlington, VA, American Psychiatric Association, 2013. Available at: www.psychiatry.org/File%20Library/Psychiatrists/Practice/Ethics/principles-medical-ethics.pdf. Accessed August 19, 2019.

Bickel J: The changing faces of promotion and tenure at U.S. medical schools. Acad Med 66(5):249–256, 1991 2025351

Israel BA, Schulz AJ, Parker EA, et al: Review of community-based research: assessing partnership approaches to improve public health. Annu Rev Public Health 19:173–202, 1998 9611617

Kingdon J: Agendas, Alternatives, and Public Policies. Boston, MA, Little, Brown, 1984

Mills CW: The Power Elite. New York, Oxford University Press, 1956

Nerlinger AL, Shah AN, Beck AF, et al: The advocacy portfolio: a standardized tool for documenting. Acad Med 93(6):860–868, 2018 29298182

Pandi-Perumal SR, Akhter S, Zizi F, et al: Project Stakeholder management in the clinical research environment: how to do it right. Front Psychiatry 6:71–89, 2015 26042053

Rogers EM: Diffusion of Innovations, 4th Edition. New York, Free Press, 1995

Stachowiak S: Pathways for change: 10 theories to inform advocacy and policy change efforts. Washington, DC, Center for Evaluation Innovation, November 2013. Available at: www.evaluationinnovation.org/publication/pathways-for-change-10-theories-to-inform-advocacy-and-policy-change-efforts. Accessed August 19, 2019.

Tajfel H, Turner JC: The social identity theory of intergroup behavior, in Psychology of Intergroup Relations. Edited by Worchel S, Austin WG. Chicago, IL, Hall Publishers, 1986, pp 7–24

U.S. Office of Special Counsel: The Hatch Act: permitted and prohibited activities for most federal employees. February 2016. Available at: https://osc.gov/Services/Pages/HatchAct-Federal.aspx. Accessed December 16, 2019.

World Health Organization: Advocacy for mental health (Mental Health Policy and Service Guidance Package). Geneva, Switzerland, World Health Organization, 2003. Available at: www.who.int/mental_health/policy/services/1_advocacy_WEB_07.pdf. Accessed August 19, 2019.

3

Where Do We Fit In?

Advocating for Our Patients and Our Profession

Eric Plakun, M.D.

R. Dakota Carter, M.D., Ed.D.

Katherine G. Kennedy, M.D.

Learning Objectives

By the end of this chapter, learners will be able to:

- Discuss five systemic health care system issues that challenge psychiatrists and their patients
- List the four key elements of medically necessary mental health care
- Recognize the main components of physician burnout syndrome and the systemic factors that contribute to its rising rate
- Describe how advocacy at different levels can address the five systemic problems in mental health care

Advocacy for Our Patients and Our Profession

This is a challenging time to be a physician, especially a psychiatrist. Regulatory demands, such as those requiring maintenance of certification and licensure, make psychiatric practice burdensome and expensive. Legislative initiatives create concerns for psychiatrists, who worry that states may enact new laws that jeopardize patient safety, such as granting prescription privileges to nonmedical or insufficiently trained personnel. Meanwhile, employers are incentivized by insurance reimbursement rates to pressure psychiatrists to reduce their time with patients to 15-minute appointments focused on medication evaluation, as if profit rather than clinical efficacy defines what is at the "top of their license." All these problems are part of a practice environment in which insurance companies and managed care entities push psychiatrists to limit goals of treatment to crisis stabilization, rather than helping patients to increase resilience, achieve long-term recovery, and establish a self-directed life within society. These issues exemplify the "moral injury" that researchers suggest may lead to burnout; it is no wonder that recent studies indicate that nearly half of U.S. psychiatrists report feeling symptoms of burnout (Shanafelt et al. 2017).

Advocacy for Our Profession Helps Our Patients

The practice of medicine has changed significantly from 50 years ago. Larger health care systems, innovations in technology, breakthroughs in medical research, and robust continuing medical education programs have advanced some aspects of health care but paradoxically have not translated into improved patient outcomes. Many physicians report feeling worn down by increasing demands on their time and energy for documentation, insurance utilization review contacts, and other obligations unrelated to face-to-face time with patients. In psychiatry, the introduction of the 15-minute "med check" means psychiatrists have far less time for psychotherapy in an outpatient setting, and inpatient stays are often brief because insurance companies deny additional coverage following acute crisis stabilization.

Retirement rates currently exceed the pace at which new graduates are entering the field, a trend that contributes to an ever-increasing nationwide shortage of psychiatrists. As a result, greater numbers of patients are straining the capacity of a diminishing number of psychiatrists, and patients are not receiving treatment early in the course of illness. In the future, these workforce tensions will likely lead to psychiatrists caring for patients with more severe mental illness, increasing the acuity (and thus the stress) of the average caseload. As psychiatrists, we need to advocate for change within our health care system to prioritize patient safety, optimize outcomes, maximize physician well-being, and decrease systemic issues leading to burnout.

Advocacy for Ourselves Helps Our Patients

Research on the complex relationship between burnout, stress, and depression underscores how poor physician health negatively impacts patient care (Shanafelt et al. 2002, 2010). Advocacy for physician wellness and self-care is in fact a form of advocacy for patients because the pursuit of meaningful activities in medicine is a well-known protective factor against burnout. In this domain, the use of our professional voices to advocate for change that addresses our own needs also improves the quality of care we provide for our patients.

Major Systemic Challenges in Psychiatry

Many serious systemic problems confront our patients and our profession. In this chapter, we focus on five major concerns:

- The lack of access to safe, quality, effective, evidence-based mental health care that is covered by payers
- An impending psychiatry workforce shortage
- The lack of parity in provision of mental health care compared with other forms of health care
- Stigma against both consumers and providers of treatment for mental disorders, including substance use disorders
- High rates of physician burnout

These five chronic systemic problems are often interrelated and, when they co-occur, may compound each other's negative impacts. For example, a worsening psychiatry workforce shortage may decrease patient access to care and increase rates of physician burnout. Concerted advocacy efforts to address all of these challenges are necessary if we are to bring about needed system-wide change, which may ultimately result in improved patient outcomes. In this chapter, we describe each of these systemic problems and suggest advocacy efforts to potentially alleviate them.

Access to Medically Necessary Mental Health Care

Access to medically necessary mental health care means access to care that is safe, high quality, evidence based, effective, and covered by the payer. Access to medically necessary mental health treatment is a fundamental concern for both patients and providers. Access may be limited by geography, by health insurance and managed care restrictions, and/or by membership in a socially marginalized or excluded group. Safe care is threatened when nonmedical personnel practice beyond the true scope of their expertise; examples include psychologists prescribing after inadequate medical training or health plan gatekeepers denying reimbursement for medically necessary care. Access to quality, evidence-based, effective, medically necessary care is threatened when insurance plans deny psychosocial treatments such as psychotherapy or restrict access to intermediate levels of care that offer treatment beyond crisis stabilization despite evidence that substantiates their role in recovery and maintaining optimal functioning (*Wit v. United Behavioral Health [UBH]/Optum* [Case No. 14-cv-02346-JCS, United States District Court, Northern District of California, 2019]).

Medically necessary care meets generally accepted standards in the field; in psychiatry, as in cardiology and other specialties, some of these standards come from research evidence, but many also come from professional society recommendations and practice patterns (Tricoci et al. 2009). Medically necessary care should be evidence based, effective, and consistent with generally accepted standards of care. Evidence-based care should also be effective and clinically meaningful. For example, care based on the demonstration of a small but statistically significant reduction in scores on a depression rating scale, as is the case with many antidepressant drug trials and short-term psychotherapies, is not effective if it leaves a patient without clinically meaningful and enduring change. Care is not effective, even if it is "evidence based," if it fails to benefit most patients most of the time. Figure 3–1 depicts the four key elements of medically necessary mental health treatment: care that is accessible, safe, evidence based and effective, and covered by the payer.

Medically necessary mental health care requires all four of these elements. Situations in which provision of medically necessary care is compromised are discussed in the following subsections. Advocacy efforts may be helpful to address and mitigate these situations.

Medically Necessary Care May Be Denied Coverage

Patients often have difficulty gaining access to medically necessary and clinically recommended mental health care because insurance companies and/or managed care entities restrict or deny coverage. This "medical necessity" criterion is usually part of the language of insurance contracts, which generally provide "medically necessary" care for med-

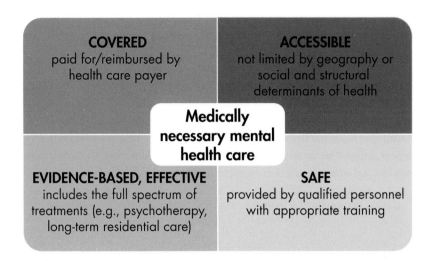

FIGURE 3–1. Key elements of medically necessary mental health treatment.

ical/surgical and mental health/substance use disorder treatment. Medically necessary care in these situations is defined as care that is within "generally accepted standards" of medical practice.

Serious problems ensue when managed care entities use flawed understanding of "generally accepted standards" to develop their own proprietary guidelines for medically necessary care. Often, this flawed understanding results in faulty guidelines that are more restrictive than generally accepted standards of care. Because managed care entities consider their guidelines to be proprietary, the processes and sources they use to develop these guidelines are often not transparent. When managed care gatekeepers use faulty guidelines to evaluate care requests in their case reviews, care that should legitimately be provided according to generally accepted standards may instead be restricted or denied. When this happens, patients often face a potentially impenetrable barrier to legitimate, medically necessary care. Advocacy directed at this problem is imperative.

Some of the most significant advocacy for addressing this obstacle of flawed medical necessity guidelines has come from patients, who have joined together to file multiple class action lawsuits against insurance entities, alleging breach of contract. These suits allege that whereas "generally accepted standards" accept recovery as the goal of treatment for psychiatric disorders, insurance companies and managed care entities focus treatment on crisis stabilization rather than meaningful, long-lasting improvement. Plaintiff patients in the class argued that this subpar goal lies outside of generally accepted standards and thus is in breach of the terms of their insurance contracts.

In 2019, Chief Magistrate Judge Joseph Spero, a federal judge in California, found the nation's largest behavioral health insurance company, United Behavioral Healthcare, to have unlawfully denied coverage of treatment for substance use and other mental health disorders to its members. Judge Spero's verdict in the liability phase of *Wit v. UBH/Optum* states the following about the company's access to care guidelines for outpatient, intensive outpatient, and residential treatment:

> Having reviewed all of the versions of the Guidelines that Plaintiffs challenge in this case and considered the testimony of the witnesses addressing the meaning of the Guidelines, the Court finds, by a preponderance of the evidence, that in every version of the Guidelines in the class period, and at every level of care that is at issue in this case, there is an excessive emphasis on addressing acute symptoms and stabilizing crises while ignoring the effective treatment of members' underlying conditions.
>
> [I]n each version of the Guidelines at issue in this case the defect is pervasive and results in a significantly narrower scope of coverage than is consistent with generally accepted standards of care." (*Wit v. UBH/Optum*)

Advocacy, especially via class action lawsuits, is necessary to effect significant change in these large, entrenched systems—for the welfare of both clinicians and patients. In this case, patient advocacy through the legal system held the insurance company to be in breach of their contracts with their insured subscribers. The court found that care is medically necessary if it meets generally accepted standards, and these standards cannot be reduced, misrepresented, or misconstrued by insurance entities. This kind of advocacy not only helps patients gain access to effective, medically necessary care but also enables psychiatrists and other mental health providers to adequately meet the needs of their patients. Moral injury from being unable to do what is right for the patient is an oft-cited contributor to burnout, and therefore, reducing obstacles to providing appropriate care may also improve provider well-being.

Medically Necessary Mental Health Care May Not Be Accessible

When Dr. Melody Goodman addressed an audience at the Dana Farber Institute in 2014, she pithily summed up the way that factors such as race, ethnicity, gender identity, income, home value, and educational level can create profound health disparities between populations in terms of disease incidence, prevalence, and mortality: "Your zip code may be a better predictor of your health than your genetic code." These factors also contribute to major inequities in how health care is delivered; racism, discrimination, and white privilege can unfairly stigmatize, marginalize, and exclude vulnerable populations. Additional contributors to health care disparities include age, gender, sexual orientation, and disability status.

Health care disparities can be further exacerbated by individual health behaviors, environmental conditions, and other sociocultural, political, and economic elements. Health care providers' implicit bias, as well as systemic bias within the health care system itself, can further worsen the quality of care for these at-risk populations. Advocacy efforts must focus on the identification and eradication of health care disparities by addressing bias, both personal and systemic, and improving social and structural determinants of health. Advocacy at every level, from the patient to the community, to the state and federal legislative levels, is necessary as are advocacy efforts to develop social and economic remedies for these intransigent systemic problems.

The contribution of geography to lack of access to mental health care is not limited to the poor who live in inner cities. Rural communities, across a range of socioeconomic statuses, also suffer from the absence of qualified mental health care providers. Additionally, incarcerated people with substance use and other mental health disorders lack access to quality mental health care and often to specialized treatment for substance use disorders, such as opioid dependence. Advocacy at the state level to permit providers to use telepsychiatry to prescribe and be reimbursed can increase access to these geographically distant or difficult locations.

Accessible Mental Health Care May Not Be Quality, Evidence Based, and Effective

Even when mental health treatment is accessible, it may not include access to such evidence-based and effective treatments as psychoeducation, psychotherapy, and treatment at intermediate levels of care (intensive outpatient, partial hospital, or residential treatment) that are essential parts of the pursuit of recovery for many patients with substance use and other mental health disorders. Psychoeducation can help patients put their suffering into context through learning about their disorders. Psychotherapy, whether psychodynamic therapy, cognitive-behavioral therapy, or another form, offers patients the opportunity to grapple with the origins of their symptoms and suffering and/or provides patients with tools to live self-directed lives. For some patients, intermediate levels of care, such as residential treatment, are critical bridges to achieving long-term improvements in functioning that subsequently allow them to better utilize outpatient services in pursuit of recovery.

Both psychodynamic therapy and cognitive-behavioral therapy are evidence-based treatments that meet generally accepted standards for a range of psychiatric disorders (Driessen et al. 2013; Steinert et al. 2017). They are known to be efficacious and cost-effective, either alone or in combination with medications, depending on the specific disorder, acuity of disease, and patient demographics (Plakun 2015). However, multiple systemic factors contribute to the low monetary value assigned to therapy by insurance companies, an issue that incentivizes psychiatrists to provide less therapy or to offer it outside insurance coverage despite its being a treatment within generally accepted standards of care. These systemic factors include the pharmaceutical industry's financial power to fund research and effectively lobby legislative bodies; psychiatry's embracing of biomedical approaches over psychosocial approaches; the public's erroneous perception of psychotherapy as not cost-effective; and society's longing for a quick-fix "magic pill" to solve problems of the human psyche.

The myth that psychotherapy is costly, "old-school," and ineffective is based on stigma, not on evidence, but this has led insurers to deny coverage for psychotherapy or to reimburse at very low rates, despite its place within generally accepted standards of care. As a result, many psychiatrists focus solely on pharmacotherapy during brief "med check" appointments, although there is no evidence base to support this practice. Also, some psychiatry residency training programs fail to train residents to provide psychotherapy to a measurable degree of competence, even though psychotherapy competence is a training requirement set forth by the Accreditation Council for Graduate Medical Education (2019).

Advocacy is needed not only to educate the public about the efficacy and cost-effectiveness of psychotherapeutic treatment but also to remind members of our own profession of its utility. Ideally, this advocacy would help dispel public misperceptions, thus increasing patient interest in psychotherapy and placing pressure on insurance companies to rightfully assess psychotherapy as an effective, clinically meaningful intervention that is within generally accepted standards. Once insurance reimbursement rates respond accordingly, clinicians would have the appropriate financial support to provide more comprehensive treatment.

Accessible, Effective Mental Health Care May Not Be Safe

In any efforts to make care more accessible, the quality of services provided should not be compromised. The recent increase of "physician extenders" may make accessing mental health care easier for patients, but it may also put patients in potential danger if these clinicians have inadequate medical training. Patient safety should remain the primary concern when considering expanding prescriptive authority to personnel without medical training. For example, some psychologists are lobbying at the state level to expand their scope of practice to include prescriptive authority. Proponents typically argue that increasing the number of prescribers will improve mental health care access for patients in underserved areas. However, although psychologists may be knowledgeable about psychological states, they have little to no training in biology, chemistry, pathophysiology, and other foundational prerequisites to prescribing medications, and only an abbreviated training experience is suggested in place of this important training. For example, typical training for a psychologist wishing to prescribe medication would include a 400-hour online course in pharmacotherapy, followed by approximately 1,000 hours spent shadowing an authorized prescriber. This training, however, is minimal compared with that of prescribers who are medically trained: physician assistants spend 5,000 hours, nurse practitioners spend 8,000 hours, and physicians spend more than 20,000 hours in clinical training.

For state legislators, who may not understand the difference in clinical training between a psychologist and a psychiatrist, the "access" argument made by proponents of psychologist prescribing creates the illusion of increased access to competent behavioral health providers. Instead, psychologist prescribing might increase the chance that psychiatric patients are cared for in a potentially unsafe system where clinicians lack the medical training and clinical experience necessary to both accurately diagnose and rule out medical conditions and to safely provide medical interventions, such as medications.

Only a handful of states have enacted psychologist-prescribing bills, and only two states, Louisiana and New Mexico, have psychologists who are actively prescribing. In these two states, where psychologists have been granted access to the full formulary, data from the Centers for Medicare and Medicaid Services (2019a) indicate that they have also prescribed antihypertensive, cardiac, and other nonpsychotropic medications for which they have no training at all. This behavior suggests that prescriptive authority in the hands of inadequately trained prescribers could have dangerous implications for patient safety.

This prescribing issue requires both legislative advocacy and education. Advocacy at the state government level has been somewhat effective at curbing psychologist-prescribing legislation. However, further advocacy efforts are needed. Psychiatrists can also increase awareness by educating state legislators and the public about the safety and health concerns related to granting prescriptive authority to psychologists and other non-medically trained personnel. In addition, psychiatrists can work to develop stronger coalitions and alliances with other medically trained prescribers: physician assistants, advanced practice registered nurses, and primary care physicians.

Psychiatry Workforce Shortage

The United States is experiencing a worsening physician workforce shortage and may face a shortfall of more than 100,000 physicians by 2030 (Dall et al. 2018). Primary contributors to this potential health care crisis include an aging, sicker U.S. population; physician retirements; and a bottleneck in physician training at the residency level. The training bottleneck has been created by the lack of Medicare funding for additional graduate medical education (GME) slots. Since 1997, the U.S. Congress has failed to increase funding for the additional 3,750 physicians needed to avert this impending shortage. Training a physician takes approximately 10 years, so legislative advocacy to fund additional GME slots is a time-critical imperative.

The psychiatry workforce is no less affected: between the opioid epidemic and the rising rates of depression and suicide, the demand for mental health services is growing. Although there has been a strong uptick in medical students entering psychiatry in recent years (Goldenberg et al. 2017), given the inadequate number of residency positions in psychiatry and the retirement rate of psychiatrists, the influx of newly trained psychiatrists has not kept pace with demand. New models of team-based, integrated behavioral health care, such as the evidence-based Collaborative Care Model (American Psychiatric Association and Academy of Psychosomatic Medicine 2016), may help mitigate this shortage, expand mental health screening and services, and improve outcomes in a cost-effective way. However, health care models like these will require new reimbursement codes for these services and may require new state laws. Advocacy at the state level will be needed to promote such change.

Lack of Parity of Mental Health Care

For decades, insurance restrictions via "care management" were much tighter for mental health and substance use treatment than for medical and surgical services. It was also typical for patients to face higher deductibles and out-of-pocket costs for behavioral health care than for other types of health care. In 2008, the Mental Health Parity and Addiction Equity Act (MHPAEA) was signed into law (Centers for Medicare and Medicaid Services 2019b). It requires that all health insurers and group health plans for more than 50 employees have substantial parity in access to treatment for substance use and other mental health disorders compared with medical/surgical treatment.

Parity is evaluated across a range of dimensions, which are classified in terms of whether they are quantitative or qualitative (often referenced as non-quantitative treatment limitations, or NQTLs). Quantitative dimensions are more easily measured; these include deductibles, copays, limits in days or dollars for mental health care, and other care management tools. NQTLs are more difficult to measure, resulting in difficulty making fair comparisons between psychiatric and medical/surgical services. Examples of NQTLs include the nature of prior authorization and concurrent review hurdles, such as the problem of access-to-care criteria that fail to meet generally accepted standards (addressed in the section "Access to Medically Necessary Mental Health Care").

Although many quantitative limitations to behavioral health care access have been removed, qualitative limitations continue to be substantially more restrictive for behavioral health care than for medical and surgical care—such as use of access-to-care criteria that limit the goal of mental health treatment to crisis stabilization. In contrast, insurers would not limit medical or surgical treatment in an individual with underlying lung cancer to treating the pneumonia without also addressing the underlying malignancy. Hence, despite the legislative achievement of MHPAEA, full parity remains unrealized. States, which are responsible for monitoring and evaluating insurers' compliance with MHPAEA, have generally been ineffective at identifying and addressing these qualitative inequities. There is still much work to be done by psychiatrist-advocates, at both the federal and state legislative levels, to address the ongoing disparities in coverage.

In 2019, a promising piece of bipartisan legislation was introduced: the Mental Health Parity Compliance Act (H.R. 3165). It would require insurance entities to make public their degree of compliance with MHPAEA requirements. Sunlight, as the saying goes, is the best disinfectant. As noted earlier (see subsection "Medically Necessary Care May Be Denied Coverage"), there has also been some success in "bottom-up" patient-led advocacy around these issues through class action lawsuits that target insurers' fiduciary responsibility to their subscribers as codified by insurance contracts.

Stigma

Many of the problems faced by our patients and our profession are rooted in long-standing stigma toward patients with substance use and other mental health disorders. Stigma can be directed toward any aspect of mental illness: the diagnosis, the treatment, the payment, the treater, the patient, and family members. Origins of stigma stem from unrealistic fears, not unlike ancient fears that demonic possession caused mental illness and that the possessed should be kept away from the rest of the population. Added to this misperception are the realities of negligent treatment of institutionalized psychiatric patients (such as occurred at Willowbrook State School) as well as media portrayals of intentionally cruel psychiatric treatment (as personified by Nurse Ratched in Ken Kesey's 1962 novel *One Flew Over the Cuckoo's Nest* and the 1975 film adaptation). In addition, many people envision psychiatrists as the embodiment depicted in *New Yorker* cartoons: a bearded, bespectacled, silent therapist who offers tangential, mother-blaming perspectives. Hence, fears, fantasies, and—unfortunately—at times real horrors fuel ongoing public distrust of psychiatry, which promotes stigma and leads to systemic distrust, dehumanization, and segregation of psychiatric patients and their providers.

Stigma can manifest in many forms. One of the most pernicious is the view that mental disorders are less significant than medical or surgical disorders. This form can present as lower compensation for psychiatrists. In fact, according to a Milliman Report (Melek et al. 2017), psychiatrists are paid on average 20% less than when the same service and Current Procedural Terminology (CPT) code are provided by a nonpsychiatric physician, such as an internist. As psychiatrists, we need to advocate for equitable reimbursement policies via state legislation and, sometimes, the courts.

Dehumanizing treatments of patients with psychiatric disorders that fuel stigma include needless use of seclusion and restraint. In addition, more subtle forms of stigmatizing treatments exist. These include pressures to focus on symptom checklists and computer screens rather than attend to the humanity of our patients. Our patients bring us their human suffering. They deserve to be met with our compassion and concern. The opportunity for patients to tell their story is recognized as part of the healing process. However, employers' financial demands often place pressure on psychiatrists to work at the financial "top of their license." These demands are a perversion of what we actually know about the most effective treatments, which often include a combination of biopsychosocial components, such as medication and psychotherapy, and represent the top of a psychiatrist's license from a clinical perspective. These pressures constitute implied directives that psychiatrists should limit their practice only to prescribing medications, often in 15-minute medication appointments, despite the lack of an evidence base supporting this model for provision of care. Psychiatrists cannot allow these directives to reshape patient interactions into checklist reviews of symptoms that fail to follow patients' affects or hear their stories. Advocacy is necessary to promote a full biopsychosocial approach to treatment.

Physician Burnout Syndrome

As the health care system has changed, so have the medical and residency education experiences. More time is spent teaching basic medical knowledge, learning efficiencies, and improving computer-based patient management at the expense of teaching quality patient-centered care (Neumann et al. 2011). Trainees are entering clinical environments with increased levels of stress, depression, sleep deprivation, harassment experiences, and other negative factors that lead to career dissatisfaction and less ability to express compassion toward patients (Neumann et al. 2011). As they enter a medical era in which medical record keeping and communication are primarily electronic, medical students and residents describe feeling exhausted by information overload. In addition, the persistence of the intimidating medical hierarchy—in which attending physicians rank above residents who rank above medical students—can result in trainees' modeling of behaviors of poor self-care and the valuing of efficient work over patient-centered care (Hojat et al. 2009). Williams et al. (2009) report that an "increasingly stressful medical workplace brought on by changes in contemporary medical care that include disparities in access and quality, inequities in compensation, and increased work demands with decreased control over multiple aspects of daily work life" can negatively impact patient care (p. 4).

Increased stress from medical training at all levels can lead to the development of a syndrome termed *burnout*. Burnout is characterized by a triad of 1) emotional and mental exhaustion; 2) an increasingly depersonalized attitude, with decreased empathy for patients and colleagues; and 3) a low sense of personal accomplishment and self-efficacy. Additional symptoms include a sense of helplessness and lack of control over stressors; secondary traumatization from bearing witness to others' stress; and lower levels of professional gratification (e.g., as a result of documentation demands or poor work-life balance). Burnout can result in increased medical errors, poorer patient health outcomes, and increased workplace turnover. Burnout can also worsen the risk for physicians' substance use, divorce, and suicide.

How Medical Training Fosters Burnout

Hojat and colleagues (2009) noted that burnout often begins early in the third year of medical school. Their appropriately titled study, "The Devil Is in the Third Year...," highlights a trend of increasing burnout, depression, and faltering empathy in medical students due to the massive changes in medicine, technology, health care systems, and day-to-day obligations of physicians. Although formal research regarding stress in medical students is dated, limited, and controversial, Chang et al. (2012) noted increased levels of suicidality in medical students who were stressed and suffering from burnout. In their study, which used the Primary Care Evaluation of Mental Disorders (PRIME-MD) and Maslach Burnout Inventory (MBI), students had the highest level of depression and burnout in their third year of medical school, but these averages continued through training. More than 60% of students surveyed had depressive symptoms, and 55% were noted to have burnout on one of the three subscales of the MBI. In one study, 10% of medical students met DSM-5 criteria for depression (Stecker 2004). In another study (Moffat et al. 2004), first-year medical students' stress levels more than doubled over the course of the year, as found using the 12-item General Health Questionnaire (GHQ-12). In a review of 40 articles, researchers found high prevalence of affective disorders among medical students, with "levels of overall psychological distress consistently higher than in the general population and age-matched peers by the later years of training" (Dyrbye et al. 2006, p. 359). Later studies by this group noted that stress, burnout, and depression in medical students led to a poorer quality of life, a lower level of professionalism, thoughts of leaving medical school, and higher rates of suicidal ideation (Dyrbye et al. 2006, 2008, 2010).

Notably, as training continues, burnout usually increases; the percentages of medical students, residents, fellows, and early career physicians experiencing burnout are also increasing (Bellini and Shea 2005; Bellini et al. 2002; Neumann et al. 2011; Rosen et al. 2006; Shanafelt et al. 2005; Stratton et al. 2008; West et al. 2006). Many of these individuals report that they are becoming cynical, feeling a lesser sense of accomplishment, and experiencing high levels of emotional exhaustion and depression. Replicated studies show that as trainees progress through medical training, the burnout syndrome that began in medical school persists in specialty training and early careers (Bellini et al. 2002). The burnout syndrome frequently transitions into depression in cohorts of this population of physicians who struggle with burnout. Many experience a decline in empathy and interest in their careers, despite the years they invested in training to be physicians. Sadly, many of these physicians complete training and enter their careers without addressing their experience of burnout. Many report feelings of depression and "going through the motions" of treating patients at any cost, even if that cost is to their own well-being.

Some researchers suggest that this traumatic deidealization, dehumanization, or lack of self-advocacy and wellness results from a range of systemic and individual differences, including lack of role models, increased adverse influence of electronic devices, education volume, health care market changes, time pressures, patient and environmental factors, and the potential belief that self- and patient-focused empathy may be outside of clinical- and evidence-based medicine (Hojat et al. 2009). Hojat and colleagues (2009) discuss the notion of the "battered child syndrome" or the "heart hardening" that develops during medical school, residency, and medical careers: health care providers become so stressed that they need to be "rehumanized" and learn to take better care of themselves if they are to be effective providers for their patients (Hojat et al. 2009).

Trainees and early career physicians who do not seek treatment for burnout or depression may still have these symptoms when they become attending physicians and specialists in their fields. These physicians may give up on their medical careers and leave medicine entirely. Another smaller but significant portion may contemplate or even die by suicide (Schernhammer 2005). Often, the highest levels of burnout and depression occur in those physicians on the "front lines" of care access, including primary care physicians, psychiatrists, and emergency department providers. Changes in education models have occurred in efforts to mitigate these trends (Accreditation Council for Graduate Medical Education 2019; Liaison Committee on Medical Education 2019). A focus on wellness and well-being is now often added to medical training curricula in response to the increased number of trainees experiencing burnout and depression. However, more advocacy and further change on this front are imperative to combat these pervasive problems.

The Downstream Impact of Burnout

Among health care workers, and compared with the general population, physicians are the most likely to experience burnout and be dissatisfied with their work-life balance (Shanafelt et al. 2012). In a study by Shanafelt et al. (2002), three-quarters of internal medicine physicians exhibited burnout symptoms and reported providing suboptimal care. Burnout in trainees and physicians leads to poorer patient outcomes and has significant impacts on service quality and job performance (Halbesleben and Rathert 2008). Although professionals with advanced degrees are generally unlikely to experience burnout, this is not the case for physicians (Dyrbye et al. 2014). Stress and burnout have been identified as factors that erode professionalism and promote a negative culture of self-care (Wallace and Lemaire 2009). They can also negatively influence the quality of patient care (Dyrbye et al. 2010; Shanafelt et al. 2002), increase medical errors (Shanafelt et al. 2010), promote early retirement (Shanafelt et al. 2014), lead to broken interpersonal relationships (Balch et al. 2011), result in higher levels of substance use (Jackson et al., 2016; Oreskovich et al. 2012), and increase suicidality (Dyrbye et al. 2008).

Case Example: Dr. Y's Burnout

Dr. Y, an early career psychiatrist, discusses with her mentor the ongoing stress that her new position has brought. She laments that since training, her patient volume has increased immensely while time with patients has been reduced. She is spending more energy after work to complete documentation or finish phone calls related to the day's work, often a result of insurance companies denying services, care, medication, or payment. Appeals take more time and too often confirm the original rejection of payment or coverage. Most days Dr. Y feels a diminished connection to her patients and her colleagues, which worries her because it was her deep empathy for others that drew her to psychiatry as a specialty. She never has enough time for trainee education, committee and grant meetings for career advancement, or her research interests. The department is looking for ways to increase revenue through her clinical role, so she is concerned about managing increased demands in the future. Dr. Y does not reveal the following information to her mentor: most evenings, she finds herself unwinding with several glasses of wine, feels distanced from her partner, and contemplates leaving medicine. She often feels despair and hopelessness. From time to time, thoughts of suicide enter her mind.

Managing Burnout

Two processes counteract the effects of physician burnout: prevention and alleviation. These efforts need to occur both on a personal level and through advocacy for systemic changes to our profession and the health care system as a whole.

Prevention of Burnout

Advocacy aimed at reforming medical education is a vital component of preventing burnout on personal, systemic, and professional levels. "For physicians, burnout is the inevitable consequence of the way that medical education is organized and the subsequent maladaptive behaviors that are reinforced in healthcare organizations via the hidden curriculum. Thus, burnout is an important indicator of how the organization itself is functioning" (Montgomery 2014, p. 50). Empathic training, awareness, screening, and intervention for those experiencing burnout are all part of the solution.

In medical education, it is important to acknowledge the various problems and discuss them on an ongoing basis. Fortunately, organizations such as the American Medical Association and the American Psychiatric Association offer education and other resources on burnout and physician wellness, and the Liaison Committee on Medical Education and the Accreditation Council for Graduate Medical Education have begun to embrace educational standards on wellness to incorporate into medical and residency programs. Burnout has been shown to be ameliorated with positive support and stress reduction programs in trainee programs (Santen et al. 2010). Other recommendations include team-building initiatives and trainee focus on teamwork, aimed at creating a culture of appreciation and support, and inclusion of seminars that address physician sleep deprivation, substance abuse, and mental health, along with resources and means to address these issues in a compassionate manner (Maslach and Leiter 2016).

Modeling and mentoring are other vital ways to impact medical culture. Medicine is hierarchical in nature, with much of clinical training, including empathic care and self-care modeling, passed down from "top to bottom." When senior physicians do not model empathic care or self-care, they communicate to trainees and colleagues that these behaviors lack value. Therefore, transformational change happens when attending physicians and upper-level residents embrace wellness and model self-care. The practice of wellness can be transformative for the individual, for the profession of medicine, and for patients; that is, self-care is a pivotal component of patient care.

Burnout can also be prevented by advocacy to address the systemic problems that plague the medical profession, as discussed earlier, such as improving access to medically necessary, quality, effective, and safe mental health care; addressing workforce shortage issues; improving mental health parity; and decreasing stigma. When we are able to minimize the potential for moral injury, we will also lessen the frequency of a burnout response.

Alleviation of Burnout

Research has identified innovative ways to help mitigate burnout and its effects through self-care. These include learning and wellness education, teamwork, modeling of positive behavior, and physician support. Numerous person-oriented proposals have been tried and validated. These include workshops and educational activities; changing negative work patterns; increasing coping skills, utilizing relaxation strategies; initiating therapy and/or treatment; refocusing on health and fitness; and finding social support from colleagues or friends (Maslach and Leiter 2016).

Advocacy for systems-based changes to mitigate burnout often focuses on contributions by hospitals and health care systems. Research demonstrates that efforts to increase workplace civility and embrace positive social behavior in organizations are useful. In fact, most research points to interpersonal connections as key to ameliorating burnout, especially in health care professions based in teams (Montgomery 2014). Further advocacy at the organizational level might include a review of a hospital's or health system's organizational structure, resources, regulations, and procedures, with the goal of identifying practices and factors that may be responsible for contributing to burnout. Including stakeholders in the task of identifying possible solutions is key.

Case Example: Two Potential Scenarios for Dealing With Dr. Y's Burnout

Any number of possible outcomes could follow from Dr. Y's meeting with her mentor, presented earlier. Two possibilities are described here.

Scenario A: Dr. Y's mentor cautions Dr. Y about complaining and tells her to "suck it up." He acknowledges that he also feels this way but has "learned to live with it" and assures her that she will as well. However, Dr. Y becomes increasingly depressed and sometimes drinks so heavily at night that she oversleeps and is late for work in the mornings. Her longtime partner moves out. Eventually, the hospital puts her on notice for her tardiness. Her work with patients becomes increasingly perfunctory. One day, she fails to adequately inquire about a patient's psychotic symptoms; later that night, he is psychiatrically hospitalized after stabbing his mother. Dr. Y feels increasingly worse but is also ashamed, so she tells no one about her feelings. One year later, Dr. Y is admitted to the intensive care unit after being involved in a motor vehicle accident she caused while driving under the influence.

> **Case Example: Two Potential Scenarios for Dealing With Dr. Y's Burnout *(continued)***
>
> *Scenario B:* Dr. Y's mentor recognizes that she is exhibiting signs of burnout and inquires about depressive symptoms or suicidal ideation. Although Dr. Y denies these symptoms to her mentor, his questions prompt her to examine her feelings more closely. Dr. Y decides to seek a psychiatric consultation and soon after begins a course of treatment. Eventually, Dr. Y feels relief from her symptoms, stops drinking, and begins to take stock of the issues in her hospital that are contributing to her frustration. She speaks with colleagues and learns that they share similar views. In response, she organizes her colleagues to form a team to work with departmental administrators to address problems with workloads, insurance authorizations, and the electronic health record. One year later, Dr. Y feels much more satisfied with her work-life balance and is considering marriage to her longtime partner.

Advocacy Recommendations and Conclusion

The issues described in this chapter reflect major systemic issues that face our profession and impact our patients. These issues include how insurers deny and restrict access to medically necessary care, workforce shortage issues, mental health parity concerns, stigma, and physician burnout. Advocacy at all levels can help to either prevent or mitigate these problems and can result in higher-quality patient care and improved psychiatrist well-being. In Table 3–1, we provide examples of how advocacy across all levels can be used to potentially address these serious systemic issues.

Psychiatrists can be leaders for change when we understand and address the complex issues facing our profession. We need to take ownership of our own well-being in order to be healthy providers to our patients and to model self-care behavior to our trainees and colleagues. We must also advocate for better access to quality care, better pay for services, and more funding and resources to educate and train new providers. When we advocate for ourselves, our patients, and our profession, we are helping to improve the quality of patient care. Our hope is that by engaging in advocacy at every level to address these difficult and complex systemic problems, we will take steps forward to improving the health care outcomes of our patients and reducing the rate of burnout in ourselves.

TABLE 3–1. Examples of advocacy across all levels to address major systemic issues in psychiatry

	Burnout	Access to care	Workforce shortage	Mental health parity	Stigma
Self-advocacy	Self-monitor, seek self-care, and set limits with peers and colleagues	In the face of pressure to limit treatment to pre-scribing, strive to offer psychotherapeutic interventions	Identify ways to work in interdisciplinary teams to alleviate burden; advocate for patient caps when necessary for well-being	Recognize self-worth and value in the care that is provided; advocate for equal pay for equal services	Continually evaluate your own internalized stigma toward psychiatry
Patient-level advocacy	Continually address your own deficits in empathic capacities for patient care	Address health disparities experienced by patients	Use time and resources efficiently; determine which patients can be served through other providers (i.e., stable patients who can return to primary care physicians)	Assist patients with burdensome preauthorizations; support patients in their legal advocacy efforts	Continually address your own stigma toward patients
Health-system and community-level advocacy	Speak out about workplace issues and advocate for change	Understand local systems and resources for referrals, partner with primary care, and advocate for local funding	Advocate for local funding/resources for consultation lines, work-share programs, and physician-led teams	Join local, city, or county coalitions for advocacy days; educate trainees on important topics such as parity	Educate colleagues about stigma

TABLE 3–1. Examples of advocacy across all levels to address major systemic issues in psychiatry *(continued)*

	Burnout	Access to care	Workforce shortage	Mental health parity	Stigma
State legislative advocacy	Advocate for new state laws to protect trainees and providers	Advocate for new state laws to enable telehealth, improve patient transportation, promote network adequacy, and limit prescriptive authority to medically trained providers	Advocate for state laws to enable integrative and collaborative care	Advocate for state laws to promote mental health parity by insurers	Educate state legislators about stigma
Nationally focused/federal-legislative advocacy	Advocate for LCME and ACGME educational requirements; work with national organizations, such as the APA, for more resources on well-being	Advocate for full implementation of the mental health parity law and federal laws to limit prescriptive authority to medically trained providers	Advocate for Medicare to increase funding for more GME slots	Join advocacy organizations to support advocacy efforts to promote federal legislation that advances parity implementation	Educate federal legislators about stigma

Abbreviations. ACGME = Accreditation Council for Graduate Medical Education; APA = American Psychiatric Association; GME = graduate medical education; LCME = Liaison Committee on Medical Education.

References

Accreditation Council for Graduate Medical Education: Common program requirements. Chicago, IL, Accreditation Council for Graduate Medical Education, 2019. Available at: www.acgme.org/What-We-Do/Accreditation/Common-Program-Requirements. Accessed: April 23, 2019.

American Psychiatric Association; Academy of Psychosomatic Medicine: Dissemination of integrated care within adult primary care settings: the collaborative care model. Arlington, VA, American Psychiatric Association, 2016

Balch CM, Shanafelt TD, Sloan J, et al: Burnout and career satisfaction among surgical oncologists compared with other surgical specialties. Ann Surg Oncol 18(1):16–25, 2011 20953718

Bellini LM, Shea JA: Mood change and empathy decline persist during three years of internal medicine training. Acad Med 80(2):164–167, 2005 15671323

Bellini LM, Baime M, Shea JA: Variation of mood and empathy during internship. JAMA 287(23):3143–3146, 2002 12069680

Centers for Medicare and Medicaid Services: Medicare provider utilization and payment data: Part D prescriber. Baltimore, MD, Centers for Medicare and Medicaid Services, 2019a. Available at: www.cms.gov/Research-Statistics-Data-and-Systems/Statistics-Trends-and-Reports/Medicare-Provider-Charge-Data/Part-D-Prescriber.html

Centers for Medicare and Medicaid Services: The Mental Health Parity and Addiction Equity Act (MHPAEA). Atlanta, GA, Centers for Disease Control and Prevention, 2019b. Available at: www.cms.gov/cciio/programs-and-initiatives/other-insurance-protections/mhpaea_factsheet.html. Accessed August 29, 2019.

Chang E, Eddins-Folensbee F, Coverdale J: Survey of the prevalence of burnout, stress, depression, and the use of supports by medical students at one school. Acad Psychiatry 36(3):177–182, 2012 22751817

Dall T, West T, Chakrabarti R, et al: 2018 update: the complexities of physician supply and demand: projections from 2016 to 2030. Final Report. Washington, DC, Association of American Medical Colleges, March 2018

Driessen E, Van HL, Don FJ, et al: The efficacy of cognitive-behavioral therapy and psychodynamic therapy in the outpatient treatment of major depression: a randomized clinical trial. Am J Psychiatry 170(9):1041–1050, 2013 24030613

Dyrbye LN, Thomas MR, Shanafelt TD: Systematic review of depression, anxiety, and other indicators of psychological distress among U.S. and Canadian medical students. Acad Med 81(4):354–373, 2006 16565188

Dyrbye LN, Thomas MR, Massie FS, et al: Burnout and suicidal ideation among U.S. medical students. Ann Intern Med 149(5):334–341, 2008 18765703

Dyrbye LN, Thomas MR, Power DV, et al: Burnout and serious thoughts of dropping out of medical school: a multi-institutional study. Acad Med 85(1):94–102, 2010 20042833

Dyrbye LN, West CP, Satele D, et al: Burnout among U.S. medical students, residents, and early career physicians relative to the general U.S. population. Acad Med 89(3):443–451, 2014 24448053

Goldenberg, MN, Williams, DK, Spollen, JJ: Stability of and factors related to medical student specialty choice of psychiatry. Am J Psychiatry 174(9):859–866, 2017 28618855

Halbesleben JR, Rathert C: Linking physician burnout and patient outcomes: exploring the dyadic relationship between physicians and patients. Health Care Manage Rev 33(1):29–39, 2008 18091442

Hojat M, Vergare MJ, Maxwell K, et al: The devil is in the third year: a longitudinal study of erosion of empathy in medical school. Acad Med 84(9):1182–1191, 2009 19707055

Jackson ER, Shanafelt TD, Hasan O, et al: Burnout and alcohol abuse/dependence among U.S. medical students. Acad Med 91(9):1251–1256, 2016 26934693

Liaison Committee on Medical Education: Function and structure of a medical school: standards for accreditation of medical education programs leading to the M.D. degree. Washington, DC, Association of American Medical Colleges, 2019. Available at: https://lcme.org/publications/#Standards. Accessed April 25, 2019.

Maslach C, Leiter MP: Understanding the burnout experience: recent research and its implications for psychiatry. World Psychiatry 15(2):103–111, 2016 27265691

Melek SP, Perlman DJ, Davenport S. Addiction and mental health vs. physical health: analyzing disparities in network use and provider reimbursement rates. A Milliman Report, 30 November 2017

Moffat KJ, McConnachie A, Ross S, Morrison JM: First year medical student stress and coping in a problem-based learning medical curriculum. Med Educ 38(5):482–491, 2004 15107082

Montgomery A: The inevitability of physician burnout: implications for interventions. Burn Res 1(1):50–56, 2014

Neumann M, Edelhäuser F, Tauschel D, et al: Empathy decline and its reasons: a systematic review of studies with medical students and residents. Acad Med 86(8):996–1009, 2011 21670661

Oreskovich MR, Kaups KL, Balch CM, et al: Prevalence of alcohol use disorders among American surgeons. Arch Surg 147(2):168–174, 2012 22351913

Plakun EM: Psychotherapy and psychosocial treatment: recent advances and future directions. Psychiatr Clin North Am 38(3):405–418, 2015 26300031

Rosen IM, Gimotty PA, Shea JA, Bellini LM: Evolution of sleep quantity, sleep deprivation, mood disturbances, empathy, and burnout among interns. Acad Med 81(1):82–85, 2006 16377826

Santen SA, Holt DB, Kemp JD, Hemphill RR: Burnout in medical students: examining the prevalence and associated factors. South Med J 103(8):758–763, 2010 20622724

Schernhammer E: Taking their own lives—the high rate of physician suicide. N Engl J Med 352(24):2473–2476, 2005 15958803

Shanafelt TD, Bradley KA, Wipf JE, Back AL: Burnout and self-reported patient care in an internal medicine residency program. Ann Intern Med 136(5):358–367, 2002 11874308

Shanafelt TD, West C, Zhao X, et al: Relationship between increased personal well-being and enhanced empathy among internal medicine residents. J Gen Intern Med 20(7):559–564, 2005 16050855

Shanafelt TD, Balch CM, Bechamps G, et al: Burnout and medical errors among American surgeons. Ann Surg 251(6):995–1000, 2010 19934755

Shanafelt TD, Boone S, Tan L, et al: Burnout and satisfaction with work-life balance among U.S. physicians relative to the general U.S. population. Arch Intern Med 172(18):1377–1385, 2012 22911330

Shanafelt TD, Gradishar WJ, Kosty M, et al: Burnout and career satisfaction among US oncologists. J Clin Oncol 32(7):678–686, 2014 24470006

Shanafelt TD, Dyrbye LN, West CP: Addressing physician burnout: the way forward. JAMA 317(9):901–902, 2017 28196201

Stecker T: Well-being in an academic environment. Med Educ 38(5):465–478, 2004 15107080

Steinert C, Munder T, Rabung S, et al: Psychodynamic therapy: as efficacious as other empirically supported treatments? A meta-analysis testing equivalence of outcomes. Am J Psychiatry 174(10):943–953, 2017 28541091

Stratton TD, Saunders JA, Elam CL: Changes in medical students' emotional intelligence: an exploratory study. Teach Learn Med 20(3):279–284, 2008 18615305

Tricoci P, Allen JM, Kramer JM, et al: Scientific evidence underlying the ACC/AHA clinical practice guidelines. JAMA 301(8):831–841, 2009 19244190

Wallace JE, Lemaire J: Physician well being and quality of patient care: an exploratory study of the missing link. Psychol Health Med 14(5):545–552, 2009 19844833

West CP, Huschka MM, Novotny PJ, et al: Association of perceived medical errors with resident distress and empathy: a prospective longitudinal study. JAMA 296(9):1071–1078, 2006 DOI: 10.1001/jama.296.9.1071 16954486

Williams ES, Lawrence ER, Campbell KS, Spiehler S: The effect of emotional exhaustion and depersonalization on physician–patient communication: a theoretical model, implications, and directions for future research, in Biennial Review of Health Care Management: Meso Perspectives. Advances in Health Care Management Vol 8. Edited by Savage GT, Fottier MD. Bingley, UK, Emerald Group, 2009, pp 3–20

Advocacy Role Model Interview: Julie Chilton, M.D.

Advocacy Through Self-Disclosure

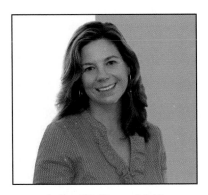

Julie Chilton, M.D.

Board-certified child, adolescent, and adult psychiatrist in private practice in Asheville, North Carolina; Assistant Clinical Professor, Yale Child Study Center

How did you come to be an advocate?

I didn't become an advocate until medical school. But the story behind my advocacy started during my freshman year of college, when my older sister killed herself. It wasn't until after I graduated from college and came home that I really grieved for the first time. I became depressed and saw a psychiatrist and started to feel better with medications and therapy.

However, even after I felt better, I judged myself a lot for having been depressed. I thought I couldn't be successful after that. Who would hire me? Who could love me, or want to date me? I had no role models who had been through this before to tell me, "You can get through it. You *can* be successful."

My mom noticed this, so she gave me a copy of *An Unquiet Mind* by Kay Redfield Jamison. Reading about Kay Jamison's journey with bipolar disorder and her success inspired me to see a future for myself. I decided that I wanted to be a child psychiatrist, since I'd had positive experiences with psychiatry. So I applied to medical school and got in.

Medical school could have been a fresh start for me: no one knew about my mental health history, and I didn't plan to draw attention to it. But beginning my second year, I realized that a lot of people were struggling. A beloved anatomy professor of mine killed himself, and around the same time, a medical student acquaintance of mine tried to kill herself, too. I came to see that I couldn't keep quiet about my own struggles if I wanted to help other people, so I started talking. I told my class about my history with depression and then set up a confidential dinner at my house for anyone experiencing mental health issues who wanted support.

I expected to be eating dinner by myself that first night, but to my surprise, seven people showed up. Before long, over 40 people were coming to these dinners during the 3 years I hosted them. We called ourselves the Redfield Group, after Kay Redfield Jamison. Eventually, Kay Jamison herself caught wind of our group. She came to our medical school to give grand rounds on suicide, donated her entire honorarium to the Redfield Group, and attended one of our meetings.

Could you describe the kind of advocacy work you do now?

I continued to tell my story throughout the rest of my training and beyond. I also got involved with the American Foundation for Suicide Prevention during residency and started a fellows' wellness program during fellowship. Currently, I'm continuing to travel nationally and internationally, giving talks and sharing my experiences with trainees.

So that's my form of advocacy. The reason I go around telling my story is this: with all the focus on burnout and wellness now, medical students and residents are being told that they *must* seek help for their mental health issues. Yet they don't have any role models, especially more senior physicians, who did the same thing. When that's the case, how can we expect them to feel comfortable with seeking help? My goal is to give them a role model and to encourage them to be role models for each other.

What advice do you have for other psychiatrist advocates?

1. You have to really believe in the issue you're fighting for. That's how you form authentic connections with people who feel similarly, which is so rewarding and results in more effective advocacy.
2. A huge barrier to advocacy is fear—fear of getting your message out there, fear of whether others will accept your message. When you're feeling this, remember that none of that stuff matters. Just focus on what's happening and on what you need to do to make things better.

4

How Do I Become an Advocate?

Onyi Ugorji, M.D., M.B.A.
Mary C. Vance, M.D., M.Sc.
Jessica S. Bayner, M.D.

Learning Objectives

By the end of this chapter, readers will be able to:

- Identify the essential factors needed for effective advocacy
- Understand the importance of mentorship and recognize pathways to mentorship
- Examine examples of how to integrate advocacy into the psychiatrist's career path
- Identify strategies that encourage lifelong advocacy

As physicians practicing in today's increasingly complex health care environment, it important that we not only "talk the talk" but also "walk the walk" when it comes to advocacy. The importance of becoming more intentional in the ways that we incorporate advocacy into our professional obligations cannot be overstated. Despite the growing consensus of the importance of advocacy within the physician's role, it remains difficult for many of us to find a place for advocacy in our psychiatric work.

The two subroles within advocacy are *agent* and *activist*. Some articles highlight how these seemingly contrasting subroles are a source of confusion and controversy. The physician as agent is one who "acts on a patient's behalf in order to secure access to resources, facilities, and support (such as specialist care, diagnostic testing, and ancillary services)" (Dobson et al. 2015, p. 214). In other words, the physician-agent *works within the established system* to help the patient. In contrast, the physician as activist uses their "expertise and influence…[to] change specific practices or policies on behalf of those served" (Dobson et al. 2015, p. 214). Consequently, the physician as activist focuses on *changing the system*.

A common barrier to becoming an advocate, for both trainees and practicing physicians, is the limited understanding of what exactly an advocate is and how an advocate acts, in addition to inexperience with the factors required to become an effective advocate. These barriers can be linked to the nature of medical training (for more information, see Chapter 1, "What Is Advocacy, and Why Is It Important?" and Chapter 8, "Education as Advocacy") in that the essential factors needed to become an effective advocate across a broad spectrum of advocacy levels are often not taught or developed, and in fact may be overlooked during medical education, training, and practice. The effect is that physicians can feel poorly prepared to work outside of the more familiar clinical arena, where they feel competent following their countless hours of medical training. Physicians need to find ways to manage their anxiety regarding inexperience in order to more effectively incorporate advocacy into their professional lives and into their roles as clinicians, administrators, and other health care leaders. In this chapter, we provide an overview of the essential factors for effective advocacy, examine strategies to identify and optimize mentorship, and look at opportunities to integrate advocacy into one's career.

Essential Factors for Effective Advocacy

Educating and Addressing Potential Knowledge Gaps

Any skill that is not used or called on frequently will no longer be useful. The same is true regarding the factors needed for effective advocacy. Beginning during medical education and training, many of us have developed the habit of ongoing, self-motivated learning. After training, we must remain experts in our field by staying up to date with current research findings, diagnostic updates, treatment revelations, changes to practice parameters, and even review of the basics of psychopathology and/or psychopharmacology. Fortunately, there are many ways to access medical information, depending on personal preference. In addition to an abundance of traditional resources, such as books and journals, that are available via print, online, and via apps, there are audio lectures, videos, podcasts, and other educational forums to engage us as lifelong learners. Remaining up to date helps us to fulfill certification and continuing medical education (CME) requirements, as well as to deliver the best possible patient care, which serves as a form of advocacy at the patient level. When we educate patients and their families about their conditions and recommended treatments, we empower them to take on an advocacy role regarding their own health.

Remaining up to date will also better prepare us to educate fellow health care providers (especially those in other medical specialties) and the community at large. We should take every opportunity to dispel misconceptions related to mental health disorders and address associated stigma tied to mental health concerns. Simply relating mental illness to other illnesses with a biological basis and conveying that mental illness is not the result of something wrong or defective with the person are important to repeat over and over again to patients, families, and the community at large. The stigma of mental illness is common and prevents many individuals from seeking help or acknowledging mental health concerns in themselves or family members.

It is important to identify non-illness-based knowledge gaps that are essential to the role of an effective physician advocate. Sometimes these gaps can be identified immediately from one's own experiences, but many times these knowledge gaps become evident as a result of questions from patients, system inadequacies, or policy failures, any of which can provide the inspiration to delve into a topic that is relevant to the role of an advocate but not yet understood by the burgeoning advocate. For example, someone might ask, "How is health care financed?" Knowledge of this topic is crucial to understanding health care as a whole, yet often neither physicians nor patients know much about it. To learn about this enormous topic, it is helpful to start with looking at a specific payer (Medicaid, Medicare, or private insurer) and the specific aspects that are most pertinent to your patient population or a specific patient in question. There are countless resources online that succinctly summarize many of the important points to be aware of in regard to a specific payer. Although the goal is not to be an expert when it comes to health insurers, becoming more familiar with health care financing can prove to be an asset for you when navigating the financial aspects of health care and can also better position you to advocate for improve-

> ### Case Example: Counteracting Stigma
>
> Dr. S recently became the medical director of a community health center's inpatient adult psychiatric unit. He frequently noticed that other medical personnel (e.g., medical consultants, nurses for cross-coverage, social workers to assist in disposition difficulties) appeared wary about visiting the unit or receiving psychiatric patients from the unit for medical stabilization. He decided to host an open house for the psychiatric unit and invited staff members from other hospital departments to see the psychiatric unit firsthand. During the open house, Dr. S, together with the unit staff members, took special care to explain some of the routine unit procedures, common diagnoses encountered, and basic inpatient treatment modalities. Some patients also volunteered to contribute by speaking to the visiting staff about their mental health improvements due, in part, to the help of the psychiatric unit staff and the inpatient treatment. Dr. S believed that inviting a diverse array of staff members from different departments could help dispel problematic and false images of mental illness and psychiatric care fostered by stereotypes and instead develop a more realistic view of the psychiatric unit and ways it might help a range of patients with various psychiatric illnesses. The open house event was so well received that it became a biennial event and recently hosted almost 300 staff members. The hospital staff's overall opinions about the psychiatric unit improved, and nursing staff members from multiple other departments requested experience on the inpatient psychiatric care unit.

ments in remuneration as well as availability of and access to needed resources and services for patients and their families.

Many of the essential factors for effective advocacy described in the following subsections incorporate an aspect of education and addressing knowledge gaps, demonstrating that these factors are not isolated abilities and attributes but instead typically flow together and can potentially form a formidable skill set for an effective physician advocate.

Awareness of the Sociopolitical Contexts

Analyzing the larger picture is crucial when assessing and treating a patient's health status. In other words, you need to consider the social, economic, and political influences that impact your patient's diagnosis, presentation, prognosis, access to treatment or services, and so on. You can ask yourself questions such as "How did this person land in my office?" and "What are the broader social factors at play?" (Law et al. 2016). These non-illness-related factors that impact health status are called the determinants of health. The Centers for Disease Control and Prevention (2014) provide the following definitions, which clarify the close relationship between determinants of health, social determinants of health, and health inequities.

- *Determinants of health:* "Factors that contribute to a person's current state of health." The five factors or determinants of health of a population are detailed in Table 4–1.
- *Social determinants of health:* "The complex, integrated, and overlapping social structures and economic systems that are responsible for most health inequities. These social structures and economic systems include the social environment, physical environment, health services, and structural and societal factors. Social determinants of health are shaped by the distribution of money, power, and resources throughout local communities, nations, and the world."
- *Health inequity:* "A difference or disparity in health outcomes that is systematic, avoidable, and unjust."

Figure 4–1 illustrates how vastly impactful determinants of health can be and how they affect most if not all aspects of a patient's life. Differences in social determinants of health can result in health inequities and increased morbidity and mortality. Having a general understanding of determinants of health provides the physician with the ability to see the patient and/or a patient population in a more comprehensive way. Focusing on specific social determinants of health can inspire numerous advocacy opportunities that span the entire spectrum of advocacy.

Communication

Active Listening and Nonverbal Cues

An effective advocate needs to master the art of communicating effectively. When thinking about improving communication skills, you might easily fall into the trap of focusing on how to verbally relay your ideas to a variety of individuals and/or groups in an engaging and persuasive way. However, before focusing on how to "win" people over with the gift of gab, consider sharpening your listening skills. Active listening is the ability to give your full attention to the concerns of others (fellow students, trainees, and physicians; patients and their families; hospital staff; policy

TABLE 4–1. The five determinants of health

Determinants of health	Examples
Biology and genetics	Sex, age
Individual behavior	Psychological assets (e.g., self-efficacy)
	Negative mood/affects (e.g., hopelessness)
	Risk-related behavior (e.g., alcohol use, unprotected sex)
	Physical activity; sleep and diet habits
Social environment	Social connectedness
	Race, ethnicity, culture
	Discrimination
	Work conditions
	Gender identity
Physical environment	Residence quality
	Crowding conditions
	Educational opportunities
	Pollution
	Exposure to firearms
Health services	Access to health care
	Quality of health care
	Patient engagement
	Health literacy

Source. Adapted from Centers for Disease Control and Prevention: Definitions. Atlanta, GA, Centers for Disease Control and Prevention, March 21, 2014. Available at: www.cdc.gov/nchhstp/socialdeterminants/definitions.html. Accessed August 24, 2019.

makers) to determine what issues are most important to your patients and the community and what the various current opinions are.

Many people assume that psychiatrists excel at listening, which may be the case for some but not for all. Unfortunately, because of the nature of health care today, with increasing requirements for documentation eroding the time spent with patients, even in psychiatry we struggle to engage in active listening. For example, it is commonplace (and in some settings seen as an asset) for a physician to document notes while seeing a patient. It is unfortunate how we have "adapted" to the demands of the

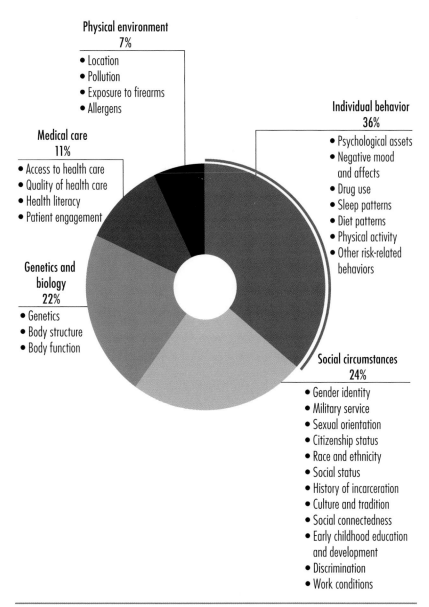

FIGURE 4–1. Determinants of health.

Source. For a more detailed map of all factors correlated with health outcomes for an individual, see GoInvo: Determinants of health. Arlington, MA, Goinvo, 2019. Available at: www.goinvo.com/vision/determinants-of-health. Accessed August 24, 2019.

electronic health record, and being a psychiatrist does not protect us from being ineffective listeners. Like most skills, communication (and, by extension, active listening) is a skill that requires consistent practice for a person to become proficient.

Physician communication expert Kenneth Cohen has been quoted as saying, "Active listening is…listening with one's eyes as well as one's ears. [Only a small amount] of communication is related to content—the rest pertains to body language and tone of voice" ("Developing Effective Communication Skills" 2007). With active listening, you should focus completely on the speaker. Pay attention with your eyes and ears. Take note of the speaker's nonverbal cues, such as body language and tone of voice, that may give insight into any emotions underlying and/or driving the speaker's message. To do this effectively, avoid both mental multitasking and judgment. Withholding judgment does not mean that you must agree with the views of the speaker; rather, it means avoiding the urge to criticize, negate, or blame the speaker if their opinions or words do not coincide with yours. By putting aside judgment, you can better understand the speaker, both verbal and nonverbal cues, and take in new perspectives and insights that may prove valuable in your potential advocacy.

Finally, encourage the speaker to speak openly or to explain a topic in more depth by using phrases such as "Can you tell me more?" Try not to say too much or to hijack the speaking position. Reflecting a speaker's message by asking questions that briefly summarize the speaker's points not only demonstrates to the speaker that you are listening (which also builds rapport) but also helps both parties to be absolutely certain that the received message was understood as the speaker intended. Examples of phrases and questions could include, "What I'm hearing is…?" or "What do you mean when you say…?" (Robinson et al. 2018).

Effective listening applies to anyone and everyone, from patients and their families to colleagues, attending physicians and supervisors, hospital or clinic leadership, professionals in other medical and nonmedical fields, and so forth. At the level of the individual patient, improving listening skills can improve diagnostic accuracy, physician-patient partnership, and patient treatment adherence (by choosing an appropriate treatment regimen that is in line with the patient's goals and socioeconomic capabilities). As you can already see, the potential breadth and depth of insights obtained by effective listening habits are numerous and invaluable.

Conveying Your Message

Now that you understand the importance of active listening, the next steps are aimed toward building your message. As discussed earlier in this chapter (see subsection "Educating and Addressing Potential Knowledge Gaps"), it is important to recognize knowledge gaps and to research the topic of concern (i.e., by reviewing current literature) so that you can speak knowledgeably about the identified topic. Research will help you identify valuable facts, patterns, and details of the issue, such as the following (Dobson et al. 2015; Law et al. 2016):

1. Who the key stakeholders are
2. What progress has been made on the issue
3. Who or what is involved in addressing or contributing to the issue
4. What may be the best ways to disseminate your message

After researching the issue, it is time to develop your message. The message may be refined across time as circumstances associated with the issue change and even your own opinions or strategies evolve. The following are key aspects that should be addressed in an effective message (Dobson et al. 2015; Law et al. 2016):

1. Your key audience
2. Your key messages
3. Your talking points
4. Your story

Keep in mind that the words and phrases you choose for your message are important. Ultimately, you should make sure that your message will be received as you intended. Asking different people to review your message and provide feedback about what they interpret your message to be can help to identify personal blind spots and make sure that your message is as clear as possible. Some readers might still remember this 2004 statement from then-President George W. Bush: "Too many good docs are getting out of the business. Too many OB/GYNs aren't able to practice their love with women all across the country." The President likely had good intentions with this statement, but it is easy to see how the message can be misconstrued. Although this is a lighthearted example, it serves to support the point: the words in any message, especially from a psychiatrist, are important and garner significant attention, so choose your words carefully.

After developing an effective message, you can decide how to disseminate your message. Means of conveying a message include, for example, a newspaper op-ed, newsletter, radio, social media (e.g., Twitter, Facebook, Instagram), podcasts, presentations, letters or phone calls to legislators, research papers, town halls, lectures, and forums of social groups of like-minded individuals. For more information on the essential elements of communication when engaging in legislative or media advocacy, see Chapter 7, "Legislative Advocacy," and Chapter 10, "Engaging the Popular Media."

Leveraging Social Position

As physicians, "we often find ourselves at the crossroads of a unique and sometimes intimate knowledge of patient needs, intersecting with the ability to leverage influence to change health care system delivery, social barriers, and even impact political policy" (Luft 2017, p. e109). In advocacy work, use your professional status as a physician, your network, and your access to resources to assist in addressing the issue or to jump-start your efforts to address it. When you are working on an advocacy issue, leveraging your professional identity can prove helpful when translating your ideas into action plans.

Working in Teams and in the Community

There is strength in numbers. Although some advocacy activities can be done without a team or community involvement, these are often limited to patient-level interventions, such as ensuring that your treatment plan is realistic and affordable. Even certain activities that can be done individually, such as contacting local legislators via letters or phone calls, are more effective when a larger group collaborates to deliver the same message—in this example, to convey to legislators that this group represents an even larger group of potential voters.

When working at the community level, we should take care not to underestimate what we can learn from the community—or to overestimate what we can teach the community.

> It is essential to have the humility to recognize many physicians come from a background of relative privilege, and thus may not be able to directly relate to how a person without social privilege experiences illness or need. Being educated professionals, physicians ought to be reflective, self-aware, and cautious in assuming they know or understand the socially disadvantaged patient's priorities. (Luft 2017, p. 110)

If we are self-aware about possible blind spots, we should want to receive feedback from community members who are close to the problem that we are trying to address. By creating a safe space for bidirectional communication, education, and the sharing of ideas, we can strengthen ties to the community that can prove valuable for advocacy activities.

Forming a team is another way to bring together like-minded individuals and groups. One example of how to do this is presented in the

American Academy of Child and Adolescent Psychiatry's (2012) guide *Organizing Forums on Children's Mental Health*, which highlights the necessary aspects of coming together to build an effective team. Some of the recommendations are summarized here:

- Be organized and strategic when forming a team or participating in one.
- When considering your team, reach out to your professional network for members or join local groups, task forces, committees, coalitions, and so on. If there is no group that quite addresses the specified problem, create your own.
- Name your network and make it clear and brief. This is a small snapshot of what the group will be doing or advocating for.
- Identify a clear and achievable goal. This will allow you to streamline strategies and also allows potential members to be clear about whether their goals align with those of the team.
- Identify roles and strategies or tasks for each member's role. Try to "divide and conquer" but also support collaboration and support each other's work at every step.
- With the goal in mind, create a timeline that is neither overly aggressive (to prevent setting up the team for failure) nor too slow or relaxed (which may squander the inspiring momentum that may have built up at the initial stage of team formation and development).

Mentorship

As mentioned at the beginning of this chapter, some of the anticipated barriers to becoming an advocate can be attributed to the nature of medical education and training. Advocacy training is not emphasized or taught in a formal manner for most physicians during medical school, residency, and fellowship. Directly related to this is the fact that it can prove difficult for trainees to identify mentors without being involved in a formal training curriculum (e.g., one that includes lectures on advocacy by attendings) in which potential mentors participate and therefore are more easily identifiable. Physicians should attempt to identify an advocacy mentor, although doing so is not as straightforward as identifying mentors during medical education, training, and practice. In fact, research conducted by interviewing physician-advocates revealed that participants considered mentorship to be one of the critical experiences that led to a "transition from an inclination towards health advocacy work to active engagement in such activities" (Law et al. 2016, p. 1394).

If you have observed an individual engage in effective advocacy in a way that you would like to emulate, consider contacting that person, either directly or through established channels. When you speak with a potential mentor, you may feel awkward about requesting mentorship at the initial meeting. Ideally, arrange to meet with your potential mentor, and during the meeting ask about the mentor's career trajectory. Eventually, it may feel appropriate to directly ask for guidance and mentorship, especially if you are able to highlight your shared goals and any similarities in your careers. Keep in mind that the work is not done after a mentorship relationship commences. A common pitfall is that mentees may be too passive, expecting that mentors should initiate topics. This is how many mentor-mentee relationships fail or fade with time. Be proactive (without being overbearing) and follow up after every meeting.

Conferences and networking events with like-minded individuals provide additional opportunities to find mentors. There are also organized groups and fellowships that match members with mentors on the basis of career interests. For example, the American Psychiatric Association's (APA's) resident-fellow fellowship programs offer multiple opportunities for guidance through networking with many professionals during the fellowships and also match members with experienced APA mentors (for more information, see subsection "Integrating Advocacy Through Organized Medicine").

Depending on your current role, after you have benefited from a mentorship experience, you might consider becoming involved in guiding or mentoring students, trainees, and/or early career psychiatrists. If you work in an academic setting, there are many avenues for identifying students and/or trainees with whom to work. Many groups and associations, including the APA and other psychiatric subspecialty organizations, also eagerly welcome volunteer mentors. Individuals and organizational support personnel who do not serve as traditional mentors are viewed as *facilitators*. They provide resources, time, and other opportunities that help to sharpen essential advocacy skills and develop strategies that turn ideas into action (Law et al. 2016).

Integrating Advocacy Into Your Career

Even with a well-developed advocacy toolbox and a strong mentor or team of mentors, it can be difficult to sustain advocacy efforts and keep up your enthusiasm if you have not found a way to integrate advocacy into your career in a way that is sustainable and rewarding. Instead of doing advocacy as a "side gig," which decreases the time available for advocacy and increases the risk of burnout, you can consider implementing strategies to help to integrate advocacy into your career, such as by pairing advocacy with involvement in organized medicine or by learning more about advocacy during medical school, residency, and fellowship training.

Integrating Advocacy Through Organized Medicine

Becoming involved with a professional medical advocacy organization provides an excellent introduction to physician advocacy. These organizations include, but are not limited to, general medical organizations such as the American Medical Association; specialty medical organizations such as the APA; and subspecialty medical organizations such as the American Academy of Child and Adolescent Psychiatry, the American Society of Addiction Medicine, the American Academy of Addiction Psychiatry, the Academy of Consultation-Liaison Psychiatry, the American Association for Geriatric Psychiatry, and the American Academy of Psychiatry and the Law. After you determine that an organization's advocacy goals align with yours, you might consider becoming an active part of it. In the following box, ways to become involved specifically with the APA are described to illustrate how you can become involved in organized medicine in general. Additionally, at the end of this chapter, an advocacy role model interview with Dr. Jeffrey Akaka is provided as an example of a long and successful career involving advocacy through organized medicine.

Becoming Involved With the American Psychiatric Association

Trainees, early career psychiatrists, private practitioners, community psychiatrists, and providers integrated in academic settings all have the ability to collaborate with APA and address their concerns. As of 2018, APA is divided into seven areas for North America, and these areas are further subdivided into district branches that represent smaller subsections within each geographic location. Identifying one's district branch within a given area and becoming involved with that district branch provides an opportunity to be involved in a network of like-minded colleagues who are aware of the community's needs. Furthermore, such peers have insight about how to navigate the political landscape in order to tackle issues on local and state levels.

Becoming Involved With
the American Psychiatric Association *(continued)*

Once you have become involved with APA, there are numerous ways to engage in efforts to effect change. Officially becoming a member of a district branch and attending meetings will help you to become aware of various legislative issues. If members express a desire to receive guidance about a particular topic, APA is an excellent resource for information, including relevant resource documents, action papers, or position statements on the topic. If no information is available about the issue, the district branch can enlist members to write suggestions to the area council. Once a cohesive document is created, it moves forward through proper channels for review by specific councils and committees, with the potential to be adopted by APA. Moreover, district branch members can opt to be on a task force or run for various elected positions and thereby further their participation in the governance of APA. Please reference the diagram below for more details about APA's structure, keeping in mind that understanding an organization's governance structure can go a long way in helping you to steer your advocacy efforts within that organization as well as to eventually become an organizational leader.

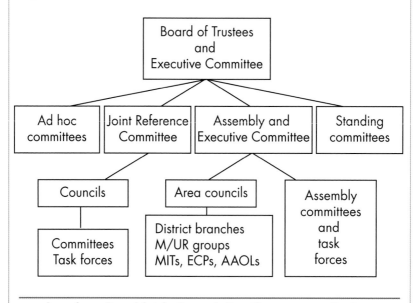

American Psychiatric Association Governance System

Abbreviations. AAOLs=Assembly allied organization liaisons; ECPs=early-career psychiatrists; MITs=members in training; M/UR=minority and underrepresented.

**Becoming Involved With
the American Psychiatric Association *(continued)***

Psychiatry residents and fellows have special opportunities to broaden their advocacy efforts and find advocacy mentorship within APA through its APA/APA Foundation fellowship programs. For example, trainees throughout North America who are dedicated to combating disparities in health care are considered for a fellowship in public psychiatry. Ten people are chosen each year for the 2-year program, which is done in tandem with training. Over the course of the fellowship, the designated participants have monthly teleconference calls, receive a stipend to attend conferences, become connected with leaders who are passionate about working in the public sector, and participate in an APA council to become familiar with the governance of the organization. Other fellowships sponsored by APA emphasize other aspects of mental health, but all are intended to foster leadership and promote advocacy among trainees.

Integrating Advocacy Through Medical School, Residency, and Fellowship Training

Although there will be opportunities to integrate advocacy into an established or burgeoning career, one might also engage in such work as a student before beginning to practice. Certain medical schools have organized tracks for those looking for a more experiential approach to becoming a community physician (see "Training Resources" at the end of the chapter). An example of this is the University of Texas Southwestern's community action research track, which encourages students to be a part of the local patient population while gaining clinical knowledge. George Washington University also offers students a chance to train in the community and urban health track. Participants in the program are educated about the challenges in treating the underserved and ways to overcome associated obstacles. In the event that such curricula have not been developed in a given medical school, students may consider creating a track of their own and tailoring it to address the needs of their community.

Getting involved in national organizations as a medical student is another way to intertwine advocacy with medical education. The American Medical Student Association has a Community and Public Health Action Committee that promotes activism and aims to motivate future physicians to become passionate about public health issues. Likewise, the Student National Medical Association has chapters in allopathic and osteopathic schools in the United States that support underrepresented minority medical students and are committed to developing cultural competence among providers across the country. Participation in such groups facilitates community outreach, and this effort helps to reduce health inequities and stigma against mental illness.

During psychiatry residency, budding psychiatrists may be exposed to social justice work through advocacy-oriented training programs. Similar to community tracks at medical schools, some residency programs have curricula designed to promote advocacy and to provide hands-on experiences with underserved populations. For example, the rural psychiatry track at Upstate Medical University was developed to ensure that quality treatment and research is available at affiliated sites in scarcely populated regions in New York State. Residents may also choose to train in a community hospital and/or a more urban setting to obtain greater clinical exposure and learn practical aspects of treating another at-risk demographic. The psychiatry residency at Bergen New Bridge Medical Center is an example of this type of program, which has developed services for the county at large, in response to the substance abuse, behavioral health, and medical needs of its patients.

Apart from working in a specific track or training in a community hospital, psychiatry residents can act as advocates in a variety of ways. As described in the previous subsection, joining the local APA district branch allows members to become cognizant about issues of concern in their demographic area. The Committee of Interns and Residents, which is the largest house staff union in the United States, also provides unique opportunities for leadership. Residents may serve as representatives from their training programs and also may expand their participation by running for elected positions at the national level. Other members have founded union chapters in programs that were not previously affiliated with the Committee of Interns and Residents. Such efforts help to build leadership skills and to create a unified voice for trainees, with resulting improvements in workplace quality.

For individuals who would like to acquire more training after residency, fellowships are an opportunity to become subspecialty qualified and to broaden areas of expertise within which to advocate. Not all types of fellowships are accredited by the Accreditation Council for Graduate Medical Education (ACGME), however, so psychiatrists considering a fellowship experience to broaden their advocacy skill set should weigh program accreditation, among other factors. For example, multiple programs in the country offer official public psychiatry fellowships. Although ACGME does not yet include public psychiatry as an accredited specialty, the American Association of Community Psychiatrists has been approved to offer a certification exam for community psychiatry (Moran 2018). Public psychiatry fellowship training has the advantages of providing rich clinical experience with marginalized populations who would benefit from physician advocacy, as well as offering many opportunities to practice advocacy skills.

Case Example of Advocacy in Action

The need for greater access to mental health care has been a long-standing issue throughout the nation. Challenges range from limited insurance coverage to stigma associated with seeking psychiatric and psychological care. The shortage of mental health professionals is of particular concern. Depending on the region in the country, people may have to wait months before they can schedule an intake appointment or may limit their follow-up sessions because of the inconvenience of traveling far distances to see a practitioner. Mental Health America (2018) reported that 24 million individuals with mental illness are not in treatment.

The following case example illustrates how medical education can serve as both a tool for advocacy to improve access to care and an end product of advocacy by creating a new pipeline of psychiatrists to address workforce shortages. More information on using education as advocacy can be found in Chapter 8, "Education as Advocacy."

Case Example: Education and Advocacy

One approach to increasing the workforce is to create more training opportunities for future psychiatrists. This was evident to the psychiatry department at the Billings Clinic in Montana. Everyone recognized the challenge of recruiting physicians to the underserved region in one of the three states without a psychiatry residency program (Alaska, Montana, and Wyoming), which was due, in part, to the lack of people who felt comfortable and familiar with the systems in place. As part of the leadership council in the hospital, the chair of the department petitioned to start a program for psychiatry trainees. The board members agreed to move forward with the idea, but the department had to procure funds to support his proposal. Local leaders were included to advise how to utilize mental health resources in the area, and financial backing was also provided by philanthropists. The ACGME was a part of the process in order to ensure that the prospective curriculum was in line with the core competencies.

> ### Case Example: Education and Advocacy *(continued)*
>
> The program's first three psychiatry residents started in July 2019, and the program will continue to have three slots per year. The Montana track at Billings Clinic will officially be a part of the University of Washington's psychiatry residency program and will offer the chance for residents to learn about community-based systems in frontier medicine (www.uwmtpsychtrack.org). The psychiatry department's efforts illustrate the impact that people can make in their environment by identifying a problem and advocating for meaningful solutions.

Strategies That Encourage Lifelong Advocacy

The realities of health advocacy are that change, especially on a large scale, can be slow and that small successes may be followed by a series of setbacks. These can be frustrating for physician-advocates and cause many to limit their advocacy work and/or experience feelings of burnout. Despite these frustrations, many physicians have embraced advocacy for many years. Law et al. (2016) describe three "more elaborate skills" that "lifelong advocates" reported as significantly contributing to their advocacy persistence and stamina.

1. *Placing a premium on continuous learning and improvement:* The lifelong physician-advocates regularly invested in their commitment to advocacy work by routinely assessing their prior advocacy efforts and actively learning from them. To describe this process, the authors use the term *constructive discontent*, which means to be "constructive and positive, but to never be satisfied with where we're at, and to always be looking for and striving for ways to do things better [at all levels of advocacy]" (Law et al. 2016, p. 1395).
2. *Practicing self-reflection and self-reflexivity:* These actions foster self-awareness, humility, and the ability to learn from one's mistakes.
   a. Self-reflection focuses on critical thinking, personal reflection, and the integration of new learning into existing cognitions.
   b. Self-reflexivity focuses on recognizing one's social location or place in a situation and the capacity to intuit how these attributes may affect others.

3. *Embracing collaboration:* Lifelong advocates identified social connectedness as a way to "weather the storm together" and to help cope with anticipated frustrations and setbacks that are characteristic of the typical winding path of advocacy work. They viewed advocacy as an "inherently social endeavor.... For some, the social dimension of advocacy was also the element that made it possible to endure the unavoidable disappointments and stay committed over time" (Law et al. 2016, p. 1395).

Conclusion

There are many avenues to advocacy in mental health. For both beginning and experienced advocates, numerous opportunities are available to acquire an advocacy skill set. Medical students, residents, fellows, early career psychiatrists, and seasoned professionals can all benefit from becoming aware of local and national resources, learning about advocacy issues, and working in concert with others to address these issues. Through mentorship, we can all inspire others to become advocates, help to develop collaborative advocacy networks by urging colleagues to join medical advocacy organizations, and address and improve today's urgent mental health care concerns.

Training Resources

American Medical Student Association, Community and Public Health Action Committee: www.amsa.org/advocacy/action-committees/cph. Accessed June 27, 2019.

Bergen New Bridge Medical Center: www.newbridgehealth.org. Accessed June 27, 2019.

Committee of Interns and Residents: www.cirseiu.org. Accessed June 27, 2019.

George Washington University School of Medicine and Health Sciences, Office of Student Professional Enrichment, Community/Urban Health: https://smhs.gwu.edu/oso/track-program/community. Accessed June 27, 2019.

Student National Medical Association, Community Outreach: https://snma.org/page/programsoutreach. Accessed January 9, 2020.

University of Texas Southwestern Medical Center: Community Action Research Track (CART): www.utsouthwestern.edu/edumedia/edufiles/departments_centers/fam_comm_med/cart-overview.pdf. Accessed June 27, 2019.

University of Washington Psychiatry Residency Training Program, The Montana Track at Billings Clinic: www.uwmtpsychtrack.org. Accessed June 27, 2019.

Upstate Medical University, Psychiatry, Rural and Community Psychiatry Tracks: www.upstate.edu/psych/education/residency/rural_community_psych/index.php. Accessed June 27, 2019.

References

American Academy of Child and Adolescent Psychiatry: Organizing forums on children's mental health. Washington, DC, American Academy of Child and Adolescent Psychiatry, 2012. Available at: www.aacap.org/App_Themes/AACAP/docs/medical_students_and_residents/residents_and_fellows/organizing_forums_on_childrens_mental_health.pdf. Accessed August 24, 2019.

Centers for Disease Control and Prevention: NCHHSTP Social Determinants of Health: Definitions. Atlanta, GA, Centers for Disease Control and Prevention, March 21, 2014. Available at: www.cdc.gov/nchhstp/socialdeterminants/definitions.html. Accessed August 24, 2019.

Developing effective communication skills. J Oncol Pract 3(6):314–317, 2007 29436953

Dobson S, Voyer S, Hubinette M, et al: From the clinic to the community: the activities and abilities of effective health advocates. Acad Med 90(2):214–220, 2015 25470309

Law M, Leung P, Veinot P, et al: A qualitative study of the experiences and factors that led physicians to be lifelong health advocates. Acad Med 91(10):1392–1397, 2016 27438157

Luft LM: The essential role of physician as advocate: how and why we pass it on. Can Med Educ J 8(3):e109–e116, 2017 29098052

Mental Health America: Mental Health in America—Access to Care Data. Alexandria, VA, Mental Health America, 2018. Available at: www.mentalhealthamerica.net/issues/mental-health-america-access-care-data. Accessed on June 27, 2019.

Moran M: AACP offers certification exam in community psychiatry. Psychiatric News, November 9, 2018. Available at: https://psychnews.psychiatryonline.org/doi/10.1176/appi.pn.2018.11b2. Accessed June 27, 2019.

Robinson LJS, Segal J, Smith MMA: Effective communication improving communication skills in your work and personal relationships. September 2018. Available at: www.helpguide.org/articles/relationships-communication/effective-communication.htm. Accessed August 24, 2019.

Advocacy Role Model Interview: Jeffrey Akaka, M.D.

Advocacy Through Organized Medicine

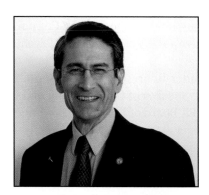

Jeffrey Akaka, M.D.

Clinical Professor of Psychiatry, University of Hawai'i School of Medicine and Former Medical Director, Diamond Head Community Mental Health Center, Honolulu, Hawaii; Past President, Hawaii Psychiatric Medical Association; Board of Trustees, American Psychiatric Association (2006–2008, 2012–2018)

How did you come to be an advocate?

At 6 years old I marched around the Hawaii State Capitol carrying a sign that said "Vote NO!" on a bill that would have harmed Native Hawaiians. My father and his torch led that march for 3 dark nights against powerful interests against us, but we won by a 13 to 12 vote in the Hawaii State Senate. My father, the late Reverend Abraham Akaka, taught me that no matter what the odds, always strive to do the right thing; ask first politely and strategically, but do not be afraid to make your point assertively if necessary.

Advocating means taking action to uplift the lives of others. If something isn't right and needs to be stopped, or when something good needs to be created, then no matter how formidable the odds against you may look, advocate anyway, and you just might win!

Could you describe the kind of advocacy work you do now?

In congress and in Hawaii I have testified in formal hearings as well as lobbied behind the scenes—including for parity at the turn of our century, legalization of gay marriage in Hawaii in 2011 (the first piece of legislation signed by the newly elected Governor and friend Neil Abercrombie), and more recently educated over a dozen elected and appointed public officials to push forward collaborative care and wrote a bill to have Hawaii Medicaid cover collaborative care the same as Medicare (which almost passed).

From my first appointment to the APA Committee of American Indian, Alaska Native and Native Hawaiian Psychiatrists by past President Joseph English, M.D., I served as Chair of the Committee of Minority and Under Represented Representatives, Recorder, and Parliamentarian, Speaker of the Assembly and two terms as Area 7 Trustee on the APA Board of Trustees. I continue as Vice Chair of the APAPAC for over a dozen years since shortly after its creation in 2001 and as Delegate to the AMA. As past President of the Hawaii Psychiatric Medical Association, I continue to chair its Legislative Committee and its Political Action Committee, HIPPAC.

Involvement in organized medicine can facilitate big advocacy goals you can't achieve by yourself. You have to join, or gather together, like-minded people. The bigger your goals are and the more people you organize and persuade, whether APA, AMA, your community, or your elected representatives, the greater your likelihood of accomplishment. That's how we won parity in Congress in 2008.

Finally, just as I had great mentors, I've tried to help the next generation of advocates succeed and was surprised to be presented by the Assembly of the APA in May 2019 the Assembly Resident-Fellow Member Mentor Award for Outstanding Mentorship of Residents/Fellows and/or Medical Students in Psychiatry.

What advice do you have for other psychiatrist-advocates?

1. The more specific you are in defining what you want to accomplish, the better your chance of success. Read *Good to Great* by Jim Collins, *The Seven Measures of Success* by ASAE, and *The 360 Degree Leader* by John Maxwell.
2. Think outside the box to create win-wins: In 1998 we asked Hawaii legislators to lobby APA leadership to bring the Annual Meeting to Hawaii, had the best meeting ever in 2011, and stopped bad prescribing legislation for decades!
3. Have fun!

PART II
Practicing Advocacy

5

Patient-Level Advocacy

J. Corey Williams, M.D.
Mary C. Vance, M.D., M.Sc.
Kristin S. Budde, M.D., M.P.H.

Learning Objectives

By the end of this chapter, readers will be able to:

- Define patient-level advocacy
- Understand the rationale for patient-level advocacy, especially as it relates to health disparities and the social realities of historically marginalized groups
- Identify opportunities for patient-level advocacy in daily clinical practice
- Describe how patient-level advocacy can advance social justice and equity in health care

The bulk of this volume addresses advocacy in the wider world, yet we as psychiatrists spend most of our time treating individual patients. Moreover, many psychiatrists are looking to bring a sense of social justice and equity to their clinical practice, especially given that patients with mental illness have a long history of being disenfranchised and mistreated by the medical system as well as by society at large—and that they fare even worse when the presence of mental illness intersects with other historically marginalized identities. How do we bring the spirit of advocacy and social justice to our everyday clinical encounters? In this chapter, we discuss advocacy at the level of individual patients, especially in the context of promoting social justice and equality for historically marginalized groups (i.e., groups that have been marginalized and even oppressed in the United States on the basis of race, sexual orientation, religion, psychiatric or physical disability, or other minority or underrepresented status), and provide a series of clinical vignettes to demonstrate what patient-level advocacy looks like in action.

What Is Patient-Level Advocacy?

Patient-level advocacy centers on individual patients and the societal forces that shape their life and health. (For more background on the social determinants of health and how health care systems impact patients' care, see Chapter 1, "What Is Advocacy, and Why Is It Important?") But rather than focusing merely on the clinical encounter, therapeutic relationship, and medications prescribed, patient-level advocacy takes into account the frames of care and services that patients usually navigate alone, as well as patients' social, cultural, and historical context. Importantly, we believe that patient-level advocacy should also seek to ensure equitable and just care for all, with special attention to advocacy for historically marginalized groups, who are often at a disadvantage when advocating for themselves because of a myriad of factors, including cultural barriers and discrimination (as discussed in the next section). Also, because patient-level advocacy requires us to be responsible for representing the interests of diverse individuals who may have very different backgrounds and values from ourselves, we must stay attuned to our own biases when engaging in patient-level advocacy and not allow such biases to impact whether and how we advocate.

The role of the patient-level advocate can be split into two parts: clinical agency and paraclinical agency (Dobson et al. 2015). *Clinical agency* (i.e., within the health care system) begins with a patient's immediate medical needs (e.g., therapeutic relationship and medicine) but takes an extra step to ensure that the recommended treatments are available and affordable. *Paraclinical agency* also grows out of the clinical needs of a patient but expands to address the societal factors that affect health and wellness (e.g., housing status, discrimination, neighborhood violence). Both parts are related to the direct clinical care of an individual patient but broaden the scope of the clinician's role beyond a traditional approach to medical care.

There are many ways in which we can implement patient-level advocacy in our daily clinical practice. Patient-level advocacy can potentially occur in every encounter that we have in the clinic or hospital, including during office visits, team rounds, administrative meetings, and consultations. For example, clinical team rounds and other group meetings are often daily or weekly responsibilities for many psychiatrists. These can be particularly effective settings in which to disrupt discriminatory frameworks and conversations, thereby influencing patient care toward more equitable and just practices.

Principles of Advocacy for Historically Marginalized Groups

In this chapter, we place a special emphasis on advocacy for historically marginalized groups—which includes individuals with mental illness from all backgrounds—because there is a large body of evidence that demonstrates that U.S. medical institutions, including the mental health care system, are not effective in treating these diverse populations (Pumariega et al. 2013). Researchers have found evidence of discrimination and disparities in care across all phases of the health care system, from prehospital management (Hewes et al. 2018) and emergency department care (Goyal et al. 2015) to diagnostic and treatment practices (Bradley et al. 2004; Haeri et al. 2011; Morgan et al. 2013). In all phases of medical care, historically marginalized groups are worse off. Although ensuring access to health care for all is fundamentally important, this research suggests that even when they have access to care, patients from historically marginalized groups are treated discriminatorily within the health care system on a daily basis.

Patients with a psychiatric diagnosis are already part of a historically marginalized group. Accordingly, psychiatrists play a crucial role in advocacy for historically marginalized groups, especially in those cases when the intersectionality of mental illness and other historically marginalized statuses creates additional barriers for these groups. The stigma surrounding patients with mental illness within the medical system is well known to contribute to a variety of negative outcomes (Acosta et al. 2012; Jones et al. 2008; Thornicroft et al. 2007). An additional issue documented in the literature is *diagnostic overshadowing*, in which patients' physical complaints are misattributed to mental illness, especially when physicians on the treatment teams hold stigmatizing attitudes (Shefer et al. 2014). (For more information on diagnostic overshadowing and other challenges that patients with mental illness commonly face in nonpsychiatric medical settings, see Chapter 18, "Advocacy for Patients in Medical Settings"). Given these findings and the long history of mistreatment of individuals with mental illness, all providers must be careful not to stigmatize individuals with mental illness and to ensure that these patients receive equitable care as compared with their nonpsychiatric counterparts. As psychiatrists, the physicians most often responsible for representing patients with mental illness to the rest of the medical community as well as the larger world, we must be particularly aware of this evidence of past and present mistreatment and vigilantly guard our patients against future mistreatment.

Within psychiatry and other medical fields, much work is needed to ensure equitable treatment of marginalized groups in daily clinical practice. To successfully advocate for them, we as physicians must be aware of the patients who belong to marginalized groups, understand these patients' history and culture, and be mindful of our own biases and knowledge gaps. A historically and culturally informed approach takes into account how the accumulation of past experiences, spanning not only the patient's own lifetime but also the lives of previous generations, may inform a patient's current experiences of and reactions to treatment providers. Maintaining an ongoing, present-day awareness of the ways in which people are discriminated against, both in the medical system and in broader society, is also necessary in order to be able to correct these injustices when presented with the opportunity.

A physician's extensive medical education and knowledge do not necessarily translate into expertise on complex issues such as the intersections of mental illness, race, gender, sexuality, and more. Therefore, physicians who wish to be advocates for patients should approach this task with an attitude of continual learning and humility, which includes continually striving to acknowledge and address their own biases. We encourage the reader to examine the suggested readings and references at the end of the chapter, which may be helpful to those looking to hone their critical lens in order to be better advocates.

Case Examples of Patient-Level Advocacy

In the rest of this chapter, we present and discuss four clinical vignettes that demonstrate effective patient-level advocacy. We hope to illustrate through these examples how psychiatrists can advocate for their patients from all backgrounds in historically informed, culturally competent ways that successfully navigate the murky waters of the current health care landscape while also advancing health equity and social justice.

Advocating for Ethnic-Based Treatment Equality

Case Example 1

A medical intern is admitting patients to the hospital's inpatient medical service overnight. The first admission of the night is a 28-year-old white woman with a history of cystic fibrosis presenting with severe, acute abdominal pain related to pancreatitis. The patient describes the pain as a 10 out of 10 shooting pain in the epigastric region. The intern calls the attending physician to review the treatment plan, and the attending recommends pain management with an intravenous opioid medication (morphine).

The next admission of the night is a 26-year-old African American woman with a history of type I diabetes mellitus complicated by gastroparesis presenting with severe, acute abdominal pain. She describes the pain as a 10 out of 10 stabbing pain in the epigastric area. When the intern calls the attending physician for this admission, the attending does not recommend pain management with opioids and instead offers the patient an intravenous nonsteroidal anti-inflammatory medication (ketorolac).

The intern realizes that the two patients' subjective complaints of abdominal pain are similar in description and severity, but the two pain management regimens are much different. The intern wonders to what extent the underlying pathophysiology was a consideration when these decisions were made and to what extent the team is actually treating these two women differently because of their race. During clinical rounds the next morning, the intern presents both patients to the team and notes this discrepancy. The intern then asks for clarification on the hospital's pain management guidelines. The attending physician explains that there are no clear policies on pain management and that each regimen is decided on a case-by-case basis.

Case Example 1 *(continued)*

The intern then calls the team's attention to the robust evidence that the pain of racial minorities is often treated less aggressively in hospital systems and that perhaps the team needs to take steps to ensure that the same process does not occur at this hospital. The attending appreciates that the intern is being thoughtful about these admissions and has done extensive research to ensure that patients receive equitable care. The team works together to revise the two patients' pain management plans so that both pain complaints are adequately treated. After rounds, the intern and the attending discuss the pain management policy in more detail and decide to propose an acute abdominal pain pathway or standardized algorithm to help ensure consistency and equality for future patients in the hospital's care.

In this vignette, an intern physician strategically used clinical rounds to draw attention to the inequality of pain management between a white patient and an African American patient. To ensure that the team was treating the African American patient in an equitable and just manner, the intern cited the large body of evidence that pain in African American patients is treated less aggressively than pain in patients of other ethnic groups across treatment settings (Goyal et al. 2015; Hewes et al. 2018; Rasooly et al. 2014). Additionally, the intern used this research evidence to evoke a long, fraught history of disregard for African American subjectivity that still plays out today. A historical example of this phenomenon is drapetomania, a mental illness diagnosis given to African slaves who ran away from slave owners that clearly neglected to take into account the suffering that slaves endured (Myers 2014). A contemporary example of treatment inequality is the research demonstrating that in emergency departments, on average, complaints from African American patients are coded as less serious than similar complaints from white patients (Schrader and Lewis 2013).

Medical internship, a rite of passage for all physicians, is among the first instances in our careers when we might be exposed to these kinds of glaring inequities in the health care system. However, interns who wish to challenge such inequities might face an especially uphill battle, given the hierarchical nature of medical culture and their low status in this hierarchy. Nevertheless, in order to break the cycle of injustice and discrimination, it is vital for all physicians, including physicians in training, to speak out when they see patterns that must be corrected (as this intern did) and, furthermore, for more senior physicians to support their junior colleagues who do speak out (as this attending physician did).

Specifically, the intern took several steps when making the case for equitable treatment that both demonstrated cultural competence and successfully engaged the team. First, the intern acted in a historically informed manner, knowing that to disregard the pain of this African American patient was to reproduce centuries of racism. Second, the intern held the team accountable for examining their racialized decision making, by directly addressing the topic with the entire team at clinical rounds. Finally and importantly, the intern took care not to sound accusatory because that approach is usually met with defensiveness and resistance. Instead, the intern used objective research evidence to frame the discussion and encourage critical thinking. In these ways, the intern used the clinical case to encourage shifts in institutional culture and policy that will ensure equity of care in the future.

Advocating for a Patient With a Subtle Presentation

Case Example 2

Dr. G, an outpatient psychiatrist working in a community center, is sitting down to some paperwork between appointments when a psychologist rushes in to say that a woman and her daughter are making a scene in the lobby. Dr. G arrives to find an exasperated middle-age woman with a black eye and her daughter, who is in her mid-twenties and has an intellectual disability. Dr. G asks a few questions and learns that the woman brought her daughter in today after weeks of worsening behavior. This morning, the patient had punched her mother after an argument about cereal. The patient is now smiling sweetly, waving at staff, and not giving any indication that she needs an inpatient psychiatric admission.

Dr. G recognizes the need for a full conversation with the family, despite the fact that this means an unscheduled appointment during an already overbooked day. He takes the patient and her mother into the office, where a full history reveals that the patient definitely needs to be admitted. However, because the patient currently looks well, Dr. G predicts that the emergency department (ED) team is likely to send her home rather than admit her. But he believes that the patient is getting worse and worries that waiting until she is at imminent risk might cause her or her mother to get hurt in the meantime. Dr. G decides that the best way to keep this patient safe is to go to the ED with her and advocate for an admission.

> ### Case Example 2 *(continued)*
>
> Dr. G writes an emergency commitment certificate, calls ahead to the ED attending physician, and escorts the patient and her mother to the ED. After the patient is triaged and ushered safely to the locked psychiatric ED, Dr. G escorts the mother to the waiting room and provides her the direct phone number to his office in case any issues should arise. He then heads back to the office to catch up on paperwork and appointments.
>
> Hours later, Dr. G has not heard back from the ED. He calls the ED attending physician to ask what happened. The ED physician, after explaining hurriedly that there has been a code as well as multiple other pressing matters in the ED, then expresses surprise and skepticism that the patient needs to be admitted. Therefore, Dr. G explains to the attending physician the detailed rationale for admission. After this exchange, the attending agrees with Dr. G's impression and decides to admit the patient. Shortly thereafter, Dr. G receives a call from the patient's mother, thanking him for helping her family navigate the ED system to secure this needed admission.

In this vignette, a psychiatrist advocated for a patient with a subtle presentation to be admitted to the hospital. This is a common scenario that many of us face in our daily clinical practice, wherein the combination of long wait times, a lack of availability of psychiatric beds, overburdened ED staff, and sometimes stigmatizing or dismissive attitudes toward patients with mental illness can result in disposition decisions that are not in the best interests of the patients. In these cases, it often falls to psychiatrists to ensure that patients receive the treatments they need.

The psychiatrist in this vignette demonstrated both an astute understanding of how to navigate the health care system and a patient-centered approach to clinical care and advocacy. First, the psychiatrist knew the local care system well enough to recognize this patient's slim chance of admission without the psychiatrist's help. This in itself involves mastery of a tremendously complicated interplay of clinics, hospitals, and cultures—but one that is crucial to learn because it is nearly impossible to be successful as a patient-level advocate if one is not familiar with the system in which one works. Second, the psychiatrist took time out of a busy workday to advocate for the family and effectively argued a case for admission directly to the ED attending. Finally, the psychiatrist showed respect for the patient's and family's needs and wishes throughout this process, including taking adequate time to obtain a full history and anticipating any future needs by providing the mother with a way to reach the psychiatrist.

The psychiatrist's efforts in this vignette are laudable, but at the same time the vignette reminds us that patient-level advocacy can require a significant amount of work. Although we challenge here and throughout the book the notion that attention to the complexities of the health care system and to patients' unique psychosocial, cultural, and historical circumstances is "beyond" the scope of medicine, we also recognize that there are surely days when this sort of advocacy would not be realistic. However, on days when time and clinical demands permit, we can make a tremendous difference in our patients' lives by advocating for them.

Continuing to Advocate When Team Members Disagree

Case Example 3

An inpatient psychiatrist, Dr. P, is leading a team treating a patient with borderline personality disorder after a suicide attempt. She believes that the patient needs another few days in the hospital before discharge, but the rest of the team disagrees. At morning rounds, Dr. P describes the patient's ongoing suicidal thoughts and lack of adequate outpatient follow-up. Other members of the care team respond with how "difficult" the patient is to work with and observe that he rarely follows up with aftercare planning anyway.

Seeking to understand the team's perspective and enlist support for the idea of keeping the patient a bit longer, Dr. P asks the other team members why they feel that the patient is ready to go home. The response is close to 10 minutes of complaints about the many ways in which the patient frustrated the staff this past weekend. Dr. P understands and sympathizes with the challenges of caring for this patient but also worries that he is more depressed now than during previous hospitalizations.

Case Example 3 *(continued)*

Dr. P reminds the team about the patient's history of serious suicide attempts, multiple intensive care unit admissions, and utter lack of outpatient supports. Although the other team members are still hesitant about having the patient stay longer, they acknowledge these concerns. Dr. P tries to convey an understanding of the staff's frustrations while recognizing that it is the staff and not Dr. P who must manage this patient moment to moment. Ultimately, she decides not to discharge the patient yet and hopes that in another few days the patient will feel better and be ready to go with an improved outpatient plan.

The advocacy in this vignette, as in the first vignette, took place during clinical team rounds, demonstrating the importance of this setting as a space for patient-level advocacy. Of note, no patient appeared in this vignette, although a patient was discussed at length. Especially in a hospital setting, many of the discussions and decisions that determine approaches to patients take place without them being present. Therefore, it is particularly important to advocate for patients in these situations, in which they do not have the ability to advocate for themselves.

Furthermore, "difficult" patients raise particular challenges from both clinical and advocacy perspectives. In that sense, this vignette reminds us to be aware of our own feelings and/or countertransference responses about particular patients as well as any biases we may have against certain mental illness diagnoses that tend to be more stigmatized (e.g., borderline personality disorder or other personality pathology, substance use disorders). Advocacy for these patients can take the form of recognizing the role that diagnosis and behavior play in their presentation and interpersonal style and then helping other members of the treatment team recognize this as well. These actions will ensure that clinical decisions are made in the best interest of each patient.

Finally, the vignette illustrates that when psychiatrists serve as medical leaders of treatment teams, we must often attend to the morale and dynamics of the team as well as the clinical status of the patient. And sometimes, despite our best efforts to maintain team unity, we must make decisions that other team members disagree with. The psychiatrist in this vignette took care to express understanding of and respect for the team's difficulties but ultimately made a decision that the team may have disagreed with in order to ensure equitable patient care.

Advocating for a Patient With Culturally Different Views

Case Example 4

An inpatient psychiatry consultation-liaison (CL) team is asked by an inpatient nephrology service to see a 62-year-old man with kidney failure who is refusing the initiation of lifesaving dialysis. The primary team requests that the CL team assess the patient's capacity to refuse medical treatment. The nephrology service explains that the patient is refusing treatment because he does not want to be a "victim of the white man's health care system."

The psychiatric team speaks with the patient at length about his culture, values, and perspectives using the Cultural Formulation Interview (American Psychiatric Association 2013) as a guide. Over the course of the evaluation, the patient discloses that he identifies with an American Indian tribe, lives within an American Indian community, and adheres closely to his tribal traditions. He regularly follows the advice of his tribal elders and healers for his medical decision making. The patient explains that he and his tribe continually mourn the violent erasure of the land, history, and heritage of their native people at the hands of white colonizers. He states that the tribe's collective grief has caused him to avoid medical institutions for decades because the hospital institution is a representation of the "white man's oppressive systems."

The patient expresses that the thought of interacting weekly with a dialysis center, where staff and physicians would be disproportionately white and where he would be a vulnerable patient within that system, is too much to bear. He states that he understands that refusing dialysis would result in his death and that he is resigned to having lived a fulfilled life within his tribe. Ultimately, the CL team determines that the patient is able to communicate a clear choice, understands the consequences of the medical decision at hand, and expresses a culturally consistent rationale for his decision. Thus, the patient is deemed to have capacity to refuse dialysis, and the CL team recommends a consultation from palliative care.

In this vignette, the CL team took the time to understand the patient's background and cultural values, during which process the Cultural Formulation Interview (American Psychiatric Association 2013) was a useful tool. Using this approach, the CL team was able to demystify the patient's decision to refuse life-sustaining treatment. This case illustrates how the inherent vulnerability of being in the patient role is compounded for those who belong to communities that have historically been victimized by American institutions. American Indians and other native groups have experienced massive losses of lives, land, and culture as a result of European contact and colonization, resulting in a legacy of chronic trauma and unresolved grief across generations (Brave Heart and DeBruyn 1998).

To understand patients' experiences of medical institutions and their reactions to those institutions, the physician must have some working knowledge of the concept of historical trauma. *Historical trauma* is a psychic wound that people of color and indigenous people carry with them daily as they navigate the modern world, with the knowledge that the suffering of their predecessors has contributed to the making of the current world. The historical trauma construct was a salient part of the case presented here, in which the patient expressed that the pain of historical trauma would be exacerbated by undergoing intensive medical treatment (i.e., dialysis). All patients are vulnerable to experiencing indignities and disempowerment in the health care system, but for historically marginalized groups, those experiences may interact with the memory of historical events to make such experiences even more stressful or traumatic. Despite the health care system's stated goal of providing care for the patient, hospital systems are inevitably associated with broader institutions (e.g., political, military) that have historically oppressed and suppressed many communities, especially indigenous communities. Furthermore, there are numerous historical examples in which American medical institutions enacted violence against racial and ethnic minority groups such as in the case of forced medical experimentation and sterilizations (Washington 2006).

We acknowledge that allowing for the withdrawal of care in this case was likely uncomfortable for the medical team because the act goes against the training of physicians to use medical technologies to treat disease and prolong life. However, we must recognize and respect that patients have deeply held values and beliefs that may conflict with those of the physician. Ultimately, the CL team's decision that the patient had capacity to refuse life-sustaining treatment was historically informed and culturally sensitive because it recognized the impact of historical trauma on the patient's current experience and allowed the patient to live out his remaining days more authentically according to his cultural values.

This vignette also illustrates that patient-level advocacy does not always mean advocating for *more* medicine or *more* treatment. Indeed, patient-level advocacy may not, and does not necessarily need to, result in better health outcomes. Rather, advocating for individual patients can sometimes mean supporting patients in living out their culturally and historically consistent values, which requires attention to each patient's unique preferences and beliefs. A physician wanting to advocate for a patient must always consider the broader historical, social, and political position of the patient and adjust accordingly and be especially careful not to allow their biases to affect the care of the patient. This approach diverges dramatically from that of a "color-blind" mentality, in which one attempts to treat every patient in the same way.

Conclusion

In this chapter, we have conceptualized patient-level advocacy as a necessary component of a physician's professional responsibility, given the fragmented and discriminatory health care system that is currently in place. The chapter's vignettes have illustrated how patient-level advocacy can occur in a variety of settings and how physicians, including psychiatrists, at different career stages can be effective as advocates for patients. In particular, we have stressed the importance of advocating for patients from historically marginalized groups, including individuals with mental illness, who are underserved on the basis of their historical positionality and ongoing discrimination within the medical system.

Psychiatrists who wish to be patient-level advocates must at times do extra work to subvert oppressive frameworks, disrupt discriminatory discourses, and navigate convoluted systems to meet the needs of patients. It may indeed be challenging to go above and beyond the traditional standards of professional responsibility to ensure that patients receive high-quality care, especially in this age of increasingly overwhelming demands on our clinical time. However, the path to social justice and equity begins and ends with patient-level advocacy, and psychiatrists, as the physicians providing much-needed mental health care to patients from all walks of life, should be among the trailblazers in this journey.

Suggested Readings

Anderson E: The White Space. Sociology of Race and Ethnicity 1(1):10–21, 2015

Bassuk EL, Carman RW: The Doctor-Activist: Physicians Fighting for Social Change. New York, Springer, 2013

Brave Heart MY: The historical trauma response among natives and its relationship with substance abuse: a Lakota illustration. J Psychoactive Drugs 35(1):7–13, 2003

Brave Heart MY, DeBruyn LM: The American Indian Holocaust: healing historical unresolved grief. Am Indian Alsk Native Ment Health Res 8(2):56–78, 1998

Byrd WM, Clayton LA: An American Health Dilemma: Race, Medicine, and Health Care in the United States 1900–2000. New York, Routledge, 2001

DiAngelo R: White Fragility: Why It's So Hard for White People to Talk About Racism. Boston, MA, Beacon Press, 2018

Roberts D: Fatal Invention: How Science, Politics, and Big Business Recreate Race in the Twenty-First Century. New York, New Press, 2011

Roberts DE: Killing the Black Body: Race, Reproduction, and the Meaning of Liberty. New York, Vintage Books, 1999

Vincent B: Transgender Health: A Practitioner's Guide to Binary and Non-Binary Trans Patient Care. Philadelphia, PA, Jessica Kingsley, 2018

Washington HA: Medical Apartheid: The Dark History of Medical Experimentation on Black Americans From Colonial Times to the Present. New York, Doubleday, 2006

References

Acosta FJ, Hernández JL, Pereira J, et al: Medication adherence in schizophrenia. World J Psychiatry 2(5):74–82, 2012 24175171

American Psychiatric Association: Diagnostic and Statistical Manual of Mental Disorders, 5th Edition. Arlington, VA, American Psychiatric Association, 2013

Bradley EH, Herrin J, Wang Y, et al: Racial and ethnic differences in time to acute reperfusion therapy for patients hospitalized with myocardial infarction. JAMA 292(13):1563–1572, 2004 15467058

Brave Heart MY, DeBruyn LM: The American Indian Holocaust: healing historical unresolved grief. Am Indian Alsk Native Ment Health Res 8(2):56–78, 1998 9842066

Dobson S, Voyer S, Hubinette M, et al: From the clinic to the community: the activities and abilities of effective health advocates. Acad Med 90(2):214–220, 2015 25470309

Goyal MK, Kuppermann N, Cleary SD, et al: Racial disparities in pain management of children with appendicitis in emergency departments. JAMA Pediatr 169(11):996–1002, 2015 26366984

Haeri S, Williams J, Kopeykina I, et al: Disparities in diagnosis of bipolar disorder in individuals of African and European descent: a review. J Psychiatr Pract 17(6):394–403, 2011 22108396

Hewes HA, Dai M, Mann NC, et al: Prehospital pain management: disparity by age and race. Prehosp Emerg Care 22(2):189–197, 2018 28956669

Jones S, Howard L, Thornicroft G: "Diagnostic overshadowing": worse physical health care for people with mental illness. Acta Psychiatr Scand 118(3):169–171, 2008 18699951

Morgan PL, Staff J, Hillemeier MM, et al: Racial and ethnic disparities in ADHD diagnosis from kindergarten to eighth grade. Pediatrics 132(1):85–93, 2013 23796743

Myers BE II: "Drapetomania": rebellion, defiance, and free black insanity in the antebellum United States. Unpublished doctoral dissertation, UCLA, Los Angeles, CA, 2014

Pumariega AJ, Rothe E, Mian A, et al; American Academy of Child and Adolescent Psychiatry (AACAP) Committee on Quality Issues (CQI): Practice parameter for cultural competence in child and adolescent psychiatric practice. J Am Acad Child Adolesc Psychiatry 52(10):1101–1115, 2013 24074479

Rasooly IR, Mullins PM, Mazer-Amirshahi M, et al: The impact of race on analgesia use among pediatric emergency department patients. J Pediatr 165(3):618–621, 2014 24928697

Schrader CD, Lewis LM: Racial disparity in emergency department triage. J Emerg Med 44(2):511–518, 2013 22818646

Shefer G, Henderson C, Howard LM, et al: Diagnostic overshadowing and other challenges involved in the diagnostic process of patients with mental illness who present in emergency departments with physical symptoms—a qualitative study. PLoS One 9(11):e111682, 2014 25369130

Thornicroft G, Rose D, Kassam A, Sartorius N: Stigma: ignorance, prejudice or discrimination? Br J Psychiatry 190(3):192–193, 2007 17329736

Washington HA: Medical Apartheid: The Dark History of Medical Experimentation on Black Americans From Colonial Times to the Present. New York, Doubleday, 2006

6

Organizational Advocacy

Luming Li, M.D.
Thomas N. Franklin, M.D.

Learning Objectives

By the end of this chapter, readers will be able to:

- Define organizational advocacy and differentiate it from other types of advocacy efforts
- Describe models for change for navigating complex organizations
- Develop a better understanding of the different levels of leadership and organizational hierarchy, and describe how to create measurable change efforts by navigating these
- Describe special case scenarios, pitfalls, and tips to consider in organizational advocacy
- Use case example to contextualize and learn about organizational challenges faced by individuals

> ### Case Example: Dr. C's Dilemma
>
> Dr. C is a junior attending physician in the psychiatry department of Downtown Medical Center (DMC) in charge of the 15-bed acute inpatient unit. This is her first position out of residency, and she is only just now settling in after 18 months on the job following a bewildering transition from her training program in another city, where she was lauded for her no-nonsense leadership ability as chief resident. Dr. C's team and her patients can tell how much she genuinely cares about her work with a mainly indigent population. As she looks at her patient list today, she sees that there were several admissions overnight of homeless individuals who cycle in and out of her busy unit with regularity. These patients, whom she knows well, have often endorsed suicidality on admission but rarely had any acute psychiatric symptoms after a period of observation. Dr. C understands that in the absence of adequate housing options for individuals experiencing homelessness, these individuals might understandably turn to the hospital system for a respite from the streets. She has been thinking about this problem ever since she started working at DMC and feels ready to advocate for changes that will both serve this population and keep desperately needed beds open for acutely ill patients who might benefit more from the care provided.

Organizational Advocacy: Context and Definition

Advocacy at the level of organizations is challenging. Organizations are based on identified values and missions, which may or may not align with the physician-advocate's own personal values and missions. In addition, the personal differences and workplace dynamics that result can be especially frustrating and difficult to address. However, in organizational contexts, it is critical to find ways to work meaningfully with others toward optimal outcomes and solutions, especially in settings that deliver health care.

There are many definitions of *organizational advocacy*. In her article titled "Organizational Advocacy 101," Jane Galloway Seiling (2001a) defined organizational advocacy as the "spontaneous activities of workplace members that are significant to expanded achievement and furthering the well-being of themselves, their co-members, and the collective workplace community" (p. 42). In this definition, *organizational advocacy* relates an individual or group's performance and achievement to an overarching principle of organizational accountability. In the context of health care, organizational advocacy can be defined as advocacy within an organization, such as a hospital system, to effect change that in the best-case scenario advances the health and well-being of patients and populations while also furthering the organizational mission.

In this chapter, we provide an overview of how to engage effectively in organizational advocacy within health care. The case example woven throughout this chapter provides a typical organizational advocacy scenario. As you contemplate how to be a more effective advocate within organizations, you can learn from Dr. C's story.

What Is the Advocacy Goal?

Before you set out to advocate at an organizational level, it is important to take time for self-reflection in order to identify the specific aims and goals of your advocacy efforts. These advocacy efforts can involve various types of change: in policy, in process, or in the allocation of resources. It is important to identify specific aims and goals in order to limit confusion, to minimize challenges of overly ambitious scope, and to facilitate measuring successful outcomes. For example, immediately asking individuals in roles of power to fix a problem will likely be viewed as a complaint, especially without the offer of a formulation of potential solutions. Sharing poorly prepared ideas may affect your reputation and credibility and may impact future interactions. Typically, ideas that have been well formulated and thought out with intention are better received than those that are presented in an ill-conceived manner.

Some strategies for developing ideas about an issue include brainstorming and research. For example, creating a list of different problems and solutions is an important starting point. From there, research about the issue can take place by asking others for feedback, by asking about solutions from other parts of the organization, and by inquiring at peer institutions. You can talk to trusted mentors and colleagues about the issue and perform an honest self-appraisal about your individual role, influence, and impact within the organization. Self-reflection includes awareness of personal qualities that can help or hinder your ability to influence other people.

General Framework for Organizational Advocacy

For anyone thinking about how to advocate for change, the eight-step model developed by John P. Kotter might be a helpful tool. In this model, which was described in an article published in the *Harvard Business Review* (Kotter 1995/2007) as well as a book on the subject (Kotter 1996), Kotter identified eight steps to help organizations transform and included descriptions of "lessons learned" around the natural progression when the model is not followed (Kotter 1978). The eight steps are as follows: 1) establishing a sense of urgency, 2) forming a powerful guiding coalition, 3) creating a vision, 4) communicating the vision, 5) empowering others to act on the vision, 6) planning and creating short-term wins, 7) consolidating improvements and producing still more change, and 8) institutionalizing new approaches. Although Kotter developed the model for companies and businesses, you can use ideas from the model to advocate on behalf of organizations within mental health settings.

Table 6–1 exemplifies how the elements of Kotter's original steps can be applied to a case involving a psychiatric care setting. The case is an example of organizational advocacy in the form of a quality improvement initiative. It is important to note that Kotter's proposed stages of change can be used to solve a variety of challenges requiring modification and organizational momentum. What is particularly powerful about the concepts proposed by Kotter, which have been tested and used with success since the article's original 1995 publication, is the ability to use different component pieces of the model to sequentially achieve powerful outcomes and transformations within organizations. The model allows for individuals and groups to start developing a specific strategy for effective organizational advocacy.

Case Example: Dr. C's Concerns

Dr. C had complained several times to her supervisor, Dr. M, the chief of psychiatry, about the fact that individuals experiencing homelessness without acute psychiatric symptoms were receiving psychiatric admissions, which meant that more acute patients sometimes had to wait several days for a bed. Dr. M would throw up his hands and remind her that this was a problem that had been going on for longer than the 12 years he had been there. He suggested faster assessments and discharges of these patients. Dr. C tried this but remained frustrated about the situation. Clearly, however, simply pointing out the problem to her superiors did not result in any changes.

Case Example: Dr. C's Concerns *(continued)*

Dr. C began to research how other area hospitals dealt with similar issues. She also familiarized herself with the local advocacy groups for psychiatric patients and for people experiencing homelessness. In addition, she discussed the problem with a mentor of hers from residency and with trusted members of her team. One longtime DMC social worker recounted a past failed effort to deal with the issue: A committee that was formed to study the problem met three times over a few months, but the administrator involved got a new job and the group never met again. That effort had been 7 years ago. Dr. C knew that although she disliked speaking in front of large groups, she had been effective in one-on-one interactions in the past, and her current position gave her significant credibility around this issue.

Building Urgency

Although Dr. C recognized the urgency of the issue given the frequent readmissions of individuals experiencing homelessness, others around her did not feel this same sense of urgency. Dr. C realized that if she failed to create a sense of urgency within the organization about homelessness, she would likely be the sole crusader on this issue for years, and with stagnant results. She might find other individuals who passively endorse interest in this issue but do not act to create meaningful change. For example, her supervisor had thrown up his hands, and the long-term social worker had described the committee that had stopped after a few meetings. To be an organizational advocate, Dr. C would need to develop a sense of urgency (step 1). Accomplishing this can be challenging within busy health care contexts, but this sense of urgency is critical in order to set the stage for the next stages of change.

The cyclical process in which homeless patients without acute psychiatric illness present over and over again to the hospital can be a difficult organizational advocacy issue because it can be challenging to build momentum for a large problem that involves multiple stakeholders and systems beyond the hospital setting, including state and federal government programs, laws, and regulations and complex reimbursement processes for mental health services. Many psychiatric hospitals and mental health outpatient clinics are unable to keep up with costs because of poor insurance reimbursement for services. Managed care may limit treatment for patients without serious mental illness, who may be

TABLE 6–1.   Kotter's eight stages of change

Stage	Case example: formation of a new patient safety/quality committee at Yale New Haven Psychiatric Hospital
1. Establishing a sense of urgency	Clinical leaders recognized the need for a new patient safety/quality committee (PSQC), which had been in the idea phase for 2 years. However, the arrival of two personnel to colead the committee led to an urgency to form the new committee.
2. Forming a powerful guiding coalition	In preparation for the formation of a new committee, the vice president, director of nursing, and medical director became sponsors and advisors.
3. Creating a vision	The two coleaders for the new committee met with multidisciplinary groups and individuals to identify a vision for the committee aligned with the values of the psychiatric hospital and discussed the appropriate membership for the new committee.
4. Communicating the vision	The PSQC's vision and missions were initially sent by e-mail to the entire psychiatric service line in a document stating the goals of the new group. In addition, the psychiatric leadership helped guide presentations about PSQC at multiple staff meetings and approved multiple rounds of communication about the new effort in the form of newsletters, e-mails, and face-to-face meetings.
5. Empowering others to act on the vision	A competitive application process was used to solicit membership and participation in the new committee. Members were selected on the basis of preestablished criteria for interest in engagement and commitment to act on the PSQC's vision and mission.
6. Planning and creating short-term wins	After selection, the committee worked for several months to identify short-term win projects in quality improvement for the psychiatric service line, including projects on improving communication during care transitions, assessing completion rates of laboratory reports, and establishing a pharmacy technician to help medication reconciliations in the psychiatric emergency setting.

TABLE 6–1. **Kotter's eight stages of change** *(continued)*

Stage	Case example: formation of a new patient safety/quality committee at Yale New Haven Psychiatric Hospital
7. Consolidating improvements and producing still more change	During educational and communication initiatives, the PSQC asks the service line staff to recommend additional improvements and future projects to help with shifting psychiatric practice and care delivery. Ideas provided by staff and leaders are stored on a project tracker, which helps organize future project selection and implementation.
8. Institutionalizing new approaches	Since its inception, PSQC has become an important part of quality improvement, with members helping with education, communication, and projects. Projects are selected and implemented on the basis of factors of feasibility and importance. Project progress is transparently shared with the psychiatric service line, both at leadership meetings and with the frontline staff through monthly newsletters.

Source. Adapted from Kotter 1995/2007, 1996.

discharged soon after hospital admission to a lower-level treatment setting, such as a homeless shelter or a rehabilitation facility. In addition, patients may have difficulty navigating complex regional and local services.

Nevertheless, although Dr. C is a new attending physician, she is a vital stakeholder who can create urgency around this issue. She has an important perspective to present to health care administrators, even if her direct supervisor recognizes, but has not acted on, the problem of readmissions for homeless individuals without serious mental health conditions. One important approach to building urgency is gathering data, such as developing a rudimentary cost analysis and using measurement-based tools to further study the problem (Jensen and Bojeun 2017; Seiling 2001b). For example, Dr. C can consider working with individuals in the organization, such as the utilization manager or data analyst, to identify the characteristics and cohort of patients who frequently present to the hospital with homelessness as one characteristic. With tangible data, Dr. C can create urgency for hospital administrators who take notice when a small group of patients disproportionately generate large health care costs for the hospital. Hospital administrators may then decide that patient homelessness is necessary to address in order to manage costs and improve access to the acute inpatient unit for all patients.

After building urgency, Dr. C can create a group or structure within the organization to share the work of reaching out to the different organizations and stakeholders involved (step 2). Because prior attempts to create a lasting committee had failed, it would be useful to understand why these earlier attempts had not succeeded. For example, staff members who were on the committee and are still working for the organization could be contacted, and their first-hand experiences could be recounted. Possible reasons for the committee failure might be that there were no champions or powerful allies able to effectuate change or that the committee met too infrequently to build momentum and create a vision. Dr. C also needs to assess who in the organization can help and to identify powerful allies with leverage who are able to find the resources and tools needed for meaningful change. After others with shared interests have been identified, they can form a group and start developing a vision (step 3).

In order to advocate successfully within an organization, scope is an important consideration. It is easy to have an extensive vision and identify more problems than individuals who can take responsibility for them. When starting out, one should aim small and create early wins to garner credibility within an organization. However, having a defined vision is important to help communicate to others about the initiative and goals (steps 4 and 5).

Of note, it is better to successfully complete one small project than to have a grand idea and no end results (step 6). For example, Dr. C could develop metrics to identify the types of patients who have a "homeless" designation and create a procedure to rule out more serious conditions (e.g., homeless patients with schizophrenia who have an acute psychotic episode, homeless patients with severe alcohol use disorder who present to the emergency department with a head bleed).

After developing this process, Dr. C can use this information to engage hospital policy makers and administrators, who can then help brainstorm, design, and update policies regarding admission and readmission criteria. Dr. C can engage with these diverse stakeholders in an iterative manner until the goals are successfully reached (step 7).

Finally, it is important for efforts to be institutionalized so that effort is sustained (step 8). In Dr. C's case, she might be able to work with her institution to designate patients with "homeless" as part of the electronic medical record or highlight these patients through an alert when they are seen in the emergency department on future visits. Having these efforts be automated through the electronic medical record can help providers recognize patients with special needs and offer the appropriate treatment

How Much Should an Advocate Ask For?

In order to advocate successfully within an organization, scope is an important consideration. It is easy to have a grand vision and identify more problems than individuals who can take responsibility for them. When starting out, you should aim small and create early wins to garner credibility within an organization. It is better to successfully complete one small project than to have a grand idea and no end results. For example, Dr. C could develop metrics to identify the types of patients who have a "homeless" designation, and create a procedure to rule out more serious conditions (e.g., homeless patients with schizophrenia who have an acute psychotic episode, homeless patients with severe alcohol use disorder who present to the emergency room with a head bleed). After developing this process, Dr. C can use this information to engage hospital policy makers and administrators, who can then help brainstorm, design, and update policies regarding admission and readmission criteria.

Whom Must the Advocate Engage?

Difficult organizational issues often involve multiple departments or responsibility areas. An important question for any advocate to ask is why the issue has been hard to solve from the beginning. Understanding the organizational chart and understanding who has decision-making power across multiple departments and service lines can help bring about the change being sought.

The organizational chart, which details the different roles, reporting structures, and leadership positions within an organization, is a good place to learn how an organization functions, in order to identify which leader to approach to assist with a potential policy change. However, overreliance on the organizational chart is not recommended. For example, the organizational chart may not be fully updated. More importantly, the person nominally responsible for a specific role may not have the influence, the skills, or the administrative training to help address the concern. This limited transparency of the organizational chart makes organizational advocacy challenging. One safe approach is to start with your immediate supervisor, especially because it can be problematic to go over or around your supervisor without their approval, and often your direct supervisor may be helpful. In fact, developing a strong working relationship with your supervisor can be tremendously helpful because your supervisor may know more organizational history and can be a powerful advocate within the organization. At the very least, you can ask your supervisor for a lesson on the organizational chart to gain a better understanding of the structure of the workplace.

In addition to your direct supervisor, there may be other people or subgroups who are important stakeholders. These individuals or groups may be involved in setting the organization's mental health policy, determining quality standards, allocating resources toward new services or projects, and/or creating a vision for the organization's direction. Consider those responsible in the organization who allocate resources and/or set policy. They may include a department chair or chief, a vice president or operations officer, or, in smaller organizations, the chief executive officer.

Case Example: Dr. C's Advocacy as Viewed by Her Supervisor

Dr. M, chief of psychiatry and Dr. C's supervisor, was happy to find out that Dr. C wanted to advocate around the issue of repeat admissions for homeless individuals without ongoing serious mental illness. He suggested that she begin by meeting with the chief of emergency medicine, who he knew shared many of Dr. C's concerns about this issue. Any solution would need to involve the emergency medicine department.

Meanwhile, Dr. C's research had uncovered a local advocacy group for homeless individuals that oversaw the bulk of shelter beds and other services, and these beds and services were under a contract from the city. Dr. C, in her zeal, had already begun an e-mail correspondence with the chairwoman of this group, Ms. H, who wanted to meet and discuss the issue. Ms. H had been trying to work more closely with DMC for years around the issue of health care for homeless individuals.

Dr. M was generally a pretty low-key supervisor, but his eyes got big when he heard Dr. C was already in touch with Ms. H. Evidently, Ms. H's organization had been a thorn in the side of the DMC for several years, suggesting that the DMC didn't provide quality care for indigent patients. Ms. H had given several interviews highly critical of DMC to the local paper. Dr. M suggested that Dr. C back off on networking in the community around this issue until she had the blessing of DMC's leadership.

Internal Versus External Advocacy

Notably, organizational advocacy should almost always be internal, or rooted *inside* the organization. Advocates often choose to work as administrators in order to be able to effect change within the system. Dr. Ken Duckworth, whose interview is provided at the end of this chapter, is an excellent example of this trend. If at all possible, you should refrain from creating external pressure on your own organization through public criticism or negative publicity, either deliberately or inadvertently, as Dr. C risked doing by networking with Ms. H. This behavior can be detrimental to both the advocate and the organization.

For example, if Dr. C approaches the local news channel about the recurrent readmissions for the homeless population and the anchor decides to cover the story with a negative portrayal of DMC, the hospital may experience negative consequences. These may include reduced government funding or reduced public usage of hospital services, especially in a fairly competitive health care environment. A more serious consequence for the hospital would be the potential loss of credentialing by national credentialing organizations or state-level public health organizations, which are required to maintain standards of practice. These outcomes would harm the organization and its employees without effecting meaningful change for the issue at hand. (For more information on external advocacy, including the limited instances in which it may be useful or necessary, see the subsection "Going Outside the Organization" later in this chapter.)

On the other hand, creating a coalition of organizations can be useful, especially for a complex issue such as homelessness. For example, other stakeholders involved in the homelessness problem that Dr. C is facing include the state and local mental health authorities, the town or city aldermen and congressmen (to help with advocating for more services for homeless individuals), homeless shelter administrative leadership (to help build collaborations for thoughtful hospital postdischarge planning), and staff members from social services and other state-level benefits offices.

Contextualizing Organizational Advocacy Across Roles

In any organization, there are multiple layers of hierarchy and reporting structures. In the medical professions, these include a frontline provider, who is then supervised by a unit chief or clinic director. All the unit chiefs and clinic directors are typically governed by a specialty-specific division chief or chair. These individuals then report to another individual, who is likely someone who oversees a multidisciplinary group of chiefs or chairs in various specialties. At different levels, the necessary resources requiring advocacy may be different. However, the skills used can be similar. For example, a unit chief may want to request the hiring of one attending psychiatrist. A division chief, by extension, may need to request 15 extra psychiatrists during the hiring period. Considering this volume of requests, important organizational advocacy skills at every stage include 1) communicating a specific ask, 2) conveying urgency and need associated with the request, and 3) providing context that relates to the organizational mission. It can be helpful to have prior relationships that are built on trust and knowledge about one another, especially in health care settings where trust can be low (Shore 2007). However, even without specific knowledge of the other individual or individuals involved, the issue itself can be deemed to be relevant and important in order to generate willingness to work toward its solution.

Moreover, most organizations have structures in place to solve problems. The structures take many forms, such as workgroups, staff meetings, or committees, but they generally have the same broad mandate to make necessary and important changes. It can be helpful to uncover and understand which administrators are the key influencers and decision makers with respect to these groups within the organization. These administrators may offer individual meetings or conduct walking rounds throughout the organization. Having regular and frequent interactions with the groups and individuals who are powerful decision makers can help drive advocacy momentum.

Case Example: Dr. C's Emergency Medicine Connection

Dr. C backed off from Ms. H for the time being and reached out to Dr. J, the chief of emergency medicine, who was thrilled to have a partner in dealing with an issue that vexed her as well because psychiatric patients were often held in her emergency department for days waiting for an inpatient bed to become available. They agreed to have lunch away from the hospital to discuss the issue and brainstorm solutions. After their lunch, Dr. C was energized. She had found a critical like-minded ally in Dr. J, an older woman who had been a trailblazer in emergency medicine when it was primarily an all-male specialty. Dr. J was on the ill-fated committee that had disbanded years ago without offering solutions. She also had deep institutional knowledge about how things got done at DMC and knew from experience the necessary strategies for approaching the personalities involved.

> ### Case Example: Dr. C's Emergency Medicine Connection *(continued)*
>
> The primary decision maker was the chief operating officer, Dr. K, a nonclinician health care administrator who had been hired several years ago to stop the flow of red ink that had almost led to the sale of DMC to an out-of-town conglomerate. The layoffs that were necessary to maintain their independence still were talked about even 3 years later. Dr. J let Dr. C know that any solution to the problem would have to be revenue neutral and proposed to Dr. K in the language of business. Dr. J suggested that they arrange a meeting with Dr. K to discuss next steps.

Pitfalls

Organizational advocacy can be more delicate work than broader extraorganizational efforts. Individual personalities must be negotiated, and opaque organizational politics must be navigated. The personal stakes may be high. As such, the organizational advocate should take note of the following potential pitfalls: loss of credibility, going outside the organization, and setting unrealistic or unclear goals.

Loss of Credibility

A cautionary note is that credibility and perception are key to organizational advocacy efforts. For example, if a direct supervisor perceives an advocacy effort to be meaningless and the advocate continues to push for the change despite being told "no," this behavior can lead to negative perceptions about the advocate's capability and rational decision making. These optics can result in prolonged stagnancy in a role, limited opportunities for job advancement, or even job elimination. Therefore, the adage to "pick your battles" is key in organizational advocacy.

Going Outside the Organization

One of the major pitfalls for organizational advocates is their tendency to take the issue outside the organization (i.e., external advocacy). Putting pressure on the organization from the outside is fraught with danger and is often less effective than working from the inside. Generally, the most effective organizational advocates work from within the organization, using its current structures and getting buy-in to create new structures to address issues. Although you may want to gather allies from outside the organization, especially if individuals within the organization do not seem supportive about your advocacy efforts, you should resist this impulse in the vast majority of cases.

Working successfully in organizational advocacy requires trust, a positive reputation, and a collaborative attitude. You can lose the potent advantages of being deemed "an insider" if you ally with people or groups outside your organization. Leaders within the organization must trust that an advocate is loyal to the organization. Organizations, both public and private, can be protective of their public image and have both legal and fiduciary responsibility to maintain or enhance this public image.

An advocate who has a negative or critical perspective to offer about the organization should exercise care and sensitivity. For example, you may frame an advocacy initiative as a quality improvement project or as a series of smaller projects, especially when organizations (and supervisors) may be more receptive to smaller-scale projects.

It is important to understand the appetite for change within the organization. If advocacy ideas are brought to leaders not interested in change, then you might be met with hostility, resentment, or, at the least, ambivalence. If all internal options are exhausted, you may consider external avenues of advocacy, such as involving the media. However, in these instances, it is important to be aware that when going outside the organization, the outcome may be worse, and you may be asked to leave the organization.

One rare exception to this general rule to avoid external advocacy concerns whistle-blowing, or exposing unethical or illegal organizational practices. As reported in media stories (e.g., Adams 2017; Kowalczyk 2017), the mental health care system is not without the potential for corruption. When cases of corruption endanger patient safety and/or defraud the public and there is no recourse to correct the situation from within the organization, whistle-blowing is arguably necessary to prevent or stop grave harm from occurring. Advance planning, extreme caution, and sound judgment are critical when considering whistle-blowing because whistle-blowers often face reprisal, despite various laws and regulations aimed to protect them.

Setting Unrealistic or Unclear Goals

Another major pitfall in organizational advocacy is the proverbial "biting off more than you can chew." Often, advocates approach leaders with a solution for a problem that is unrealistically large in scope. For example, if you propose to "solve homelessness" to avoid inappropriate readmissions, the solution may involve multiple organizations and health systems, as well as factors that involve political and consumer-driven trends beyond the control of any single organization. Thus, in working on organizational advocacy, an important approach is to think of small initiatives to implement.

Similarly, if you present a problem without a solution, many administrators will not sense the urgency for action. Therefore, you need to be specific about the ask, the goals for change, and the process for change. You need to have a clearly identified solution early on. This means that more research, including gathering interview information from coworkers and staff members about the issue and potential solutions, is an important first step before asking for anything to be changed.

Gaining Influence

Advocacy requires the ability to be persuasive. This comes more naturally to some, but it is a skill that can be learned and improved on. Knowing the individuals and groups to be influenced is critical (Neiva et al. 2015; Review et al. 2017). Below are some general tenets to consider in persuasion and influence:

1. Establish credibility
2. Be passionate about a specific facet being advocated for.
3. Tell an emotionally valent story to illustrate the problem.
4. Vary tone of voice, facial expressions, and gestures during advocacy efforts.
5. Back up the story with facts and figures.
6. Make the ask in a straightforward way because it can be difficult to achieve results without being specific and clear.
7. Offer a way to measure the results.
8. Offer a pilot project or working group and have a range of possible ideas and solutions in mind that would keep the issue relevant and help the organization reach the goal.

Conclusion

Dr. C's story illustrates many of the steps needed to negotiate effective advocacy at the organizational level, as well as a few of the potential pitfalls. Although she is off to a promising start, this is likely only the beginning of Dr. C's advocacy journey.

Case Example: Dr. C's Storytelling Success

Dr. C and Dr. J met several times and proposed a meeting with Dr. K to "improve bed use efficiency" in both the emergency department and the inpatient psychiatric unit. The fact that two unit directors wanted to meet about improving efficiency got Dr. K's attention, and he offered a meeting time several weeks later. Dr. C told a detailed story that she had practiced about Joe, a patient she knew well who lived on the streets and often presented to the emergency department complaining of suicidal ideation but after 24 hours would say he was okay and wanted to be discharged. She related the resources expended to evaluate and take care of Joe from the moment he walked in to the time he was discharged, while more acute patients were waiting days for a bed at the DMC emergency department. Dr. C suggested that there needed to be a way to more appropriately offer people like Joe a place for respite from the street while keeping the psychiatric beds open for people with serious psychiatric emergencies. She proposed a task force made up of various stakeholders, including DMC and the city, to create additional shelter space and services for homeless individuals and to develop a process to divert patients like Joe into this social service system and away from the emergency medical/psychiatric system.

Dr. K was moved by Dr. C's story and the amount of direct costs and lost revenue resulting from this problem. He let Dr. C and Dr. J know that DMC was in talks with the city around care for individuals experiencing homelessness but no one from any clinical service was involved in the discussion. Dr. K then invited them to join the current working group. Dr. K decided to take Dr. C and Dr. J's insights to the chief executive officer and ask for authorization of a larger financial commitment to this advocacy initiative. Dr. C suggested that they begin to systematically track "social service admissions" so that they would be better able to understand the impact of these admissions on the system and to identify baseline data to study the impact of future interventions. Dr. C and Dr. J both left feeling that their organizational advocacy had been effective and that their dream of connecting people to social services through the emergency department to divert patients from inappropriate psychiatric admissions was off to a good start.

Advocacy Is Not One Moment in Time but the Story Arc of an Entire Career

At the organizational level, advocating for patients' best interests while being mindful of organizational goals can help address issues in a meaningful manner. When advocacy is intentional, the work can help develop skills in leadership and accountability. Credibility and trust gained can help advance the mission of the organization and also improve the lives of both patients and people in the workplace. Organizational advocacy has a ripple effect that can yield significant gains for individuals, communities, and entire organizations.

Summary Points and Important Ideas

- Find like-minded individuals from *within* the organization and try to evaluate how the problem has been dealt with in the past.
- If past efforts have been made on the issue, ask, "What happened?" and/or "Why have they failed?"
- Establish a sense of urgency as the first step and use Kotter's (1995/ 2007, 1996) model steps to transformational change within organizations.
- Do research and gather pilot data about the issue at hand, which could mean reaching out to data scientists and analysts within the organization.
- Go to your supervisor with a thoughtful solution to the problem (if possible) because vague ideas are less effective than well-thought-out plans created by single individuals or even groups within organizations.
- Develop strong internal relationships because they are key in organizational advocacy.
- Know that organizational charts can be complicated, so it is important to have allies such as one's immediate supervisor to give key lessons on current structures and practices within the organization.
- Look for collaborators from differing departments within the organization because many groups and individuals may have interest in the same problem or issue being advocated for.
- Identify individuals with power to authorize change from within the institution and get their backing.

References

Adams R: How a giant psychiatric hospital company tried to spin us—and silence its staff. BuzzFeed News, December 27, 2017. Available at: www.buzzfeednews.com/article/rosalindadams/how-a-giant-psychiatric-hospital-company-tried-to-spin-us. Accessed September 3, 2019.

Jensen D, Bojeun M: The value of emotional intelligence in transformational change. AMA Quarterly 3(1), 12–15, 2017

Kotter JP: Organizational Dynamics: Diagnosis and Intervention. Reading, MA, Addison-Wesley, 1978

Kotter JP: Leading Change. Boston, MA, Harvard Business Review Press, 1996

Kotter JP: Leading change: why transformation efforts fail (1995). Harvard Business Review 85(1):96, 2007

Kowalczyk L: Families trusted this hospital chain to care for their relatives. It systematically failed them. Boston Globe, June 10, 2017. Available at: www.boston.com/news/local-news/2017/06/10/families-trusted-this-hospital-chain-to-care-for-their-relatives-it-systematically-failed-them. Accessed September 3, 2019.

Neiva ER, Odelius CC, Ramos LD: The organizational change process: its influence on competences learned on the job. Brazilian Administration Review 12(4):324–347, 2015

Review HB, Cialdini RB, Morgan N, et al: Influence and Persuasion. Boston MA, Harvard Business Review Press, 2017

Seiling JG: Organizational advocacy 101. Journal for Quality and Participation 24(1)42–45 2001a

Seiling JG: The Meaning and Role of Organizational Advocacy: Responsibility and Accountability in the Workplace. Westport, CT, Quorum Books, 2001b

Shore DA: The Trust Crisis in Healthcare: Causes, Consequences, and Cures. New York, Oxford University Press, 2007

Advocacy Role Model Interview: Ken Duckworth, M.D.

Advocacy Through Organizational Leadership

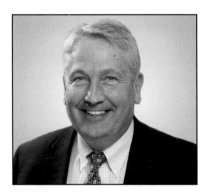

Ken Duckworth, M.D.

Medical Director, National Alliance on Mental Illness; Medical Director for Behavioral Health, Blue Cross Blue Shield of Massachusetts, Boston, Massachusetts

How did you come to be an advocate?

I grew up with a wonderful dad who had severe bipolar disorder. When he was symptomatic, he could be psychotic and disorganized. The police were at our house a lot. He went to the state hospital many times.

Watching all of this over the years, I realized around age 10 that there was something fundamentally unjust about the way my father was treated. So I got involved with the National Alliance on Mental Illness (NAMI), and that put me on track to be an advocate. I quickly realized that I wanted to advocate for people with serious mental illness, people like my father. And I thought it was very important that I work on this for the rest of my life.

By the way, when I wrote this down in my personal statement for psychiatry residency—that I wanted to be a psychiatrist because of my father—an interviewer told me that "working out your family's problems" was a bad reason to enter the field. So I asked what would be a good reason, and the interviewer said, "Because your father was a psychiatrist." That's the kind of advice you *don't* listen to.

Could you describe the kind of advocacy work you do now?

After I got out of school, I wanted to take leadership jobs early on so I could make more difference per square inch. I became a kind of "systems mechanic," taking on jobs and seeing what I could do there. And I would only take a job if I had a plan for how to change the equation, how to make things better.

One example of this is my current job as medical director for behavioral health at Blue Cross Blue Shield of Massachusetts. This of course is a job with an insurance company, which might seem unusual for someone whose passion and previous jobs were in the public sector. But I took the insurance job because, in the tailwind of mental health parity, I felt like I could do better as a Blue Cross administrator than as a Blue Cross provider.

I had goals going in: get rid of prior authorizations, eliminate co-pays, and increase access. Keep in mind, though, that when you take an administrative leadership position, you have to *do* the job. There are a lot of meetings, a lot of conference calls. But between those, pick one or two things you see as problematic and work on them with 20%–25% of your effort. That's advocacy, and it may not be your job, but it's very gratifying. For example, Blue Cross no longer requires prior authorizations overnight for mental health admissions. That's a systems change I helped to leverage.

I also have a part-time job/"love affair," though, and that's my position as medical director of NAMI. NAMI is a giant advocacy machine, and I cared about its goals, and I showed that I cared, so I was asked to be medical director eventually. In this position, I provide consultation for the board on NAMI's advocacy priorities.

What advice do you have for other psychiatrist-advocates?

1. Advocacy is a team sport. Develop your ability to work with others because a gathering of like-minded people can make all the difference.
2. Have a mission. As Nietzsche said, "He who has a why to live for can bear almost any how." Devote a lot of time to something you care about, and opportunities will come.

3. Don't hide from leadership jobs. Don't wait until you have three kids and a mortgage to take them on. Try it and see if you like it. Don't assume you can't run things because you haven't run things. Don't limit yourself.

7

Legislative Advocacy

Katherine G. Kennedy, M.D.

Learning Objectives

By the end of this chapter, readers will be able to:

- Understand the need for legislative advocacy
- List the three "basics" of legislative advocacy that every psychiatrist should practice
- Know ways to engage in legislative advocacy
- Describe common communication tools used in legislative advocacy
- Recognize common challenges to legislative advocacy

Advocating for anything at the legislative level is an art, not a science. Advocates need to be able to navigate complex political systems and negotiate transactional relationships. They need to be persuasive and persistent and to understand trends in the current U.S. zeitgeist. There is no single recipe for effective legislative advocacy, but certain guidelines can be followed that will help advocates determine what is likely to work best for their particular issue. In this chapter, I provide an overview of current approaches for advocating for mental health care initiatives at the legislative level.

Why Is Legislative Advocacy Necessary?

The U.S. health care system is undergoing substantial transformation, and decisions made today will impact how mental health care is organized and delivered for the next generation. Structural and social determinants of health contribute to multiple health disparities and health inequities, many of which require state and federal legislative interventions in order to effect systemic change. In addition, innovative legislation is needed to address many health-related societal scourges, such as the rising suicide rate and the opioid epidemic. Understanding how to advocate at the legislative level will help psychiatrists play a consequential role in developing and shaping an accessible, quality U.S. mental health care system able to meet the needs of patients and combat growing societal threats.

The Three "Basics" of Legislative Advocacy for Every Psychiatrist

Many psychiatrists imagine that legislative advocacy means "fighting city hall" and fear that they lack the time, energy, or skills to do so. However, not all legislative advocacy is time-consuming or demanding. The following three legislative advocacy "basics" can be practiced by every psychiatrist:

1. *Vote!* In the United States, voter turnout averages an abysmal 60% or less for federal elections (DeSilver 2018) and falls even lower for state and municipal elections (MIT Election Data and Science Lab; United States Election Project 2019). An important step for all advocates is to vote. If you are not able to register to vote in the United States, encourage your friends and colleagues to register. Make time to vote in every election—both primaries and regular elections—for municipal, state, and federal officials. If you are away from your polling place during an election, vote with an absentee ballot. Remind family, friends, and colleagues to vote. Studies show that posting on social media a photo of yourself voting will increase voter turnout among people who view the photo (Beck et al. 2002). Simply asking people when they plan to vote also helps to increase voter turnout (Bond et al. 2012).

2. *Know the names and backgrounds of your local, state, and federal elected officials.* As a constituent, you are well positioned to educate and make requests of your elected officials. To do this, it is helpful to understand who your elected officials are and even get to know them personally. Most lawmakers have biographies available on websites or social media. Learn about your legislative officials: What issues are they champions for? What bills have they sponsored? Do they hold a leadership position (e.g., chair a committee or hold a position within their caucus)? What committees do they sit on? Knowing these answers will help to better inform potential contacts and relationship-building efforts with your legislators.

3. *Get involved in state and national professional advocacy organizations.* Join your professional advocacy organizations, such as the American Psychiatric Association (APA) and the American Medical Association (AMA), among others. Do more than join. Get involved:

   • Familiarize yourself with the organization's federal and state legislative agenda.
   • Sign up for the organization's e-mail alerts—and then read them. Often, it takes only 2 minutes to respond to an e-mail request, which might be as simple as a quick call or e-mail to your state or federal legislator.
   • Attend an "advocacy day" organized by an advocacy organization either in your state capital or in Washington, D.C. This is often an excellent experience to advance your understanding of how to interact with legislators and their staff. Your attendance also helps the organization by adding to turnout; legislators pay more attention to organizations that demonstrate a high number of engaged members.

Beyond the Basics: Becoming an Effective Legislative Advocate

Psychiatrists who want to go beyond the basics and become more involved in legislative advocacy have a variety of avenues open to them. You might find that many of your patients face the same systemic problem over and over again, and you might want to work toward a practical legislative fix. You might learn that your state representative is working on mental health care legislation and offer to advise them in crafting and promoting the bill. Should harmful legislation be considered, you might join a campaign to stop the bill. There are several ways to use your medical expertise and contribute as a legislative advocate. In general, you can do the following:

- Research, develop, and contribute policy ideas for potential legislation.
- Serve as a resource or become a "medical expert" for your legislator.
- Help to pass a good law—or prevent passage of legislation that imperils patients or worsens care.

Finally, any committed advocate should consider the ultimate in legislative advocacy: a run for elected office. Since our nation was founded, physicians have held elected offices at the local, state, and federal levels. For example, in 1789, Dr. Jonathan Elmer, a practicing physician, was elected to our nation's very first U.S. Senate, and, more recently, Dr. Kim Schrier, a pediatrician, was elected to Congress in 2018. By virtue of the rigor of our training and skill set, we as physicians are well equipped to make highly effective legislators. If you feel passionate about legislative advocacy, you might want to do a deeper self-inventory and consider a run for office yourself. Although starting at the local or state level will give you a flavor of your area's personalities and politics, past "rules" that recommend starting locally have been upended, and new political rules are continually being rewritten. Today, there is no best "formula" for how to proceed in a political campaign, although self-awareness of your strengths and limitations often helps.

Understand Your System of Government

Before beginning any legislative effort, advocates need to learn about the structure and processes of the local, state, or federal level of government in which they plan to work. For the purpose of this chapter, the term *local* is used to designate all systems of government that exist below the state level of government. In the United States, *local* can refer to villages, towns, cities, counties, and various regional organizations, all of which have devised a multitude of structures and diverse processes for their systems of government. Regardless of the government level on which you are focused, you should take the time to study and develop a solid understanding of that system of government.

To become a legislative advocate, you will need to learn about 1) the structure of the local, state, or federal government in which you are working; 2) the specific process for how a bill within that system is transformed into a law; 3) the calendar for that process to occur; and 4) the names and political party affiliations of the current elected officials with whom you might interact. Today, this information is often easily accessible through online search engines. For the federal government, information is available at www.house.gov and www.senate.gov. Each state has a website composed of the state's abbreviation followed by ".gov" (e.g., the website for California is www.ca.gov), and many of the states' websites have a section dedicated to their legislative process. For information about local governments, website information varies, with some localities more transparent than others. You might need to pay a visit to your town hall to obtain specific information.

For example, if you choose to advocate at the state level of government, you might want to consider the following topics, which can be adapted for advocacy at other levels of government.

1. *Structure of state government:* Is the legislature bicameral (with two chambers: house and senate) or unicameral (with a single chamber)? How many senators and representatives are elected, and what are the lengths of their terms? How many committees exist, and are they joint endeavors of the house and senate?

2. *Process for passing legislation:* What are the series of hurdles that a bill must overcome before being signed into law? At what inflection points might a psychiatrist-advocate have an impact (e.g., educating an elected official about a bill, testifying at a public hearing, writing an e-mail to the governor to urge signage of a bill)? If a legislative session ends, do bills also "die," or can they be carried over into the next legislative session?

3. *Legislative calendar:* Is the legislature in session on a part-time or full-time basis? If part time, what is the time frame for the regular session? What is the current calendar, including relevant deadlines (e.g., is there a deadline for submitting a new bill)? Do committees have deadlines for advancing legislation out of committee?

4. *Your elected officials:* If you plan to engage more deeply in legislative advocacy, then you should not only know the names and interests of, as well as develop personal relationships with, your own elected officials, but also know the names, political affiliations, and interests of all key lawmakers within the branch or subbranch of the government system on which you are focused. For example, the governor of the state usually will determine which individuals are appointed to serve as state regulators, whereas the political party that holds the majority within the state senate or state house will determine which legislators are asked to lead committees and, ultimately, which bills are brought to the chamber floor for a vote.

Know That Legislative Advocacy Differs at the Local, State, and Federal Levels

Legislative advocacy efforts will be shaped by the level of government in which they are focused. Decades of gridlock in Washington, D.C., have added one more layer of difficulty to a weighty federal legislative process that already consumes considerable resources and time. Passing federal laws can be a lengthy and complicated process and requires the mobilization and engagement of many stakeholders. The process of initiating, promoting, and sustaining a campaign to pass a federal law is usually best delegated to large, well-organized national advocacy organizations, including, but not limited to, the AMA and APA, which have the requisite financial resources and personnel for these (often) gargantuan tasks. Often, these organizations network to form even larger stakeholder coalitions. Physician-advocates are advised to work as members within these large national advocacy organizations rather than risk "going it alone" or joining an ad hoc group. Nevertheless, with the rising influence of social media platforms, which enables fewer voices to better amplify differing opinions, smaller and more informal groups are finding ways to influence federal legislation. No matter how you choose to advocate, helping to pass a new federal law—with potential impacts on millions of lives—can be a deeply gratifying experience.

Passing bills at the local and state levels can also be a satisfying endeavor. Local- and state-level advocacy is usually more manageable in terms of time and resources. Advocates may choose to act alone, as part of an ad hoc group, or as a member of an informal advocacy organization. Although personnel and financial resources are always helpful, they might be less necessary. Passing laws progresses more quickly at the local and state levels than at the federal level, with more frequent markers of success. These small successes can sustain an advocate over a long-haul advocacy effort. In addition, new state laws often serve as pilot programs for future federal laws: if a state law successfully solves a widespread problem, that policy might serve as a model for future federal legislation. Also, the phenomenon of the 10-state threshold—when a minimum of 10 states pass similar laws—can open up an invisible gate to cause a flood of other states to follow suit. The mechanism responsible for causing the floodgates to open is unclear but could either reflect cultural trends or be linked to the effective dissemination of a compelling solution to a widespread problem. Regardless of why it happens, working to enact a local or state law might have a positive ripple effect on other states and in some instances might help pave the way for a majority of states to pass similar legislation.

TABLE 7–1. **Differences between federal- and state- or local-level advocacy**

Legislative level	Typical time frame	Typical advocacy organization characteristics	Typical primary relationship focus	Constituent grassroots engagement
Federal	Years, often multiple years	Nationally focused; access to substantial personnel and financial resources	Key aide; occasionally, elected official	Requires thousands of e-mails or phone calls from constituents
State or local	Months to years	State focused; can be formal or an informal, ad hoc group; level of resources vary	Elected official; can be key aide, as well	Can require as few as 10 e-mails or phone calls from constituents

Another useful piece of information for advocates to consider is the difference in numbers of constituents represented by legislators at different levels of government. A member of the U.S. Congress represents approximately 750,000 constituents, an average state representative has 60,000 constituents, and a local official might have even fewer (Ballotpedia 2019). This large difference has implications for grassroots efforts: getting a federal legislator's attention might require thousands of e-mails or phone calls, whereas getting the attention of a state or local legislator might require as few as 10 e-mails or phone calls. In addition, this difference has implications for the focus of an advocate's primary legislative relationship: at the local or state level, an advocate might be able to directly establish a personal relationship with the elected official, whereas at the federal level, this is unlikely. At the federal level, an advocate should focus on fostering a relationship with a key aide for the legislator (e.g., the aide responsible for health care policy). The differences between federal and local or state advocacy are summarized in Table 7–1.

Contribute to a Policy Proposal

Many psychiatrists possess a wealth of clinical experience that can inform and shape legislative policy. Working with patients in a variety of settings, both private and public, can lead to invaluable insights about how to better address systemic problems and mental health care disparities. In addition, psychiatrists can be effective at managing group dynamics. They are often well equipped to convene the diverse stakeholders necessary for a comprehensive evaluation of complex mental health issues. When functioning well, this stakeholder group can develop and/or support meaningful policy solutions, including potential legislative initiatives. If group members are at odds with one another, the psychiatrist, using tact, transparency, and other methods of de-escalation, has the skills to bring together a group to work for a common goal.

Case Example: Dr. R's Concerns

A psychiatry resident, Dr. R, was concerned about the rising rate of opioid overdoses in her state. She researched the topic and found studies that indicated that decreasing barriers to the availability of naloxone, a drug that reverses the effects of an opioid overdose, resulted in fewer opioid overdose deaths. She consulted with her APA district branch to learn more about the history of this issue in her state. Then she consulted the website for the National Conference of State Legislatures (www.ncsl.org) and discovered that 36 other states—but not her own—had implemented legislation for a "standing-order" model for naloxone prescription, which allowed any concerned person to bypass the burden of obtaining a naloxone prescription directly from a physician. This standing-order model eased barriers of stigma, time, and cost. Dr. R shared this model with harm prevention groups, National Alliance on Mental Illness representatives, and state regulators. They responded with skepticism and recommended modifications. Dr. R incorporated their suggestions into a new proposal and shared the update with the stakeholders, who responded with support for her legislative solution.

This case demonstrates many key steps required for an effective strategy for policy development:

- Choose an issue that you feel strongly about.
- Research the academic literature about the general history of the issue.
- Look to other states and/or countries to obtain ideas and information about their approach to problem solving around the issue. (For states, the website www.ncsl.org is helpful.)
- Review the federal, state, and local legislative history of the issue.

- Seek advice from local, state, and/or national chapters of professional advocacy organizations.
- Look for online media sources of information.
- Connect with diverse stakeholders to learn about their experiences.
- Use your research findings to modify and improve your approach and to better understand the elements of any opposition to the issue. Consider whether or not your approach helps to weaken your opposition, and take measures to ensure that your approach does not reinforce or strengthen your opposition's arguments.
- Consider convening stakeholders for a roundtable discussion to iron out differences, gain their buy-in, and cement support.

When crafting your policy solution, try to be innovative and think outside the box. At the same time, do not reinvent the wheel. For inspiration, look to how other systems of government have solved similar problems. Finally, consider advocating for incremental steps rather than sweeping reforms. Often, small steps can be easier for everyone to understand and take.

Form a Relationship With Your Legislator

The adage "all politics is local" should be amended to "all politics is relationships." Developing a relationship with your state and/or local legislators will put you in a better position to educate them about current mental health care issues, such as parity, scope of practice, and access to care. As discussed earlier, it is typically more difficult to develop a relationship with a federal legislator; however, you might be able to foster rapport with a key aide. When you help legislators, either directly or via their aides, to understand mental health issues more deeply, they will be better equipped to develop, sponsor, champion, and vote on legislation to ameliorate systemic mental health problems. In addition, a well-informed legislator will be better equipped to block a potentially harmful bill. Also, when you behave as a professional who is reliable, credible, knowledgeable, and accessible, you will gain the legislator's trust and respect. This might place you in an advantageous position to serve as a regular resource for advice and commentary about ongoing legislative and regulatory efforts.

You might feel intimidated or uncomfortable about approaching your legislator for a meeting. However, keep in mind that all elected officials—especially if they intend to seek reelection—want to know their constituents' concerns and usually want to deliver on these concerns. Lawmakers come from a range of backgrounds and experiences. Although elected officials have accepted a massive responsibility—to solve critical societal problems—they might be ill-equipped to do so. Federal lawmakers have access to staffers who can provide in-depth briefings, but many local and state elected officials do not have these staffing resources. Consequently, local and state officials often rely on others to serve as experts in areas unfamiliar to them. In addition, even the most well-informed officials will possess misinformation and have blind spots. For example, some lawmakers might not understand the difference between a psychiatrist and a psychologist, or they might express an implicit bias against the profession of psychiatry and people with substance use and other mental health diagnoses.

When working with legislators, remember that they like to hear vivid vignettes about why a law is needed. Memorable stories are more easily recalled than statistical data, and they serve to create an emotional connection to dry policy-speak. Legislators often use these stories to convince fellow lawmakers to vote for, or against, a bill. If you are involved in clinical work, you are well positioned to offer legislators poignant patient stories—with identifying information disguised or removed—to illustrate your issue and underscore why new legislation might be warranted. Legislators might be moved to action when turgid policy is animated by a lively patient story.

In sum, there are many reasons to meet with your legislators: to educate them about a mental health issue, to propose new legislation or discuss a current bill, or to offer your ongoing consultative services. The easiest way to meet your legislators is by attending one of their public in-district office hours. Most lawmakers offer these meetings at least annually, usually at convenient times and locations. Take advantage of this excellent opportunity to introduce yourself to your legislators. Even if you have no immediate concerns, you can offer your medical expertise as an ongoing service. Before the meeting, consider signing up for the legislators' e-mail updates and following them on social media. Lawmakers appreciate when constituents are up to date on their activities.

If you are unable to attend a public session, consider setting up a private meeting. Contact information is usually available online. Remember that local and state legislators might lack adequate staffing resources, so a response might take a few days. Nevertheless, be persistent and try multiple contact methods. In addition, meetings with legislators work best when you are a constituent. If you want to meet with a lawmaker who is not your elected official, consider having an actual constituent reach out to request the meeting and then accompany you to the meeting. When reaching out to schedule an in-person meeting, consider the locale, especially for federal legislators and their aides, who might have more time to meet at their Washington, D.C., office and thus appreciate the extra effort you make to meet them on Capitol Hill.

Case Example: Dr. R Meets With Her Legislator

Dr. R decided to approach her state senator to pitch the concept of a new law to support a standing-order model for naloxone. She went on Facebook and learned that she had missed his semiannual office hours at the local coffee shop a week earlier. She located Senator U's contact information online and e-mailed his office. Receiving no response after a few days, she telephoned his office and left a message. His legislative aide returned her call and set up a meeting with Senator U for the following week at his local office rather than at the state capitol office 100 miles away.

On the day of the meeting, Dr. R dressed professionally and arrived a few minutes early. When she arrived, she was cordial and thanked the senator in advance for taking the time to meet with her. She handed him a one-page printed summary of her proposal, which included her contact information. Senator U was pleasant but said he could meet for only a few minutes. Dr. R had spent time rehearsing her presentation and presented her proposal in less than 3 minutes. She answered the questions she anticipated succinctly and clearly. However, Senator U asked a question that stumped her. She offered to get back to him by e-mail. Then she made a formal request that he submit the bill to the Health Committee. Senator U responded that he would consider this possibility. As she left, Dr. R thanked the senator and mentioned that she had appreciated all of his recent work in this area. After the meeting, Dr. R found the answer to the difficult question and sent an e-mail that evening with a heartfelt thank you and a reminder of her request.

This example illustrates some helpful guidelines when meeting with a legislator and/or aide:

- Expect the meeting to be brief, meaning you might have only a few minutes to explain and discuss your issue. With this in mind, practice a succinct 3-minute synopsis of your remarks, anticipate questions, and be prepared with clear answers. Expect a private meeting to last no longer than 15 minutes.

- Dress and behave professionally. To emphasize your identity as a physician, consider wearing a white coat. If you do wear a white coat, consider covering up any institutional names or logos (e.g., an embroidered image over the pocket) unless you have received express permission from the institution to advocate about this issue on their behalf. Express thanks at both the beginning and the end of the meeting. If stumped by a question, do not get defensive but graciously offer to get back with an answer.
- Hand over a single "leave-behind" page that includes a synopsis of the issue and your complete contact information; you might also want to provide your business card.
- Be sure to include an "ask" at every encounter with a legislator. Your request should be clear, specific, realistic, and actionable—that is, ask the legislator to agree to another meeting, to cosponsor a bill, to work with leadership to bring a bill to the floor, to hold a public hearing, or to vote to support the bill. Do not miss an opportunity to advance your cause. Always aim for progress, no matter how small, and try to keep the lines of communication open. For example, if you cannot turn a "no" into a "yes," then strive for a "maybe."
- Write a thank-you note within 24 hours. Correspondence via e-mail is often preferred to written correspondence sent via the U.S. Postal Service. Include a brief summary of the meeting and reiterate your request. If a staff person was present, write a separate thank-you note to the staff member. Provide any follow-up information as quickly as possible.

There are additional considerations when speaking or meeting with a legislator. Review the legislator's online biography in advance of your meeting to ensure that you are fully apprised of the person's legislative successes and failures and of any committee roles or leadership positions related to your proposed legislation. Often, you can uncover sponsorship and voting records for previous legislation. Mine media websites and social media platforms for any history of interest or work on substance use and other mental health issues. Knowledge of this information will enhance your presentation—and help to avoid missteps. For example, if you are presenting policy ideas about substance use treatment and are unaware of the legislator's previous work in this area, your message might be discounted.

Try to consider the legislator's perspective. Lawmakers are managing multiple bills and trying to get up to speed on a range of issues; they have little bandwidth for extraneous details or minutiae. Be sure to streamline your presentation and keep it simple. In addition, most legislators are not acquainted with medical terminology or familiar with diagnoses and treatments for substance use and other mental health conditions. Try to refrain from using complex medical language, avoid jargon, and spell out acronyms. Also, many legislators are challenged by a policy dialectic: although constituents expect them to propose big ideas to address colossal problems, such as health care, most people are averse to seismic policy shifts and prefer incremental policy changes. Therefore, although many legislators might want their optics to suggest that they are producing sweeping legislation, their real efforts may in fact be bite-size. Consider this reality when you frame your proposals and make your requests.

Additionally, if you work with, or represent, an advocacy organization, you have additional tools to use to enhance your relationship with a legislator. Legislators are habitually on the lookout for ways to garner good publicity, which helps boost their image and is useful in their political campaigns. As a member of an advocacy organization, you can offer unique photo opportunities, increased social media exposure, and grassroots mobilization. Invite your legislator to speak at a meeting and post a photo of the legislator surrounded by smiling physicians. Consider having the organization offer an annual legislative award; understanding that there might be a prize will motivate some legislators to deliver results. Recognize that strong grassroots constituent support is a highly valuable commodity for legislators; indeed, powerful public support might invigorate legislators and even transform them into champions who will fight hard and prioritize the issue. Grassroots support also supplies necessary "cover fire" for legislators who may need to cast a so-called difficult vote—that is, a vote antithetical to their colleagues, their caucus, or their conscience. Legislators can employ this cover fire rationale in their explanation for why they cast a particular vote (e.g., "I had to vote nay—I received 200 constituent e-mails about this").

Finally, no matter what, the best way to strengthen a relationship with a legislator or legislative aide is to repeatedly express your gratefulness. You cannot thank legislators or their staff too many times. Legislators and their staff are the receivers of countless complaints and gripes, and a note of gratitude will stand out and be appreciated more than you might imagine.

Help to Pass a Good Law—or Stop a Bad Bill

In addition to proposing policy and offering expertise, psychiatrist-advocates can work to support good legislation or oppose bad bills. Innovative legislation is needed to create structural change within our society and health care system in order to stem the tide of health inequities and mitigate health disparities for marginalized and minority populations, such as people with substance use and other mental health diagnoses. Halting bills that deepen health inequities, worsen health disparities, and threaten public health is a critically important task.

Psychiatrist-advocates can promote or oppose legislation at key inflection points along a bill's journey through the state legislature. Although this process varies from state to state, in general, there are key moments for public input when psychiatrist-advocates can offer medical perspectives. Opportunities are also available for federal advocacy, but as discussed earlier, working in concert with a large advocacy organization is advisable at the federal level. Opportunities for psychiatrist-advocates to engage in the legislative process include the following:

1. *Provide medical expertise during the public hearing phase.* In most states, the public is invited early during the legislative process to provide comments, usually as written testimony and/or oral testimony at a public hearing. This public input can range from declarations of support to rationales for opposition to ideas for how to improve the bill. Your medical opinion and expertise are valuable contributions to the public record because legislators often look to medical science for assistance and direction. Typically, written testimony consists of a brief 1- to 2-page clear, concise document, often with a patient story to illustrate the points. Oral testimony is usually limited to 2–3 minutes, followed by an opportunity for questions from legislators. Your presence at a public hearing underscores your commitment to the issue and enables legislators to hear directly from you, which improves their comprehension and retention of the issue; however, providing oral testimony is usually more time-consuming than submitting written testimony. No matter whether you choose the oral or the written route, avoid portrayals of your institution's logos—for example, on your white coat or on your stationery—because it would be misleading to create the impression that a health system or other entity endorses your testimony unless you have been specifically engaged by such an entity to represent it.

2. *Mobilize at a grassroots level to support or oppose a bill.* There are several stages in its journey when a bill needs a majority vote in order to move forward. Although the process may vary, in general, votes on a bill are needed for the bill to a) move out of committee, b) pass in the house, and c) pass in the senate. In addition, even if a bill moves forward, there is no guarantee that the bill will go on for a vote at the next stage of its journey; in fact, many bills "die" through lack of action by the leadership to bring a bill forward for a vote. (A note here about

leadership: Usually, leadership in a chamber, either the house or the senate, is determined by which political party holds the majority. In fact, holding leadership in a chamber confers considerable power because chamber leadership appoints committee chairs and determines which bills are brought forward for a vote, in addition to other privileges.) These stages are opportunities for psychiatrist-advocates to galvanize their grassroots and have them pressure leadership to take up (or hold) a bill, and/or to lean on legislators to vote to support (or oppose) a bill. There are myriad ways to mobilize grassroots support (e.g., through phone-banking, online petitions, e-mail campaigns, social media posts). Although this task might seem daunting, if you have access to a listserv of engaged members—either one you have created through outreach to your friends and colleagues or one that you have obtained through your connection with an advocacy organization or other group—you may be surprised to discover how many members you can activate through a carefully crafted, inspirational e-mail. Keep in mind that grassroots members should be constituents of the legislators they are contacting, so your e-mail message should include links to assist members in identifying their legislators.

3. *Raise general public awareness about an issue or a bill.* As an advocate, you may want to consider outreach to raise public awareness. This can motivate a broader audience to contact their legislators. Consider creating a website or a social media page or partnering with an advocacy organization to use their website or social media platform. Other ways to raise public awareness include the following:

- Submit letters and op-eds to newspapers.
- Host educational information sessions at your hospital or in the community.
- Create events that lead to news media coverage (e.g., hold a rally, walkathon, or march).
- Reach out to journalists (e.g., call in to a local radio show).
- Use social media platforms to inform and engage a wider audience.
- Consider creative, innovative methods (e.g., the ice-bucket challenge for amyotrophic lateral sclerosis, which became an online viral sensation).
- In your outreach, be sure to provide a way for interested parties to follow up (e.g., provide a website or contact information).

4. *Work with advocacy organizations to leverage their assets.* Gaining the support of an advocacy organization can help your cause in many ways, especially if the organization includes your bill as part of its leg-

islative agenda. Besides expanding the size of your grassroots population, advocacy organizations may have personnel resources, such as a
paid lobbyist, who can go behind the scenes and obtain insight into
why a bill may or may not be moving forward. A lobbyist may also
have a better sense about the quirks of various legislators or have first-
hand knowledge about a complicated political back story. Advocacy
organizations may also have financial resources to pay for a digital ad
campaign or another form of paid advertising. Working with an organization can also help to build coalitions and alliances with other organizations, which further strengthens grassroots power.

Case Example: Dr. R's Work to Get a Bill Passed

Dr. R had several more exchanges with Senator U to answer
questions and provide additional information. Then she received
exciting news: Senator U had decided to sponsor the bill in the
Health Committee. Dr. R began to prepare for the public hearing.
She crafted her written testimony, prepared a 3-minute oral
presentation, and rehearsed with a timer. She reached out to
university pharmacists, addiction psychiatrists, and her colleagues
to ask them to provide oral and/or written testimonies. She
contacted advocacy organizations to confirm that the bill was on
their legislative agenda. She checked the state government website
daily for a public hearing notice from the Health Committee.

One day, the notice was posted: the public hearing would take
place in 3 days. Dr. R scrambled to change her clinic schedule and
notify her colleagues. On the day of the public hearing, she and
her colleagues waited 5 hours to testify. As she sat down at a large
desk facing the semicircle of 15 legislators, Dr. R felt nervous. She
took a deep breath, adjusted the microphone, looked straight
ahead, and spoke slowly and clearly. When she finished, she felt
surprisingly calm and able to answer the flurry of questions. As
she watched her colleagues testify, she felt hopeful.

Over the following months, Dr. R worked to raise public
awareness. She reached out to journalists, who produced several
articles for area newspapers. She also provided two radio
interviews, published one op-ed, and used social media to spread
greater awareness. She made a grassroots effort to organize her
fellow house of medicine colleagues to make phone calls to
legislators and rallied the stakeholder advocacy organizations to
use their listservs to engage their members to contact legislators.

Case Example: Dr. R's Work to Get a Bill Passed *(continued)*
Four months later, the bill passed the senate, and 2 weeks after that, it passed the house. Ten days later, the governor signed the bill into law. Dr. R e-mailed Senator U, her colleagues, and the advocacy organizations a note of profound gratitude for their extraordinary work.

This case illustrates a fairly ideal process, in which hard work produces a successful outcome. However, the road of legislative advocacy is more commonly paved with challenging situations. Do not be surprised to encounter unexpected roadblocks, interpersonal conflicts, shocking disinformation, e-mails that languish, and betrayals of promises. Perseverance, flexibility, resourcefulness, and resilience are essential qualities for most advocates in order to survive painful and difficult setbacks, reorganize, and move forward along new pathways.

Communication Tools for Legislative Advocacy

The overarching goal of legislative advocacy is to inspire specific actions by your targeted group, whether you are asking legislators to vote a certain way or motivating constituents to contact their legislators. Oral and written communication skills, together with effective messaging, are critical advocacy tools in these endeavors. Messaging and communications skills require rehearsal and feedback in order to develop more polished and professional skill sets. Awareness of your own strengths and weaknesses and being fearless about asking others for critiques will help you to improve the key advocacy skills of messaging, written communications, and oral communications. Chapter 10, "Engaging the Popular Media," provides additional discussion and many useful tips and resources about communication methods. Some essential legislative advocacy communication tools are listed in the following subsections.

Messaging Skills

An effective advocacy core message explains the rationale for the issue in a few sentences or less. One model suggests limiting a message to three sentences that can be stated in no more than 15 seconds (Parker 2015). A core message is essentially the "mission statement" for your advocacy issue. Effective core messaging requires two factors: 1) a psychosocial understanding of your audience, in order to identify their underlying values and moral codes, and 2) an awareness of current cultural dynamics, with a special focus on language itself and the words that unify or polarize. These two ingredients are necessary to be able to effectively frame and explain the advocacy issue to your target audience. The specific words you select, together with the feelings they evoke, will determine how your audience understands and responds to your advocacy issue. Because how an issue is perceived has far-reaching implications in terms of its success, take time to think carefully about your advocacy issue and the various ways it could be framed and messaged. Engage others in this exercise. If you overlook this crucial step, you might unwittingly frame an issue in such a way that allows opponents to poke holes in, undermine, or subvert your core message and therefore your issue.

Values inform our moral code of conduct, which is a strongly held set of beliefs about how we should behave. Values and morality are deeply connected to our sense of who we are; they resonate emotionally to gain our attention (Haidt 2013). At times, they drive us to act. For example, when we hear a story about a mother sexually molesting her son, we take notice. The scenario offends our moral sense of right and wrong. We feel disgusted and perhaps moved to justice. Our value, protection of the vulnerable, which informs our moral code for how mothers should behave, together with our emotional sense of well-being, has been disturbed.

Commonly held American values, such as protection, freedom, and opportunity, are often used to get the attention of an audience. When a value is connected to a concept—such as an advocacy issue—that concept is more likely to be noticed, responded to emotionally, and acted on. For example, consider how two opposing political parties frame and message the same 2019 U.S. House of Representatives bill, HR 986, in order to appeal to their supporters' value systems. One party posits that HR 986 would lead to "fewer health care choices and higher health care costs" and would mean "the undoing of…regulatory relief efforts designed to allow more innovative health care solutions" (Fishpaw 2019). This party frames HR 986 as the destroyer of deeply held American values, such as freedom of choice and the opportunity for innovation. Across the aisle, the opposing party labels HR 986 the Protecting Americans With Preexisting Conditions Act of 2019. This party lays claim to the value of protection of the vulnerable and also implies that this bill upholds the values of equality and fairness. Both parties, on opposite sides of the aisle, use the same tactic: attach values to a piece of legislation to garner attention, evoke feelings, and inspire action. Clearly, because opposing sides both use the same value-focused strategy, it must be powerful and effective.

When framing your advocacy message, you should also consider emerging societal themes and the language that is in vogue (Lakoff 2014). Trending words and terms are familiar and help the listener to attend more easily to the message they carry. However, be aware that trending words that serve to build a bridge to one audience may enlarge a chasm with another. For example, the words *immigrants* and *wall* may evoke polarizing and opposing responses from two different audiences.

How can you put all this together to create a core message for your advocacy issue? Although a full examination of this complex psychosocial topic is beyond the scope of this discussion, here are a few guidelines to consider:

- *Foster feelings in your audience.* Frame your advocacy issue with language that will connect emotionally with the listener. When crafting your message, think about the specific emotions you are evoking: although hate and anger are strong motivators for immediate action, it is positive, hopeful phrasing that inspires people to persevere and keep fighting, and in the long run, these positive messages are more effective than core messages that spread fear. Also, trending words that unite rather than polarize and divide will ultimately increase the size of your audience of supporters.
- *Use words that reference common values.* Consider what values motivate your audience (e.g., access, quality, equity), and use relevant language in your core message. Often, these values are highly connected to cultural "code words" that act as beacons to signal the values and the underlying moral code of conduct.
- *Try to anticipate opponents' arguments.* In your core message, avoid language that antagonizes your opponents and incites new resistance. If possible, cast doubt on your opponents' arguments and include language that refutes their assertions. Also, appreciate that your opponents' arguments might not be fair: your opponents might cherry-pick facts, use misleading data, conflate concepts, distort ideas, and outright lie.
- *Analyze each word in your core message.* Be clear and concise and use simple, accessible, jargon-free language. Replace a word if there is a better option; recognize that your choice of words will spark varied associations and subtly convey different meanings. For example, in *Words That Work: It's Not What You Say, It's What People Hear*, Frank Luntz (2007) discusses the fact that the words *does not give*

seem to be synonymous with *deny*, but they have a subtle difference in meaning when linked to the word *treatment*. If a hospital "does not give treatment," the implication is that the hospital has the right to choose whether to bestow that treatment; however, if a hospital "denies treatment," the implication is that a person is being prevented from receiving a service that is rightfully theirs.

In sum, the goal of effective advocacy messaging is to consider your target audience's values within the context of the cultural zeitgeist and to use emotionally evocative language that references these values. Once you frame your advocacy message, be consistent and use this language in all future oral and/or written communications. Regular repetition of the same message will help to reinforce your issue. Keep in mind, however, that because our society is in constant flux, what feels relevant one year may seem outmoded the next.

Written Communication Skills

Legislative advocacy uses many forms of written communication. Whether you are creating flyers to post in the hospital to advertise an upcoming information session, providing written testimony on a bill before a state legislative committee, generating grassroots support via e-mails and social media posts, or engaging the public about your issue through an op-ed, you will need to consider how to present your advocacy issue in a written manner that is persuasive and compelling and inspires readers to action. Written communications in legislative advocacy must inform, spark interest, and make a request of the reader—and ideally motivate readers to fulfill that request. Written communications should do the following:

1. *Inform.* Be selective about the facts and data that you include in your written communications. Most people have only enough "shelf space" in their working memory for up to five pieces of information about an issue. If you overwhelm a reader with too many arguments, they may lose track; instead, strive to present between three and five arguments of support for your issue. Be thoughtful about how you convey data; for example, reporting that "only 1 in 1,000,000 will develop this complication" may serve to minimize the reader's concern, whereas stating that "more than 100 state residents will suffer from this complication" may increase concern. Also, if possible, provide an acknowledgment of the opposition's arguments and your refutation of them.

2. *Spark interest.* In general, the best way to spark interest is by telling brief, vivid stories about people, especially patients. These clinical vignettes serve to humanize your issue and bring dry facts and mundane data to life. Adding even a one-sentence illustration about a patient to any written communication will increase its appeal.
3. *Make a request.* Most written communications need to include an "ask." Many advocates forget to include this simple step. If you are taking the time to provide information in whatever form—a flyer, an op-ed, a "leave-behind"—you should make sure to ask the reader to do something, even a task as simple as signing up for an e-mail listserv, going to a website for more information, or voting to support a bill. Making a request performs two functions: first, if the reader acts on your request, this will further advance the cause you are advocating for, and second, when a reader acts, they are increasing their engagement with the issue, which will increase the likelihood that they will act again in the future, should another request be made.

There are many types of written communications. Table 7–2 lists several common types of written communications and their characteristics.

The writing task may feel overwhelming. Many advocates find it helpful initially to compile their research and organize their arguments into a single coherent document, which can be used as a reference sheet for future written communications. This one-page summary, or fact sheet, on the advocacy issue often includes the following: 1) the core advocacy message, 2) the primary arguments of support, 3) a brief overview of potential opposing arguments and why they can be discounted, 4) any relevant visual images such as graphs, and 5) a "for more information" section (e.g., website, contact information). This one-page fact sheet can be especially helpful for an advocacy group, because it can assist the group in terms of identifying and clarifying the issue's core message, primary arguments, and so on and also help group members understand that they are literally on the same page. In general, all written communications should avoid medical jargon and be clear, easy to read, and visually appealing in the use of font and graphics.

Oral Communication Skills

Being able to advocate orally for your cause is an important skill. There are many opportunities to advocate orally, such as at educational activities (e.g., lectures, panel discussions, debates), in meetings with legislators, when providing oral testimony to legislative committees, and while engaging in public outreach (e.g., an elevator speech, interviews, podcasts). Basic

TABLE 7–2.   Common types of written communications used in legislative advocacy

Communication type	Purpose	Core elements	Ways to spark interest	What is your "ask"?
Informational flyers	Materials that inform an issue and/or invite attendance to a meeting, forum, etc.	Length: 1 page Include: clear description of issue and/or event details; contact information	Visual appeal is key Include graphics and photos Consider color, fonts, and logos	Examples of the "ask" include get involved or attend an informational session
"Leave-behind"	Information sheet provided to legislators during or following a meeting	Length: 1 page Include: the issue and bill number, if applicable; description of the issue and your arguments; contact information	Presentation should be clean, easy-to-read, visually accessible, and professional Use bullets and bold fonts	Be clear about what you want the legislator to do (e.g., vote the bill out of committee, oppose the bill)
Written testimony	Opinion based on medical expertise, usually given to a legislative committee in the context of a public hearing	Length: 1–2 pages (check committee rules) Include: your position on the bill (for, against, neutral); your credentials; arguments; references	Include position and bill number in header Should be clean, easy to read, and professional Use bullets and bold fonts	Be clear about what you want the legislator to do (e.g., vote the bill out of committee, oppose the bill)

TABLE 7–2. Common types of written communications used in legislative advocacy *(continued)*

Communication type	Purpose	Core elements	Ways to spark interest	What is your "ask"?
Media: op-eds, letters to the editor	Opinion based on medical expertise, written at the level of media readership (e.g., fellow health professionals, general public)	Length: Op-eds 500–800 words; letters to the editor <200 words Include: your credentials; arguments; refutation of opponents' arguments	Include a "hook" at the beginning (e.g., a clinical vignette or a reference to a recent news story) Should be easy to read, succinct, and clear	The "ask" is usually emphasized at the conclusion, often as an inspirational and gracious request (e.g., support the cause, contact your legislator)
Grassroots outreach: social media posts, e-mail listservs, blog posts	Writing intended to engage recipients and motivate action (e.g., to join a listserv, to call a legislator, to attend a rally)	Include: reiteration of the core advocacy message; request for action by the reader	Include attention-grabbing material (e.g., funny or beautiful photos, quirky vocabulary, shocking statistics)	The "ask" is a call to action and should be the focus of the outreach (e.g., sign up for e-mails, contact a legislator)

requirements for effective oral advocacy are to speak *clearly, slowly*, and *loudly* enough for your audience to understand the actual words that you are saying. Beyond that, your focus should be on trying to capture and maintain your listener's attention. To do this, you will need to modulate the tone and volume of your voice, be mindful of your gaze, and pay attention to what you convey with your body language, especially your hand gestures. Speakers who stare down at a piece of paper and rapidly read a prepared speech will hold less interest than the advocate who makes eye contact with the audience and conveys remarks with confidence and conviction.

There are varying formats for lectures, debates, interviews, and podcasts. Often, the organizer or producer will set the parameters. However, two common oral communication methods—the elevator speech and oral testimony—are less variable in structure and are useful to practice in order to develop competency. The *elevator speech* is so called because of its aim: a speaker should present the issue as quickly as it would take an elevator to move between a building's floors, or approximately 30–60 seconds. The primary elements of the issue should be included, with enough detail to ensure understanding and interest on the listener's part; often, ways for the listener to learn more, or take action, are also included. Honing an issue to its core elements and conveying it effectively in a short amount of time requires preparation and rehearsal. *Oral testimony* refers to an advocate's oral presentation to officials in a public hearing. Although rules about the length of the presentation vary according to each hearing body, these rules are usually tightly enforced, so it is important to know how much time you have in order to avoid the mishap of being ordered to stop midsentence. In addition, when providing oral testimony, state at the very beginning whether you support or oppose the issue at hand and provide your credentials upfront. It is also helpful to offer a memorable vignette and clearly explain the rationale(s) for your position. When you conclude, provide a brief summary and reiterate your hope for how officials will act. Table 7–3 describes the applications and key elements of these two methods.

Becoming an effective and engaging public speaker will take practice and experience. Embrace opportunities to advocate orally. You may discover that you perform better in some areas than in others. Try not to let fear prevent you from using your voice.

Challenges to Legislative Advocacy

Psychiatrists may also experience challenges to legislative advocacy. Learning how to work within the legislative system can be difficult and

TABLE 7–3. **Elevator speech versus oral testimony**

	Elevator speech	Oral testimony
Setting	When engaging in public outreach (look for any opportune time)	When presenting your medical opinion on a proposed bill at a legislative committee hearing
Duration	30–60 seconds	Usually 3 minutes; check with committee about how much time is allotted
Purpose	To pique your audience's interest so they will want to learn more about your cause	To engage legislators with a memorable narrative and a clear rationale for why they should support or oppose the proposed bill
Core elements	Who you are and your role in the cause The core message or mission of the cause Steps the audience can take to learn more	Who you are and your credentials What you are asking the legislator to do (e.g., support or oppose the bill) A memorable narrative (usually a patient story) Two to five reasons why the bill is helpful or harmful A statement or relevant data to diffuse opponents' arguments A final plea to support or oppose the bill

disorienting. There are many practical constraints. For example, scheduling in legislative advocacy is predictably unpredictable, with scant notice for public hearings, sudden political shake-ups, and frequent last-minute surprises. These issues can be difficult for the planning and scheduling that are common in medicine: because psychiatrists' schedules are often filled weeks in advance with patient sessions and other clinical responsibilities, changing a meeting or finding coverage at the last minute can be nearly impossible. Also, medicine focuses on putting the patient ahead of all else, and most health care professionals share this same goal of optimizing patient care. It can be challenging to engage with individuals within the legislative system who prioritize their own political needs and prefer the pursuit of optics over policy.

Integrating advocacy into your professional identity can be hard, too. For example, many psychiatrists are more comfortable keeping their opinions private. Advertising your views in a public venue may feel awkward or inappropriate. Also, how you speak to an audience might be different from how you speak to patients; finding your "outside voice" may be tough, and even when you do, switching back and forth can be jarring.

Legislative advocacy requires a sustained effort and can take years. Finding the time, energy, and internal fortitude to persist can be hard. If your day job is excessively demanding, your reserves may be compromised. To persevere, you should anticipate that progress will be incremental, so set milestones to mark your progress and celebrate each small victory. When you encounter a setback, take stock and learn from your missteps. If you hit a true roadblock, consult others, innovate, and be open to out-of-the-box solutions.

Legislative advocacy also requires the ability to compromise. Some advocates may hold out for "the perfect" and ignore "the good enough." This approach may be problematic. If your personal style is rigid or inflexible, you may have difficulty accepting a trade-off or making a deal. However, many long-range approaches require that you concede a few battles in order to win the ultimate war.

Finally, legislative advocacy requires the ability to thank many people—even when they may not deserve your gratitude. Maintaining relationships in the legislative arena means demonstrating appreciation for every action, large and small, done on behalf of your advocacy issue. Learning how to say thank you, for everything, all the time—from the aide who took your phone call to the legislator who voted your way—will stand you in good stead for the long advocacy haul.

Conclusion

Legislative advocacy can be immensely rewarding, with a myriad of ways for us as psychiatrists to participate. Legislative advocacy can help to reshape our mental health care system in ways that can greatly benefit our patients and improve their health care outcomes. Legislative advocacy not only helps us to improve our communication skills but also teaches us how to be leaders, to cope with failures, to persevere, and to innovate. Every psychiatrist should take a chance and give legislative advocacy a try—you might be surprised at the difference you make, and the difference that engaging in legislative advocacy makes in you.

Stakeholder Resources

Historically, many health care organizations have partnered with psychiatrists and psychiatry advocacy organizations to form coalitions that advocate for the best interests of patients' mental health care. The following is a list, in alphabetical order, of some of the possible stakeholder organizations to consider partnering with for future mental health care advocacy efforts.

Academy of Consultation-Liaison Psychiatry (ACLP): www.clpsychiatry.org
American Academy of Addiction Psychiatry (AAAP): www.aaap.org
American Academy of Child and Adolescent Psychiatry (AACAP): www.aacap.org
American Academy of Family Physicians: www.aafp.org/home.html
American Academy of Pediatrics: www.aap.org
American Academy of Psychiatry and the Law (AAPL): www.aapl.org
American Association for Geriatric Psychiatry (AAGP): www.aagp online.org
American College of Emergency Physicians: www.acep.org
American College of Obstetricians and Gynecologists (ACOG): www.acog.org
American College of Physicians: www.acponline.org
American Medical Association (AMA): www.ama-assn.org
American Osteopathic Association: osteopathic.org
American Psychiatric Association (APA): www.psychiatry.org
American Psychological Association: www.apa.org
American Society of Addiction Medicine (ASAM): www.asam.org
Association of Gay and Lesbian Psychiatrists (AGLP): www.aglp.org
Iraq and Afghanistan Veterans of America (IAVA): https://iava.org
Mental Health America (MHA): www.mentalhealthamerica.net
National Alliance on Mental Illness (NAMI): www.nami.org
National Association of Chiefs of Police: www.nacoponline.org
National Association of Counties: www.naco.org
National Association of Social Workers: www.socialworkers.org
National Council for Behavioral Health: www.thenationalcouncil.org

References

Ballotpedia: Population represented by state legislators. Middleton, WI, Balletopedia, 2019. Available at: https://ballotpedia.org/Population_represented_by_state_legislators. Accessed August 20, 2019.

Beck PA, Dalton RJ, Greene S, et al: The social calculus of voting: interpersonal, media, and organizational influences on presidential choices. Am Polit Sci Rev 96(1):57–73, 2002

Bond RM, Fariss CJ, Jones JJ, et al: A 61-million-person experiment in social influence and political mobilization. Nature 489(7415):295–298, 2012 22972300

DeSilver D: U.S. trails most developed countries in voter turnout. Washington, DC, Pew Research Center, May 21, 2018. Available at: www.pewresearch.org/fact-tank/2018/05/21/u-s-voter-turnout-trails-most-developed-countries. Accessed August 20, 2019.

Fishpaw M: House Democrats ready vote to undercut health care innovation. Washington, DC, Heritage Foundation, May 6, 2019. Available at: www.heritage.org/health-care-reform/commentary/house-democrats-ready-vote-undercut-health-care-innovation. Accessed August 20, 2019.

Haidt J: The Righteous Mind: Why Good People Are Divided by Politics and Religion. New York, Vintage Books, 2013

Lakoff G: Don't Think of an Elephant! Know Your Values and Frame the Debate. White River Junction, VT, Chelsea Green Publishing, 2014

Luntz F: Words That Work: It's Not What You Say, It's What People Hear. Boston, MA, Hachette Books, 2007

MIT Election Data and Science Lab: Voter turnout. Cambridge, MA, MIT Election Data + Science Lab, 2019. Available at: https://electionlab.mit.edu/research/voter-turnout. Accessed August 20, 2019.

Parker A: Digital ads sell candidates and causes, in 15-second bursts. New York Times, October 5, 2015. Available at: www.nytimes.com/2015/10/06/us/politics/digital-ads-video-campaign-2016.html. Accessed August 20, 2019.

Protecting Americans With Preexisting Conditions Act of 2019, H.R. 986, 116th Congress

United States Election Project: Voter turnout: national turnout rates, 1787–2016. Gainesville, FL, United States Election Project, 2019. Available at: www.electproject.org/home/voter-turnout/voter-turnout-data. Accessed August 20, 2019.

8

Education as Advocacy

Katherine G. Kennedy, M.D.
Falisha Gilman, M.D.

Learning Objectives

By the end of this chapter, readers will be able to:

- Identify opportunities for psychiatrists to educate their patients, the public, and their colleagues about advocacy
- Understand the challenges that psychiatrist-educators face
- Describe the benefits and barriers to developing an advocacy curriculum for psychiatry residents
- Name key advocacy skills and explain the rationale for teaching them
- Recognize that there is no one-size-fits-all advocacy curriculum

The word *doctor* derives from the Latin word *docere*, meaning "to teach." Doctors have long been expected to be educators of patients, of medical trainees, and of society. Beyond this tradition, teaching is a duty, as outlined in the American Medical Association (AMA) Code of Medical Ethics: "A physician shall continue to study, apply, and advance scientific knowledge, maintain a commitment to medical education, make relevant information available to patients, colleagues, and the public, obtain consultation, and use the talents of other health professionals when indicated" (American Medical Association 2016).

Physicians can act as educators in many ways. At the most personal level, physicians explain an illness and its treatment options to patients, which both validates patients' suffering and empowers them by providing the knowledge they need to make informed decisions about their health care. Physicians educate medical trainees by leading lectures or discussion groups, offering clinical teaching on inpatient wards, supervising in outpatient practices, and designing curricula. In society, physicians are valued as credible sources of medical expertise, and they enjoy a myriad of opportunities to educate the public through presentations (lectures, panels), the media (news articles, opinion pieces, letters to the editor, radio, TV), social media (posts, videos, podcasts, blogs), and in published works (journal articles, papers, books).

In this chapter, we describe the ways in which psychiatrists can educate their patients, colleagues, and the general public about issues that deserve—and perhaps demand—their advocacy. We also highlight approaches for developing an advocacy curriculum at the psychiatry residency training level, with the goal of training psychiatry residents to be more effective psychiatrist-advocates.

Educating others about advocacy issues means to disseminate knowledge about issues beyond a psychiatric diagnosis and its treatment; advocacy education means to educate others about the ways in which systems and structures outside of the psychiatrist-patient relationship impact the care that the patient experiences. These systems and structures include the complexities around who pays for care, the health care system in which care is delivered, the social and structural determinants of health, and the state and federal laws and regulations that impact care. Advocacy education also includes the critical task of teaching others about the range of advocacy methods that can be used to reform these systems and structures.

Psychiatrists as Educators

Many of the same qualities that contribute to competency in psychiatry are also necessary for effective pedagogy. For example, an important first step in teaching is to create a safe and comfortable learning environment, similar to the psychiatrist's creation of a safe therapeutic space for the patient. Excellent educators are personable, trustworthy, and able to form relationships based on mutual respect, characteristics that are similar to those needed for a working therapeutic relationship. Quality teaching requires actively evaluating and flexibly responding to learners' engagement with the material, which is, in many ways, how psychiatrists work with patients (Ackerman and Hilsenroth 2003; Sutkin et al. 2008).

However, psychiatrist-educators face several challenges. Whereas physicians as a group are respected by the public as objective, reliable, and evidence-based professionals, psychiatrists often experience associative stigma—that is, an extension of psychiatric stigma that is directed toward those who care for people with psychiatric illness (Verhaeghe and Bracke 2012). This may be due to the public's distortion and misunderstanding of psychiatry (Catthoor et al. 2014; Möller-Leimkühler et al. 2016). Consequently, psychiatrists may be viewed negatively, in stereotypes ranging from dispassionate intellectuals to incompetent quacks to silent sadists. These misperceptions contribute to a general mistrust and may contravene the credibility of psychiatrist-educators.

Another challenge for twenty-first century psychiatrists is finding the time to learn how to teach, which can be difficult amid the many demands we face. No longer can psychiatrist-educators recite a laundry list of facts and assume that medical knowledge has been imparted. Today, effective teaching requires experience and facility with a range of novel educational approaches that actively engage learners' abilities and interests. These approaches include the use of interactive techniques to promote broader learner participation, such as flipping the classroom (see Table 8–4 later in the chapter) and the use of digital aids. Psychiatrist-educators need to learn these new approaches and acquire new skill sets, but doing so requires time, practice, and even specialized training.

In recognition of these demands, many academic institutions have established new formalized physician-educator training programs (Searle et al. 2006; Steinert et al. 2006). Residency training programs are cultivating the next generation of psychiatrist-educators through longitudinal clinician-educator tracks, including postgraduate year 4 (PGY-4) positions with protected time dedicated to developing teaching skills (Wasser and Ross 2016), and psychiatry departments have created clinician-educator faculty tracks as pathways for promotion. However, the availability of these tracks and training programs, particularly for psychiatrists who have completed their training or who practice in community settings, remains limited. Even for psychiatrists with access to training, lack of time to practice new teaching skills can be a challenge.

Empowering Patients and Their Families

Understanding a health-related problem is often the first step toward managing it. When they are educated about an issue, patients and their families are better able to cope, devise solutions, and manage unexpected setbacks. For example, providing psychoeducation about a diagnosis of panic disorder to a patient and their family may help them to better manage future panic episodes—and prevent unnecessary visits to the emergency department.

In addition to providing patients with basic psychoeducation about the risks and benefits of various treatments, such as medication and psychotherapy, and about interventions, such as partial hospital treatment and neuromodulation, we psychiatrists can help patients and their families to better understand the range of other causes that may contribute to the onset and progression of a particular psychiatric and/or substance use condition. We might discuss issues such as stigma; difficulty accessing care; inadequate mental health parity; explicit and implicit bias against gender, race, and other minority and underrepresented groups; and social and structural determinants of health. We might explain to patients how certain systemic issues could impact their mental health outcomes or might educate families about how payers shape the quality of their health care. When patients and their families better appreciate how these factors contribute to mental health conditions and treatment, they might be more likely to take steps to advocate for their own welfare or to change a systemic problem and less likely to blame themselves or others. In these ways, we can empower patients and their families to be better self-advocates.

When educating patients and their families about systemic factors, we should consider each patient's best interests and welfare to be the highest priority and should carefully consider and always maintain boundaries. We should be wary about any motivation to engage a patient or family in advocacy about an issue in which we are involved. In general, we should follow the principle of never asking our own patients (or those in the clinic in which we work) to engage together in joint advocacy efforts. However, it is acceptable, and even encouraged, for psychiatrists to advocate in concert with persons with lived experience, as long as those individuals are not their own patients. (For more information on ethical considerations to keep in mind when engaging in advocacy, see Chapter 1, "What Is Advocacy, and Why Is It Important?").

It is not unusual for psychiatrists to encounter resistance when trying to educate patients and their families about advocacy issues, particularly about any aspect linked to substance use and other psychiatric disorders, which are cloaked in mystery and shame. Many people possess erroneous ideas about these diagnoses, and this disinformation causes them to turn away from further learning and to stigmatize people with these disorders. Advocacy around mental health issues may invite greater public exposure to patients or their families, which could worsen their experience of stigma. In addition, besides evoking negative feelings such as fear or shame, whenever an issue is complicated, people will find ways to defend themselves from learning more about it. Some may use avoidance and shy away from addressing the matter. Others may misconstrue the root cause of the problem or fabricate rationales as a way to distance themselves from, or feel mastery over, the concern. In order to soften encountered resistance, we as psychiatrists need to use the full range of our psychotherapeutic skills to engage patients and their families and establish trusting relationships.

Inspiring the General Public to Advocate

When we as psychiatrists educate the general public about advocacy issues, we have the opportunity to dispel myths and falsehoods about psychiatry, shed light on systemic problems that call out for advocacy, and tell humanizing stories to inspire empathy and decrease stigma. There are a variety of methods we can use to educate the general public's understanding about the troubling issues that plague psychiatry and its patients, including speaking at community lectures and panel discussions, writing op-eds and letters to the editor, giving radio and television interviews for news stories, contributing material to websites (e.g., blogs, podcasts), and posting on social media platforms. A deeper discussion about these various methods can be found in Chapter 7, "Legislative Advocacy," and Chapter 10, "Engaging the Popular Media."

In general, when acting in your professional identity as a psychiatrist to educate the general public, it may be helpful to keep these recommendations in mind:

1. Many people are confused, suspicious, or misinformed about the role of a psychiatrist, but they value the role of a medical doctor. In fact, many people may not understand that psychiatrists are, in fact, physicians. Clarifying that you are "a physician trained in psychiatry" may be a simple step toward decreasing stigma and increasing acceptance of your message.
2. Many people defend against their fear about psychiatry, and what it represents, by dehumanizing psychiatric patients. You can directly address that bias by providing moving patient stories that evoke empathy and humanize patient experiences. Even describing a patient using the word *mother* or *brother* will help to reposition that person as a human being with relationships.
3. Strive to pick your three best arguments or facts; do not offer more than five rationales for your position or thesis.

4. Take advantage of current news events to time the posting of educational information on social media platforms or the submission of any educational materials, such as op-eds, to media outlets. When a topic is trending, the general public is more likely to attend to your message.

5. No matter the educational method you choose, provide some form of contact method (e.g., an Internet link or a phone number) for the learner to use in order to obtain additional information or be able to take an advocacy action.

Providing Advocacy Education for the Medical Community

The same principles described above for educating the general public also apply to educating fellow physicians about advocacy issues. Additionally, we should keep in mind that most physicians place a high value on well-documented issues with a strong evidence base. When educating medical colleagues, we should be sure to use valid data and cite source material whenever possible. Traditional mechanisms, such as publishing papers and presenting at conferences, are effective methods. Also, as the digital era changes the landscape of advocacy and education, particularly continuing medical education, we should consider using webinars, on-demand courses (e.g., the American Psychiatric Association's Course of the Month [www.psychiatry.org/psychiatrists/education/apa-learning-center/members-course-of-the-month]), podcasts, and other online educational forums for advocacy presentations. Social media platforms, especially Twitter, are an increasingly popular way to provide pithy statements about advocacy issues in medicine.

A rising number of medical students are eager to learn about advocacy and health policy. Some medical schools are responding to medical students' interest in advocacy by adding classes focused on these topics (Stein 2019). However, there is no consensus within the undergraduate medical education community as to what advocacy behaviors medical students should master prior to starting residency training (Association of American Medical Colleges 2014). Although the Association of American Medical Colleges (AAMC) has a set of expected behaviors, the "Core Entrustable Professional Activities for Entering Residency," the only advocacy-related activity suggests that medical students should "advocate for patient access to community resources," and the AAMC does not enumerate the time requirements, advocacy settings, advocacy skills that should be fostered, or ways to properly assess skill acquisition (Association of American Medical Colleges 2014). Despite the absence of clear requirements, many medical schools and professional organizations, such as state medical societies, are working to engage medical students in advocacy training.

Psychiatry residents are also requesting more training and education in advocacy. As increasing numbers of psychiatry residents become aware of health disparities, especially those related to social and structural determinants of health, they also want to learn how to effect systemic change. Many have championed for the implementation of advocacy curricula in their residency training programs (Kennedy and Vance 2018). Like the AAMC, the Accreditation Council for Graduate Medical Education (ACGME) has not specified clear training requirements for advocacy education. Although their 2017 update asserts that psychiatry residency training programs should teach residents to "advocate for quality patient care and optimal patient care systems" (Accreditation Council for Graduate Medical Education 2019), no time requirements or advocacy activities are specified. Instead, the only defined expectation for advocacy is referenced in the Psychiatry Milestone Project (Accreditation Council for Graduate Medical Education, American Board of Psychiatry and Neurology 2015), which provides "frameworks for assessment" of residents' competencies. This tool recommends that by graduation from the residency training program, residents should be able to describe what is encompassed by the term *professional advocacy* but not necessarily demonstrate advocacy skills. Rather, advocacy skill acquisition is considered "aspirational," is limited to "exceptional residents," and is deemed more consistent with the practice of psychiatrists several years postresidency.

With such a limited expectation for advocacy training by the ACGME, the implementation of a more robust advocacy curriculum remains at the discretion of individual psychiatry residency training programs. Nonetheless, a wave of novel and diverse advocacy curricula has sprung up recently at several U.S. psychiatry residency training programs as an increasing number of psychiatry residency training directors respond to residents' grassroots demands for an advocacy curriculum in their educational programs (Kennedy and Vance 2018).

For these intrepid psychiatry training directors, developing an advocacy curriculum for a psychiatry residency training program can be daunting; despite the benefits, many barriers exist. One challenge for training directors is the difficulty finding time for classes within an already packed academic schedule. Another barrier is the identification of competent psychiatrist-educators with experience in advocacy; there are few, if any, "expert" physician-advocates. In addition, no evidence-based curricula exist to serve as an educational guide. These challenges stem primarily from the relative youth of advocacy as a field of focus in medicine. Despite these potential barriers, many training directors are recognizing the long-term benefits of teaching advocacy and are devising innovative solutions to finding educators, such as asking residents to develop and teach advocacy classes or looking outside psychiatry departments to legal advocates and other nonmedical advocacy professionals to assist with teaching and curricula development.

The benefits are considerable. Over the past two decades, themes involving cultural competency, social determinants of health, and systems-based practice have been incorporated into all levels of medical education (Beach et al. 2005; Dogra et al. 2010). Acquiring a deeper understanding of these systemic contributors to health outcomes has been a motivator for psychiatry residents to provide more equitable psychiatric care to their patients. However, unless training in advocacy is included, residents may feel powerless to effectively address these systemic issues. When advocacy training is connected with coursework on health disparities and social justice issues, residents acquire the skills needed to effect change.

Another benefit of formal training in advocacy during residency is the increase in residents' engagement in advocacy following residency. Even if residents were exposed to advocacy experiences during medical school, these advocacy behaviors require reinforcement during residency so that advocacy activities will continue postresidency (Minkovitz et al. 2014). Evidence suggests that although most physicians regard health advocacy as a professional duty, this attitude does not always predict advocacy behaviors (Gruen et al. 2006), perhaps because actual experience with advocacy has been limited or nonexistent.

A third benefit of teaching advocacy skills during training is the potential for a positive ripple effect on future professional behaviors. Trainees who are prearmed with advocacy skills may be more resilient and better prepared, posttraining, to combat the systemic issues that produce stigma and contribute to burnout. Rather than succumb to the depressive position that so frequently occurs in response to these common phenomena, residents empowered with advocacy skills may more effectively combat the root causes of systemic ills (Leal-Costa et al. 2015). In addition, knowing how to advocate confers an advantage and may even offer new professional pathways to leadership not only in psychiatry but in health care as a field. Table 8–1 summarizes the benefits and barriers to teaching advocacy in a psychiatry residency training program.

TABLE 8–1. **Benefits and barriers to teaching an advocacy curriculum in a psychiatry residency training program**

Benefits	Barriers
Training in how to effect systemic change: Because the primary focus of residency training is on patient and family interactions, learning about advocacy is a rare opportunity for residents to learn how to impact health problems at a systems level.	*Lack of time:* Finding time to teach advocacy skills within an already overscheduled curriculum is difficult.
Promoting lifelong advocacy: Advocacy education during residency increases the likelihood of advocacy engagement postresidency.	*Lack of experienced faculty:* Finding faculty who have experience in practicing or teaching advocacy is difficult.
Positive ripple effects: Empowering residents with an advocacy skill set may better equip them to manage stigma, lower their risk for burnout, and train them to be future leaders in psychiatry.	*No standardized curricula:* No model or standardized evidence-based advocacy curricula currently exists; residency programs need to design their own.

Advocacy Curriculum for Psychiatry Residents

With no standardized curriculum to use as a model, a psychiatry residency training program needs to design its own advocacy curriculum (Kennedy and Vance 2018). As with any curricular effort, the development, implementation, and "buy-in" of a new advocacy curriculum work best when all stakeholders are included and when there is full transparency of process. Attention should be paid to the training program's unique culture, identity, and other qualities, including strengths and weaknesses. Regional political and geographical constraints or advantages should play a role, too: for example, if a residency training program is located within a state capital, attendance at state legislative committee hearings will be more likely than for a program sited several hours away.

When creating an advocacy curriculum for psychiatry residents, psychiatrist-educators should ensure that two components are included in the residents' educational experience:

1. *A didactic component:* Provide learner-centered presentations on ways to engage in advocacy and methods to develop and foster specialized advocacy skills. Consider inviting outside speakers, such as local journalists, community activists, and elected officials, to address learners directly about their advocacy work. Ensure ample opportunities to practice advocacy skills, such as holding mock public hearings, workshops on op-ed writing, and grassroots outreach training.
2. *An experiential component:* Depending on the level of advocacy on which residents are focused, consider taking them to visit the setting for their advocacy work. For advocacy at the community level, consider a site visit to a homeless shelter or county jail. For advocacy at the legislative level, consider holding an Advocacy Day at city hall or at the state capitol and arrange for residents to meet elected officials or watch a public hearing. "Being in the room where it happens" can help to demystify government processes and ease residents' angst about future advocacy efforts.

Core Advocacy Skills

Advocacy requires the acquisition of a set of knowledge-based skills outside of the traditional medical skill set taught during medical school and psychiatry residency. These skills are independent of the specific topic that the advocacy effort is targeting. Psychiatrist-educators should not regard themselves as content experts on issues when teaching advocacy; instead, the focus of advocacy education should be on explicating and fostering advocacy skills rather than presenting a compendium of advocacy issues. This approach recognizes that the viewpoints of those within the profession are diverse. Focusing on skill building allows psychiatrists to advocate from their own perspectives and champion the causes that resonate with them. However, it is important to keep in mind that all physician-advocates work for the ultimate benefit of the patient and not for the opportunity to express their own personal political beliefs.

Effective advocates need to learn a range of core advocacy skills. For example, advocates need to learn how to frame and communicate their advocacy issue, in both oral (e.g., an elevator speech) and written (e.g., grassroots e-mails, op-eds) forms. They need to understand the complexities of systemic issues; learn how to navigate and interface with unfamiliar processes and systems, such as state legislatures and county jails; and appreciate how to network with other stakeholder organizations. Often, advocates need to provide vision, leadership, and momentum to advocacy endeavors and accomplish these advocacy tasks with maximum flexibility and a resilient capacity to regroup after failure or loss.

These advocacy skills are, in fact, complex activities, made up of even smaller subskills. Developing and mastering these larger advocacy skills requires the following:

- The breakdown of larger advocacy skills into their smaller components or subsets
- Learning about and becoming proficient in these subsets
- Having multiple opportunities for skill rehearsal ("practice makes perfect")
- Repetition over time to maintain the skills ("use it or lose it")

An exemplary advocacy curriculum offers not only descriptions of skills but also demonstrations and opportunities to practice new advocacy skills and subskills. Learners, especially physicians, may set high self-expectations ("see one, do one, teach one") and be discouraged if they do not feel proficient after only a few efforts. Some may be reluctant to practice and will need special encouragement to engage in regular skill rehearsal. Teaching advocacy skills often requires an educator to behave as an athletic coach: to provide praise when a learner achieves a new skill and to give clear direction and specific suggestions when a learner is struggling.

Table 8–2 provides full descriptions and examples of common core advocacy skills.

Elements of an Advocacy Curriculum

When creating an advocacy curriculum, psychiatrist-educators should remember the four elements of curriculum development used in medical education: 1) goals and objectives, 2) educational methods, 3) educational materials, and 4) evaluations. These four elements can serve as a guide for developing an advocacy curriculum and help to break down what can be an overwhelming process into manageable, achievable components (Kern et al. 1998; Steinert et al. 2006).

Goals and objectives are the guiding principles of a curriculum. Although these terms are often used interchangeably in popular culture,

TABLE 8–2. **Common core advocacy skills with descriptions and illustrations**

Skill	Skill description	Example
Oral communication	Engage competently in civic discourse (e.g., present a convincing argument)	Provide clear and effective oral testimony at a state committee public hearing
Written communication	Engage competently in a variety of written forms of communication (e.g., e-mails, letters to the editor, op-eds)	Write an effective op-ed that is published in a local paper
Message framing	Use underlying moral, psychological, and cognitive factors to form convincing messaging about an issue	Create an effective message that can be used across multiple platforms
Systemic issues competency	Understand how systemic societal issues contribute to health care inequities	Recognize how erratic bus schedules contribute to missed appointments and help a patient find transportation alternatives
Legislative competency	Understand the legislative process at both local/state and federal levels	Track a bill in the state legislature and identify key inflection points (e.g., when a committee's public hearing is scheduled)
Teamwork/ flexibility	Work with others to smoothly take on and/or delegate responsibilities with flexibility and fairness	Organize a rally to educate the public about an issue
Leadership/ strategizing	Make decisions; engage in short- and long-term planning; motivate and manage others with respect	Initiate and oversee a campaign to pass a bill in the state legislature

TABLE 8–2. **Common core advocacy skills with descriptions and illustrations (continued)**

Skill	Skill description	Example
Networking/ engagement	Reach out to individuals, groups, and organizations in order to engage and forge alliances	Create an attractive and informative flier and effective social media post that draw attendees to an educational forum
Perseverance/ resilience	Possess the capacity to regroup and keep moving forward despite setbacks, disappointments, and failures	Regroup and find other funding sources following the denial of critical funding by a formerly reliable source

within the discipline of education, they have different meanings, structures, and functions (Table 8–3). Creating descriptive, action-oriented learning objectives can be challenging. Fortunately, there are tools to help. Bloom's taxonomy (Figure 8–1), a hierarchy of intellectual skills, is helpful for generating verbs for learning objectives (Arizona State University 2019). There are also innovative learning objective tools online, such as Arizona State University's Learning Objectives Builder, which guides an educator through the process of identifying the information to be taught, determining the desired level of mastery, and choosing a measurable verb (Arizona State University 2019).

Educational methods are the techniques used to impart knowledge, teach skills, and change attitudes. They can be divided into two categories: teacher centered and learner centered. These methods are based on a variety of educational theories, the specifics of which are outside the scope of this chapter. Teacher-centered methods place the educator in the active role and the learner in a passive role (Harden 1986). The classic example is the lecture. With this method, the teacher, typically an expert or an authority on the topic, controls what is taught and how it is taught. Learner-centered methods place the learners in the active role, with the educator becoming a facilitator, providing guidance, synthesizing information, and delivering feedback (Harden 1986). This is often the optimal approach to use for advocacy education, especially skill development. With this method, students customize their learning by working with educators and peers to create personal learning objectives and integrate new knowledge into their own existing frameworks (Sams and Bergmann 2010). Many learner-centered methods have

TABLE 8–3.   Differentiating goals from objectives

	Goals	Objectives
Definition[a]	"*Broad* descriptions of purposes or ends stated in *general* terms *without criteria* of achievement or mastery"	"*Specific* statements setting *measurable* expectations for what learners should *know* and be able to *do*"
Function	Create foundation for the entire curriculum	Guide evaluation, inform learners about expectations, help in choosing content and designing educational methods
Example	Residents will have an enhanced understanding of the role of a physician-advocate	After learning the content of a written testimony, residents will be able to write to a legislative committee to express their opinion on a piece of proposed legislation

[a]Definitions of goals and objectives (with emphasis added) are from the International Bureau of Education 2019.

been developed. Table 8–4 outlines a selection of methods and provides case examples for an advocacy class.

An educator does not need to choose a single method of teaching. A combination of methods can yield a rich educational experience that appeals to students with different learning styles. It may be helpful to consider the following when choosing which methods to use:

- *The target knowledge, skill, or attitude:* The common advocacy skills outlined in Table 8–2 are diverse, requiring different educational methods. For example, when teaching about the structure of a legislative body, a lecture might be most appropriate. However, the same educational method may not be effective when teaching a specific skill, such as message framing, that needs practice and feedback.
- *The educator:* An awareness of one's communication style and personality allows for modification to engage all learners.
- *The audience:* Recognition of learners' existing knowledge and cultural backgrounds allows for customization of the educational experience so it is relevant and personalized.

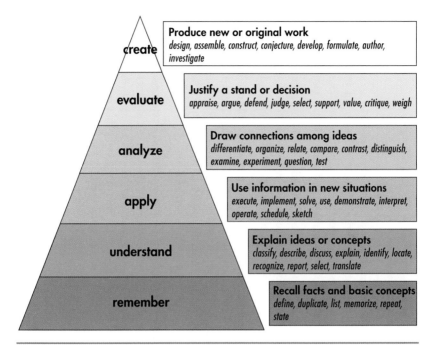

FIGURE 8–1. Bloom's taxonomy.

Source. Reprinted from Armstrong P: Bloom's Taxonomy. Nashville, TN, Vanderbilt University Center for Teaching, 2019. Available at: https://cft.vanderbilt.edu/guides-sub-pages/blooms-taxonomy. Accessed August 21, 2019. Used with permission.

- *The environment:* Despite an increasing amount of evidence supporting learner-centered methods, teacher-centered methods are still commonplace in medical education. According to Lom (2012), this is because of the following factors: 1) lectures are how most medical educators learned—we teach how we were taught; 2) lectures hold a valid place in medical education curricula, particularly if the information is not readily accessible in other formats (e.g., journals, e-books); 3) having one educator teach many students is more cost-effective than having many educators with smaller class sizes; and 4) the physical layout of schools may not be able to accommodate increased numbers of simultaneous classes.

Educational materials that are useful to integrate into an advocacy curriculum include digital aids, particularly when catering to millennial medical trainees. Audience response systems (e.g., clickers, Poll Everywhere software) allow learners to answer questions in real time, giving

TABLE 8–4. Learner-centered methods

Method	Description	Advocacy class example
Case-based learning	A relevant, complex problem is presented to students by the educator. Students learn concepts through developing potential solutions.	Students are presented with a clinical case that includes a social, economic, or political contributing factor. They break into small groups and brainstorm potential advocacy interventions. Later, the entire class comes back together, and participants share their ideas.
Flipped classroom (Ramnanan and Pound 2017)	Students engage with content at home (e.g., video, reading), then apply knowledge during class time.	Students read an opinion piece about advocacy by physicians and then participate in discussion facilitated by the educator about why and how they might incorporate advocacy into their professional work.
Community-based learning (Huntoon et al. 2012)	Students step outside of the classroom to practice skills and apply knowledge in real-world situations.	Students attend a training session that teaches skills needed when meeting with elected officials. Students choose a piece of proposed legislation and then prepare for the meeting. During the visit with the elected official, students use the techniques they have learned to effectively enlist the official's support.
Peer instruction (Serious Science 2014)	A question is posed to students, and they select an answer. Then they identify a peer who gave a different answer and meet one-on-one to explain the rationales for their responses to each other. The question is asked again, with a follow-up group discussion.	Students are given an assignment to contact their state legislator. Approximately half of the students complete the assignment. A student who completed the assignment is paired with a student who did not complete the assignment. Students discuss why they completed the assignment, what the experience was like, and what barriers existed. Students who did not complete the assignment are asked whether they think they will complete the assignment after having talked with a peer. The group then discusses the positive experiences of contacting a legislator, as well as the potential barriers they might face.

educators an opportunity to assess understanding while simultaneously bringing learners into an active role during a lecture. PowerPoint and other presentation software assist educators in communicating content visually, taking advantage of the fact that most adults are visual or visual-multimodal learners (Baykan and Naçar 2007).

Evaluations are important because advocacy curriculum development should not be a linear process but rather an iterative one, with feedback from previous curricula incorporated into future curricula. Evaluation results are used to improve the curriculum and are useful to academic departments for accreditation reviews and faculty assessments. In addition, with no standardized advocacy curricula, publications about existing curricula and their efficacy can assist other training programs in their curriculum development.

Although there are many ways to design evaluations, we find the model proposed by Gibson et al. (2008) to be particularly useful. They recommend that evaluations include the following four elements:

- *Structural components:* Evaluate the physical resources (materials, classroom, technology), as well as how the classes are structured to build a cohesive advocacy curriculum.
- *Learner experience:* Obtain students' perceptions of how the advocacy curriculum was organized and delivered.
- *Educator characteristics:* Assess the educator's level of preparation, skill and expertise in the advocacy topic, efficacy in communicating content, and enthusiasm for teaching.
- *Learner outcomes:* Give learners a pretest to assess their baseline knowledge, skills, and attitudes and a posttest to evaluate whether and how the curriculum achieved the initial objectives.

Evaluations can be completed by students, supervisors, and peers, and their responses can be collected through different modalities, such as written, online, or structured in-person feedback. (For details on evaluation instruments for these domains, as well as on designing and implementing an evaluation system, see Kogan and Shea 2007 and Schiekirka et al. 2015.)

Implementing an Advocacy Curriculum

Lao Tzu wrote, "The journey of a thousand miles begins with a single step." This perspective also applies to implementing an advocacy curriculum. The earlier discussion in this chapter about the process and content for an advocacy curriculum is intended to assist—not overwhelm.

The best advice is this: Just start. Do not be intimidated by the journey's goal, which is, ideally, a multihour, multiyear, multifaceted advocacy curriculum. Do not delay. Building the ultimate advocacy curriculum will take time and feedback and, most likely, some course corrections along the way. Take one step at a time:

Step 1: Find 1 hour, preferably somewhere early in training, either during PGY-1 or PGY-2, in which to teach an initial class in advocacy.

Step 2: Identify the teacher or teachers. Consider both residents and faculty because coteaching by residents and faculty provides a rich educational experience. Identifying a faculty member might be difficult, considering that few are likely to have advocacy experience and most programs lack an in-house expert. However, outreach to area professional advocacy organizations, such as the American Psychiatric Association's state district branch, might yield potential faculty candidates.

Step 3: During the first hour, teach advocacy basics: 1) describe the concept of advocacy by physicians, 2) provide an outline of the complex multisystem web in which patient encounters are embedded, 3) offer a brief civics lesson about how state and federal laws are passed, and 4) list the ways in which psychiatrists can advocate for their patients. If possible, place this hour following the didactic or experiential components of a curriculum focused on structural competency and/or social determinants of health.

Step 4: Keep going. Keep searching for and adding in program hours, eventually across all 4 training years. At the minimum, have at least one "reminder hour" per year to reinforce new advocacy skills and behaviors. Keep looking for additional teachers. Developing an advocacy curriculum takes time; adding incrementally may be the most practical approach. Take advantage of opportunities to workshop different methods and learn from missteps. Always make sure to offer a mechanism for constructive feedback—and then respond with substantive curriculum changes to those suggestions.

Conclusion

Psychiatrists' clinical experiences provide an advantage in developing the teaching skills needed for them to be effective educators. Like other skills learned throughout training, teaching takes practice, and the opportunities to practice are endless. We encourage all psychiatrists to include teaching about advocacy issues in their work with patients, families, and colleagues—whether by educating the general public through an op-ed or by teaching patients about the systemic issues that impact their health outcomes. We also hope that increasing numbers of psychiatry residency training programs will choose to develop an advocacy curriculum for their residents. Teaching, inspiring, and empowering advocacy in others helps to promote the well-being of patients everywhere.

Suggested Reading

Taylor DC, Hamdy H: Adult learning theories: implications for learning and teaching in medical education: AMEE Guide No. 83. Med Teach 35(11):e1561–e1572, 2013 24004029

References

Accreditation Council for Graduate Medical Education: ACGME program requirements for graduate medical education in psychiatry. Chicago, IL, Accreditation Council for Graduate Medical Education, 2019. Available at: www.acgme.org/Specialties/Program-Requirements-and-FAQs-and-Applications/pfcatid/21/Psychiatry. Accessed August 19, 2019.

Accreditation Council for Graduate Medical Education, American Board of Psychiatry and Neurology: The Psychiatry Milestone Project. Chicago, IL, Accreditation Council for Graduate Medical Education, July 2015. Available at: www.acgme.org/Portals/0/PDFs/Milestones/PsychiatryMilestones.pdf. Accessed August 19, 2019.

Ackerman SJ, Hilsenroth MJ: A review of therapist characteristics and techniques positively impacting the therapeutic alliance. Clin Psychol Rev 23(1):1–33, 2003 12559992

American Medical Association: AMA Code of Medical Ethics. Chicago, IL, American Medical Association, 2016. Available at: www.ama-assn.org/sites/ama-assn.org/files/corp/media-browser/principles-of-medical-ethics.pdf. Accessed August 19, 2019.

Arizona State University: Learning objectives builder. Tempe, Arizona State University, 2019. Available at: https://teachonline.asu.edu/objectives-builder. Accessed August 21, 2019.

Armstrong P: Bloom's taxonomy. Nashville, TN, Vanderbilt University Center for Teaching, 2019. Available at: https://cft.vanderbilt.edu/guides-sub-pages/blooms-taxonomy/. Accessed August 21, 2019.

Association of American Medical Colleges: Core Entrustable Professional Activities for Entering Residency: Curriculum Developers' Guide. Washington, DC, Association of American Medical Colleges, 2014. Available at: https://store.aamc.org/downloadable/download/sample/sample_id/63. Accessed August 21, 2019.

Baykan Z, Naçar M: Learning styles of first-year medical students attending Erciyes University in Kayseri, Turkey. Adv Physiol Educ 31(2):158–160, 2007 17562904

Beach MC, Price EG, Gary TL, et al: Cultural competence: a systematic review of health care provider educational interventions. Med Care 43(4):356–373, 2005 15778639

Catthoor K, Hutsebaut J, Schrijvers D, et al: Preliminary study of associative stigma among trainee psychiatrists in Flanders, Belgium. World J Psychiatry 4(3):62–68, 2014 25250223

Dogra N, Reitmanova S, Carter-Pokras O: Teaching cultural diversity: current status in U.K., U.S., and Canadian medical schools. J Gen Intern Med 25(2)(suppl 2):S164–S168, 2010 20352513

Gibson KA, Boyle P, Black DA, et al: Enhancing evaluation in an undergraduate medical education program. Acad Med 83(8):787–793, 2008 18667897

Gruen RL, Campbell EG, Blumenthal D: Public roles of U.S. physicians: community participation, political involvement, and collective advocacy. JAMA 296(20):2467–2475, 2006 17119143

Harden RM: Approaches to curriculum planning. Med Educ 20(5):458–466, 1986 3531778

Huntoon KM, McCluney CJ, Wiley EA, et al: Self-reported evaluation of competencies and attitudes by physicians-in-training before and after a single day legislative advocacy experience. BMC Med Educ 12(1):47, 2012 22726361

International Bureau of Education: Glossary of curriculum terminology. Geneva, Switzerland, International Bureau of Education, 2019. Available at: www.ibe.unesco.org/en/glossary-curriculum-terminology. Accessed August 21, 2019.

Kennedy KG, Vance M: Advocacy Teaching in Psychiatry Residency Training Programs. APA Resource Document. Washington, DC, American Psychiatric Association, 2018. Available at: www.psychiatry.org/psychiatrists/search-directories-databases/library-and-archive/resource-documents. Accessed August 21, 2019.

Kern DE, Thomas PA, Hughes MT, et al: Curriculum Development for Medical Education: A Six-Step Approach. Baltimore, Johns Hopkins University Press, 1998. Available at: https://books.google.com/books?id=0SOHCm CNIvYC&lpg=PA1&dq=kern&lr&pg=PP1#v=onepage&q=kern&f=false. Accessed August 21, 2019.

Kogan JR, Shea JA: Course evaluation in medical education. Teaching and Teacher Education 23(3):251–264, 2007

Leal-Costa C, Díaz-Agea JL, Tirado-González S, et al: Communication skills: a preventive factor in burnout syndrome in health professionals [in Spanish]. An Sist Sanit Navar 38(2):213–223, 2015 26486527

Lom B: Classroom activities: simple strategies to incorporate student-centered activities within undergraduate science lectures. J Undergrad Neurosci Educ 11(1):A64–A71, 2012 23494568

Minkovitz CS, Goldshore M, Solomon BS, et al; Community Pediatrics Training Initiative Workgroup: Five-year follow-up of Community Pediatrics Training Initiative. Pediatrics 134(1):83–90, 2014 24982098

Möller-Leimkühler AM, Möller HJ, Maier W, et al: EPA guidance on improving the image of psychiatry. Eur Arch Psychiatry Clin Neurosci 266(2):139–154, 2016 26874959

Ramnanan CJ, Pound LD: Advances in medical education and practice: student perceptions of the flipped classroom. Adv Med Educ Pract 8(8):63–73, 2017 28144171

Sams A, Bergmann J: The flipped classroom (video). YouTube, December 6, 2010. Available at: www.youtube.com/watch?v=2H4RkudFzlc. Accessed August 21, 2019.

Schiekirka S, Feufel MA, Herrmann-Lingen C, et al: Evaluation in medical education: a topical review of target parameters, data collection tools, and confounding factors. Ger Med Sci 13:Doc15, 2015 26421003

Searle NS, Hatem CJ, Perkowski L, et al: Why invest in an educational fellowship program? Acad Med 81(11):936–940, 2006 17065850

Serious Science: Peer instruction for active learning—Eric Mazur (video). YouTube, June 18, 2014. Available at: www.youtube.com/watch?v=Z9orbxoRofI. Accessed August 21, 2019.

Stein S: Beyond cadavers: med students learn how to dissect health policy. Bloomberg Law, February 4, 2019. Available at: https://news.bloomberg law.com/health-law-and-business/beyond-cadavers-med-students-learn-to-dissect-health-policy. Accessed August 21, 2019.

Steinert Y, Mann K, Centeno A, et al: A systematic review of faculty development initiatives designed to improve teaching effectiveness in medical education: BEME Guide No. 8. Med Teach 28(6):497–526, 2006 17074699

Sutkin G, Wagner E, Harris I, et al: What makes a good clinical teacher in medicine? A review of the literature. Acad Med 83(5):452–466, 2008 17074699

Verhaeghe M, Bracke P: Associative stigma among mental health professionals: implications for professional and service user well-being. J Health Soc Behav 53(1):17–32, 2012 22382718

Wasser T, Ross DA: Another step forward: a novel approach to the clinician-educator track for residents. Acad Psychiatry 40(6):937–943, 2016 27558628

9

Research as Advocacy

Stephanie V. Hall, M.P.H.
Jennifer Kononowech, L.M.S.W.
Andrew J. Gerber, M.D., Ph.D.
Steven J. Ackerman, Ph.D.
Kara Zivin, Ph.D., M.S., M.A.

Learning Objectives

By the end of this chapter, readers will be able to:

- Describe the differences between research and advocacy
- Define evidence-based policy and how it relates to research as advocacy
- Identify key factors that influence policy
- Explain several barriers to evidence-based policies, as well as strategies for mitigating those barriers
- Outline examples of research as advocacy in each stage of translational research
- Discuss the importance of funders and their influence on research and policy

Differences Between Research and Advocacy

Research aims to generate new knowledge. Researchers may envision themselves as neutral and unbiased actors in a quest for answers to scientific questions; however, when taken too far, this impartiality can limit the application of new evidence by creating and maintaining research silos. Advocacy, on the other hand, requires championing a particular cause rather than remaining impartial. To use research as advocacy, researchers and research consumers (defined in this chapter as individuals with close ties to the scientific community who read, interpret, evaluate, use, and/or publicize research findings), including psychiatrists, must find ways to apply their independent and objective scientific conclusions to potentially controversial topics, while working with limited time, capacity, and resources. Furthermore, the choice of research topic in and of itself could be considered an expression of advocacy for that topic; stated another way, by choosing to conduct research on a particular topic, the scientist is advocating for that topic to be researched and considered by the wider world.

Ultimately, how new evidence is or is not used lies outside the realm of research. Therefore, using research as advocacy requires translating scientific data into actionable knowledge so that the rest of society may act on the best available information. Evidence-based policies (EBPs) are generated using evidence from research to guide policy making. In this chapter, we explore common resources, strategies, and barriers to applying research to policy decisions and discuss several examples of how psychiatrists and mental health service researchers are using research as advocacy.

In general, research applies the scientific method. Scientists ask a question, generate a hypothesis, and test the hypothesis. On the basis of their findings, they either reject or fail to reject that hypothesis. Then, they might refine the question or the approach to addressing it before asking another question, ultimately beginning the cycle over again. Thus, the well-established scientific method outlines how to conduct scientific research; however, it does not establish how findings should be applied in the real world.

A central reason that research fails to translate to external fields is because of ideological and communication barriers. Academia, a major source of research, is deemed the "ivory tower" because it is more isolated from than connected to individuals outside of the scientific community. Research careers are driven by publication in journals that members of the public, including policy makers, do not read. Policy and decision makers have a difficult time consuming and applying research because there are major disconnects between how research findings are communicated and evaluated by the scientific community versus in the outside world (Table 9–1) and because implementing research can lead to both intended and unintended consequences.

TABLE 9–1. **Differences between research and advocacy**

	Research	Advocacy
Language	Unique syntax, diction, and connotations	Succinct, persuasive, declarative
	Complex, verbose	Focuses on "so what"
	Uses jargon and minutiae	
	Focuses on "who, what, when, where, why"	
	Growing number of dense, lengthy, and numerous articles (Bornmann and Mutz 2015)	
Evidence	Hedges and curtails conclusions, which can lead others to minimize the findings	Concise, impassioned
		Uses compelling anecdote or narrative over dry scientific evidence
	Cautious, precise	Considers emotion, personal connection, and intuition
Purpose	Explore unknown ideas, drill down to details, and pursue knowledge for the sake of knowledge	Have the biggest impact using the fewest available resources

Research as Advocacy: Evidence-Based Policy

The history of evidence-based medicine and EBP offers a good example of how to shift research into practice. In the last half of the twentieth century, the medical community noted inconsistencies between scientific conclusions and common medical practices. In response to this, Scottish physician and epidemiologist Archie Cochrane championed evidence-based medicine—the explicit use of the best available evidence in medical decision making (Stavrou et al. 2014). Evidence-based medicine became a guiding principle of how to apply research to medicine. Government officials in the United Kingdom took note of Cochrane's success and began exploring how to apply the principles of evidence-based medicine to policy as well.

EBP, the practice of using the best available scientific evidence to guide policy decisions, answers the question of how to use research as advocacy by offering a direct path from research to application. Under EBP, researchers may remain neutral, unbiased, and true to their experimental results as they work with policy makers to translate their findings into action. Ultimately, EBP offers a roadmap for how research consumers can apply the information generated by researchers in real-world settings.

Although EBP marries research and advocacy in an effective and efficient partnership, EBP is not routinely practiced. In *Show Me the Evidence: Obama's Fight for Rigor and Results in Social Policy* (Haskins and Margolis 2014), Ron Haskins and Greg Margolis reviewed the factors that influence legislation in the United States. They found that although the U.S. federal government spends $83 billion annually on research (American Association for the Advancement of Science 2019), research influences only 1% of policy. In other words, even with tremendous financial backing, research findings rarely get implemented, and research is rarely used to support advocacy efforts. These disconnects culminate in an isolated scientific community and limit the extent to which research consumers can translate research into action at scale.

Strategies for Using Research as Advocacy

Even if research influences only 1% of policy, studying the other factors that influence policy reveals opportunities to impact the other 99% of influence. By using research to sway the factors that influence 99% of policy, research can still indirectly affect large-scale policy changes. In this section, we review the other factors that influence policy and offer some suggestions for how researchers and consumers of research can use research as advocacy in these contexts.

Policy Makers

Influencer: Policy makers (49%)
Congressional agencies (5%), committees (8%), committee chairs (7%), committee staff (5%), congressional staff (5%), the administration (11%), political parties (8%) (from Haskins and Margolis 2014)
Ways for researchers and research consumers to have an influence: Contact legislators directly; contact your organization's office of government relations or government affairs for help with establishing a relationship with a legislator

Legislators have the largest impact on policy, with roughly 49% of policy influence coming from legislators (Haskins and Margolis 2014). To successfully reach legislators, researchers and research consumers must remain cognizant of the differences in communication identified in Table 9–1 and use channels to reach outside the scientific community. One of the best ways to do this is by contacting legislators directly to establish relationships and present evidence-based legislative "asks," such as discussing ways to change Medicaid or Medicare coverage to better reflect evidence-based population needs or how to set aside funding for public health interventions aimed at raising awareness regarding how to seek treatment or resources for substance use disorder. Although this may seem like a daunting task, many universities have an office of government affairs or government relations, and other nonacademic and professional organizations (e.g., the American Psychiatric Association) may have departments or subgroups that coordinate responses to and evaluation of policy. These offices are staffed with professionals who can guide researchers and consumers of research in forming and maintaining relationships with policy makers at the local, state, and federal levels. For more information on how to advocate effectively at the legislative level, see Chapter 7, "Legislative Advocacy."

General Population

> **Influencer: General population (22%)**
>
> The public (16%), media (6%) (from Haskins and Margolis 2014)
>
> Ways for researchers and research consumers to have an influence: Use social media to communicate research findings to the public; contact your organization's office of public affairs or public relations for help with engaging the public or media

Although legislators are responsible for writing policy, they and other elected officials will respond to the tide of public opinion. In addition to exercising their responsibility to represent their constituents, most elected officials are motivated for reelection and therefore pay attention to the optics and polling around policy issues. The general population, including the public and media, influence 22% of policy.

Sharing research with the public is a direct way to use research as advocacy. Communicating with the public can raise awareness, promote a cause, and generate support for a research agenda. Most academic and professional organizations have an Office of Public Affairs or Public Relations that can issue press releases, arrange media correspondence, and share research with the general public. Additionally, with the advent of social media, researchers and research consumers are able to communicate directly with the public through forums such as Twitter, Facebook, and even Instagram. Maintaining this type of public presence and engaging with the general population allows both researchers and research consumers to generate support for their causes. This support may ultimately affect legislators and result in policy changes. For more information on these and additional ways to engage the public and media as a form of advocacy, see Chapter 10, "Engaging the Popular Media."

Political Organizations

Influencer: Political organizations (20%)
Lobby groups (6%), policy continents (14%) (from Haskins and Margolis 2014)
Ways for researchers and research consumers to have an influence: Partner directly with lobbyists, trade organizations, or industry

Lobbyists are professional advocates who are paid to represent their clients' organizations, interests, or causes. Researchers and research consumers can form alliances and partnerships directly with lobbyists, trade organizations, and companies that share common goals with them. By providing research findings to these entities, researchers and research consumers provide the evidence that lobbyists use to formulate, argue for, and advance policy. These relationships, like relationships with legislators, take time to build, but once researchers and consumers of research gain trust and respect, they can use these partnerships to fast-track their findings from theory to action.

Policy continents are highly interrelated groupings of the forces that drive policy from a legislative or regulatory perspective, including committees, groups, and any faction with power over the policy process. Haskins and Margolis (2014) define policy continents as the complex set of statutes, regulations, lobbying groups, congressional factions, committees of jurisdiction, and so forth that affect legislation in each area of social policy.

Finances

> ### Influencer: Finances (8%)
>
> Budget (8%) (from Haskins and Margolis 2014)
>
> Ways for researchers and research consumers to have an influence: Include economic analyses in research; implement evidence-based practices in cost-effective ways

Financial constraints are a reality for any form of advocacy. Researchers have minimal ability to alter the amount of money available for a particular solution. However, by considering cost and cost analyses in their research, they are more likely to provide evidence for the affordability of their causes. There is also an opportunity for research consumers to design and initiate creative solutions to implement evidence-based practices in cost-effective ways that researchers might not yet have considered.

Research

> ### Influencer: Research (1%)
>
> Research (1%) (from Haskins and Margolis 2014)
>
> Ways for researchers to have an influence: Ask the right questions; communicate clearly

Finally, research itself has the smallest effect on policy. Translating research to advocacy requires a concerted effort. Researchers and research consumers must intentionally communicate to the public in language that is accessible, persuasive, and actionable. They must build bridges and relationships to government, industry, and the media. Additionally, if researchers want to influence policy, they need to focus their research on addressing real-world problems and identifying real-world solutions, with the ultimate goal of using their research as advocacy.

Examples of Psychiatric Research Advocacy

Adopting recommendations from the Institute of Medicine, the National Center for Advancing Translational Sciences defines the translational science classification system as "the process of turning observations in the laboratory, clinic and community into interventions that improve the health of individuals and the public—from diagnostics and therapeutics to medical procedures and behavioral changes" (quoted by University of Wisconsin-Madison Institute for Clinical and Translational Research 2018). In this context, we highlight four examples of research advocacy from each level of translational research, as applied to psychiatry: T1, translation to humans; T2, translation to patients; T3, translation to practice; and T4, translation to population health (Figure 9–1). Together, these examples illustrate a diverse collection of approaches to using psychiatric research as advocacy.

T1: Translation to Humans— Example: Neuroimaging Research

Historically in mental health, and particularly with the advent of new technologies, the translation of basic science to human applications (T1 translation) has been the most challenging aspect of applying research to advocacy. Neuroimaging provides a powerful example not only of the opportunity that exists in making such a link but also of the challenge in producing experimental findings that are relevant to understanding and treating a complex human condition. For example, in the first years of the twenty-first century, prominent mental health leaders, such as those involved in the publication of DSM-IV and DSM-IV-TR (American Psychiatric Association 1994, 2000) and in funding the National Institute of Mental Health (NIMH), predicted that within the next 10 years, the field would identify biomarkers, including neuroimaging biomarkers, that would aid significantly in clinical diagnosis and treatment planning (Kupfer et al. 2002). However, 10 years later, the president-elect of the American Psychiatric Association and director of NIMH issued a joint statement acknowledging that although research had advanced (particularly as manifested in the new research domain criteria), DSM-5 (American Psychiatric Association 2013) would not include such criteria because they were not yet clinically actionable (Psychiatric News 2013).

Even though neuroimaging findings remain more experimental than clinically actionable, there is ample evidence that images contain the

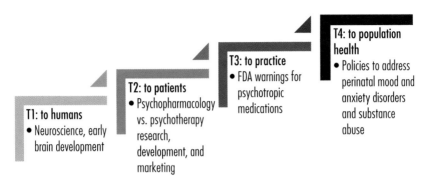

FIGURE 9–1. Translating research into advocacy: psychiatric case examples.

power to profoundly impact readers, including scientists and policy makers. Studies have shown that undergraduates rate articles with brain images higher in scientific reasoning than otherwise equivalent articles with other types of visual depiction of results (McCabe and Castel 2008). With the proliferation of neuroimaging research and technology, it is now common for mental health professionals to include at least one slide of brain structural or functional magnetic resonance imaging when presenting information about psychiatric illness to lay or professional audiences. This practice has spread to presentations by non-neuroscientists who are seeking to emphasize the "reality" of the phenomena they are trying to describe (Gerber and Gonzalez 2013). Using neuroimaging findings in this way is an example of applying research to advocacy by displaying research images to inform and influence public opinion.

Projecting into the future of neuroimaging research, we are rapidly moving in the direction of using neuroimaging to 1) diagnose and characterize mental illness; 2) identify and quantify changes in response to treatment; and 3) better understand the complex interaction between mental mechanisms and the content of mental representations, particularly as they relate to environmental experiences (Friston et al. 2017). Billions of dollars of funding, translated into hundreds of thousands of published articles, have led to an intricate web of understood relationships between brain imaging findings and psychiatric diagnoses. The projected goal for DSM-5 is now much closer to reality: it has already become clinically routine to order neuroimaging to explore possible underlying pathophysiology in first diagnoses of autism, and this use is sure to spread to other initial diagnoses in the coming years (Hampton 2017).

From the advocacy perspective, this continuing increase in neuroimaging knowledge will translate into more opportunities to use neuroimaging research as advocacy. The public, media, advocacy organizations, and policy makers all long for clarification in these areas and have already demonstrated their hunger for graphical, concrete representations of the neuroscience of mental health. It is likely that new T1 research neuroimaging findings, when used in advocacy efforts, will both satisfy this hunger and lead to more interest in this area because the results have direct implications for policy. Following this blueprint, other T1 research endeavors are also capable of influencing policy and public opinion if they are skillfully combined with advocacy messaging.

T2: Translation to Patients— Example: Psychotherapy Research

Critics assert that scientists do a poor job of translating complex social problems, including many mental health issues, to patients. Similarly, some policy makers have a distorted understanding of mental health issues, which has led to instances of misguided recommendations in federal, state, and local government. Research in general, and psychotherapy research specifically, have lacked effective ways to inform the public about many important findings. For example, even the simple notion that psychotherapy works and is cost-effective is not widely known or accepted (Leichsenring et al. 2015). It is likely that improved methods of integrating research with advocacy could bring these important findings to the attention of policy makers.

The Consumer Reports (CR) Study was a pioneering research effort and one of the most extensive attempts to hear from and share with the public their views and experiences of psychiatric treatment as it occurred in a real-world setting (Seligman 1995). The methodology included having *Consumer Reports* magazine build into its 1994 annual questionnaire a supplemental survey about psychotherapy and psychoactive medications (Seligman 1995). Approximately 7,000 subscribers responded to the supplemental survey, and more than 4,000 of them said they had sought treatment from a mental health professional, family doctor, or support group. The items in the survey represented three subscales: specific improvement, satisfaction, and global improvement. There were several unambiguous findings from this study, including that psychotherapy with a mental health provider usually helped respondents feel better. Across all types of mental health providers, of the patients who were feeling "very poor" when they started psychotherapy, 87% were feeling "so-so" to "very good" when they completed the survey (Seligman 1995).

The finding that psychotherapy works for most of the people who seek it out is one of the more important and possibly most publicly influential findings from the CR Study. Another, maybe equally important, finding supported the "dodo bird" hypothesis, named after the Dodo Bird who refereed an untimed race and declared all participants winners in Lewis Carroll's *Alice in Wonderland*—that is, the foundational idea that all forms of psychotherapy are relatively equal in effectiveness (Luborsky et al. 1975). In the CR Study, no specific form of psychotherapy had better outcomes for any specific problem. More recent research by Gerber and colleagues (Gerber et al. 2011; Thoma et al. 2012) found that psychodynamic psychotherapy and cognitive-behavioral therapy work as well as other forms of psychotherapy, findings that support the CR Study results. An additional finding of the CR Study was that individuals who chose their own therapist and stayed in therapy longer (more than 6 months) reported more improvement than did individuals who were required to attend treatment, who were assigned a therapist because of issues such as insurance restrictions, and/or who stayed in therapy for a shorter period of time (less than 6 months).

The CR Study represents one of the best scientific advocacy efforts to date in that it attempted to translate a complex social problem, mental health, into understandable terms for a large public audience. Studies like this one have a high potential to influence public opinion and policy decisions about treatment, as well as the ways in which future research may be conducted. However, a limitation of the CR Study is that although its findings were disseminated to a large public audience, the researchers failed to broadcast their results directly to policy makers. Consequently, the results did not influence a number of important policy issues, such as insurance practices or parity laws. Therefore, an advocacy lesson learned from the CR Study is that to influence policy and legislation, future studies should be designed in a methodologically sound way not only to extend the public's appreciation of the value of research but also to disseminate research in such a way that helps policy makers contextualize or relate the research findings to legislative action so that they may use the findings to ultimately shape future policy.

T3: Translation to Practice— Example: FDA Warnings for Psychotropic Medications

The knowledge gained from T3 research includes how interventions work in real-world settings. As one example of this type of research, FDA warnings for psychotropic medications can influence both prescribing behaviors and patient outcomes, such as occurred with citalopram. Prior the FDA warning, citalopram was widely regarded as a first-line agent for depression treatment because of its minimal drug interactions, demonstrated safety in older and medically ill patients, low cost, and relative effectiveness (Trivedi et al. 2006). In 2011 and 2012, the FDA warned about potential abnormal heart rhythms for patients using this medication and recommended against prescribing citalopram at dosages above 40 mg/day, or above 20 mg/day for older adults (U.S. Food and Drug Administration 2012). A subsequent large-scale study of nearly 1 million patients, however, found no dose-dependent risk of ventricular arrhythmia or mortality associated with citalopram use (Zivin et al. 2013). This study led researchers and clinicians to question the value of the warnings, as well as to consider the need to balance the risks and benefits of modifying clinical practice in response to FDA warnings (Zivin et al. 2014).

Despite these findings, the citalopram warnings influenced subsequent prescribing patterns. High-dose citalopram use declined after the 2011–2012 FDA warnings, although roughly one-third of older adults remained on higher than recommended dosages. Concomitant increases in sertraline and other antidepressant prescriptions suggested potential substitution of these medications for citalopram (Gerlach et al. 2018). However, the reduction of prescribed citalopram dosages to the new safety limits was associated with a higher rate of hospitalization in a large patient population that had been treated with substantially higher dosages. Therefore, stipulating a safety limit for citalopram dosages before the benefits and risks of doing so were firmly established appears to have had unintended adverse clinical consequences (Rector et al. 2016).

Although research did not reverse the course of the FDA warnings for citalopram, other examples show that it is possible to influence policy through research, even in the context of FDA warnings. For instance, the FDA placed a black box warning on varenicline (marketed as Chantix) in 2009 because of a potential risk for changes in behavior such as hostility, agitation, depressed mood, and suicidal thoughts or actions. (Black box warnings are the most serious type of warnings mandated by the FDA and are used to call attention to serious or life-threatening risks.) However, after new research data emerged that did not show a clear link between the drug and these reported side effects, the FDA reversed this warning in 2016 (Grover 2016; U.S. Food and Drug Administration 2016).

Research can be used to advocate both for and against policy changes, such as FDA warnings. In these two cases, as in other evaluations of FDA warnings, research can be viewed as a tool to support or refute a policy. Researchers who are concerned about the intended and unintended consequences of policies for patient health and well-being may be able to influence policy decisions by directing their research to answer these types of policy-relevant questions.

T4: Translation to Population Health— Example: Screening and Treatment for Perinatal Mood and Anxiety Disorders

Researchers and research consumers can also influence policy makers to adopt policies and legislation to improve population health. One way they can do this is by raising awareness of research findings through professional organizations, which have the ability to amass relevant scientific data on a particular topic and use this information to adopt official positions on the topic. These positions can then go on to influence policy makers.

For example, evidence has been mounting to support broad-based and systematic screening and treatment for perinatal mood and anxiety disorders (Kendig et al. 2017). This evidence base led the American Academy of Pediatrics (Earls 2010), the American Medical Association (2012), and the American College of Obstetricians and Gynecologists (2015) to recommend and promote such screening and treatment. Following the lead of these organizations, in 2016 the U.S. Preventive Services Task Force recommended screening for perinatal depression (O'Connor et al. 2016), which must be covered under the Patient Protection and Affordable Care Act of 2010 (P.L. 111-148). Finally, the Centers for Medicare and Medicaid Services issued policy guidance in 2016 to clarify that state Medicaid agencies may cover maternal depression screening, which is considered risk assessment for the child, as part of the early and periodic screening, diagnostic, and treatment benefit in Medicaid (Wachino 2016).

In these examples, researchers and research consumers working through professional societies were able to effect large-scale policy changes, which are likely to have an important impact on access to care and quality of care for women who struggle with perinatal mood and anxiety disorders. To complete the feedback loop, after these new policies are implemented, researchers can next examine how variations in state policies, as well as uptake of policy recommendations, influence patient outcomes, which can then further inform policy refinement to continue to improve public health for this population.

Barriers to Using Research as Advocacy and Proposed Solutions

The barriers to using research as advocacy are large in size and many in number (Table 9–2). These barriers may feel insurmountable, but as the examples described in the previous section have shown, researchers and research consumers can nevertheless find impactful ways to influence and evaluate policy. Moreover, numerous training programs have emerged to help researchers better explain their work to public audiences and to help public representatives be better interpreters of science. For example, the American Association for the Advancement of Science (2009) has developed programs to train early career scientists to translate research findings to public audiences and to understand the role of media in disseminating results in a way that can influence policy makers. National meetings of major professional organizations such as the American Psychiatric Association, the American Psychological Association, the American Academy of Child and Adolescent Psychiatry, and even the American Psychoanalytic Association (a group not historically known for its support of empirical research) now include programs for members interested in bringing research findings to the attention of the public, the media, and government officials in order to influence policy. Programs such as these are helping researchers and research consumers learn how to read the political winds, talk in a way that resonates with policy makers, and better understand the complex interactions between the political landscape, policy change, and research findings.

Many of the barriers described in Table 9–2 also stem from and perpetuate a culture of research that at best does not prioritize advocacy and at worst openly condescends to it as being beneath the dignity and objectivity of the focused scientist. Culture change is more complicated than a change in resources, but in the long run it is just as influential. If opinion leaders in academia, science, and nationally respected research and professional organizations indicate an interest in research as advocacy, current and future scientists may decide to tackle these formidable barriers and measure success not only in what they have learned but also in how much they have taught, communicated to, and influenced others. Although training and organization-based educational programs are beginning to systematically target many of the barriers to using research as advocacy, much more could be done, particularly by traditional academic departments, institutions of public policy, and major research funding sources. Table 9–3 provides some suggested approaches.

TABLE 9–2. **Barriers to using research as advocacy**

Barrier	Examples
Shortage of time and effort	Busy schedules make it difficult to find time to meet with legislators, prepare for interviews, or generate a social media presence
Alternative incentives	Academia rewards publications and grants, not advocacy, when awarding tenure
Legislator bandwidth	One or two legislative staffers handle all health issues, and there are many other pressing issues vying for attention
Public and media attention span	The rapid news cycle creates competition for public interest
Lack of funding and resources	National Institutes of Health budgets remain flat despite need for greater research funding

TABLE 9–3. **Suggestions to increase the use of research as advocacy**

Barrier	Proposed solution
Shortage of time and effort	Academic departments protect time for training in and use of research in advocacy and provide salary support and seed funding for these efforts
Alternative incentives	Academic departments create pathways for advancement such that advocacy is given status equal to that of publications and traditional research grants
Legislator bandwidth	Major institutions in academia and public policy create public campaigns to pressure legislators to devote the time and effort needed to understand and use research, perhaps by offering free or reduced-cost consultation in these areas
Public and media attention span	Researchers and research consumers prioritize developing ways to stay "in the news" through regular updates, clear and timely responses to public issues, and skillful use of media to compete with other sources
Lack of funding and resources	Major private and public funding sources increase funding for the use of research in advocacy

Role of Funding Sources

Despite the best of intentions of the vast majority in the research/academic complex, financial resources constitute the largest influence on the direction of research and its potential for advocacy. Therefore, the role of funding sources in influencing research as advocacy deserves special mention in this chapter. In 2016, RAND Europe published the results of Project Ecosystem, a mapping of the global mental health research funding system (Pollitt et al. 2016). Using the metric of number of research papers published between 2009 and 2014, this study showed that the U.S. government accounts for at least 39% of research funding worldwide. The top 10 funders are listed in Table 9–4.

The dominance of the U.S. government in funding research efforts means that its priorities significantly influence the careers and focus of researchers, as well as the direction and priorities of academic departments. Therefore, the most impactful way to increase the use of research as advocacy would be for U.S. government agencies to increase their support in this area. Influential voices in academia and policy can lead the way by talking with the leaders of government agencies about these issues. In addition, there are also many smaller, nongovernment charities and foundations that support mental health research and advocacy, some of which are listed in Table 9–5. However, given that their resources are more limited than those of the federal government, they often prioritize seed funding of work that will ultimately garner federal support. Thus, their resources end up supporting the same priorities as those of the federal government rather than branching out in new areas. Nongovernment charities could prioritize more funding of research as advocacy as a way to correct some of this imbalance.

Conclusion

In this chapter, we have outlined the significant challenges that researchers and research consumers face when attempting to reach and influence a broad audience such as policy makers, patients, and the general public, as well as some examples of and strategies for overcoming these challenges. As noted, most of the research community is embedded in academia, a situation that creates inherent barriers between the research being conducted and consumed and the application of that research by those in a position to effect large-scale societal change. Researchers are burdened by the competitive pressures of working in academia that make exporting study results to the general public secondary to publishing in academic journals and ob-

TABLE 9–4. **Global funders most frequently acknowledged in published papers**

Funder	Location	Number of papers published	Proportion of all papers
1. National Institutes of Health (NIH)	United States	16,716	15%
2. National Institute of Mental Health (NIMH)	United States	10,081	9%
3. National Institute on Drug Abuse (NIDA)	United States	6,231	6%
4. National Institute on Aging (NIA)	United States	5,266	5%
5. Canadian Institutes of Health Research (CIHR)	Canada	4,701	4%
6. Department of Veterans Affairs (VA)	United States	4,387	4%
7. National Health and Medical Research Council of Australia (NIHMRC)	Australia	4,033	4%
8. European Commission	European Union	4,021	4%
9. National Natural Science Foundation of China (NSFC)	China	3,836	3%
10. Medical Research Council (MRC)	United Kingdom	3,503	3%

Source. Adapted from Pollitt et al. 2016.

taining funding sources. Up to this point, limited effort has been made in the United States to develop a partnership between science and those in a position to influence public awareness. However, as more researchers, research consumers, academic departments, professional organizations, institutions of public policy, and funding sources realize the importance and impact of using research as advocacy, more opportunities will likely become available to build partnerships between research and advocacy to promote policy change.

TABLE 9–5. **Examples of Nongovernment Mental Health Charities and Organizations**

Active Minds

American Foundation for Suicide Prevention

Anxiety and Depression Association of America

Autism Speaks

Brain and Behavior Research Foundation

Dalio Philanthropies

Dana Foundation

Depression and Bipolar Support Alliance

Irving Harris Foundation

Jed Foundation

Klingenstein Third Generation Foundation

Mental Health America

National Alliance on Mental Illness

National Coalition for Mental Health Recovery

National Council for Behavioral Health

Project Semicolon

Robert Wood Johnson Foundation

Simons Foundation

Stanley Medical Research Institute

Treatment Advocacy Center

Trevor Project

William T. Grant Foundation

References

American Association for the Advancement of Science: Science and policy resources. Washington, DC, American Association for the Advancement of Science, 2009. Available at: www.aaas.org/programs/science-technology-policy-fellowships/fellowship-resources. Accessed August 21, 2019.

American Association for the Advancement of Science: Historical trends in federal R&D. Washington, DC, American Association for the Advancement of Science, 2019. Available at: www.aaas.org/programs/r-d-budget-and-policy/historical-trends-federal-rd. Accessed August 21, 2019.

American College of Obstetricians and Gynecologists: ACOG committee opinion: screening for perinatal depression. Washington, DC, American College of Obstetricians and Gynecologists, May 2015. Available at: www.acog.org/Clinical-Guidance-and-Publications/Committee-Opinions/Committee-on-Obstetric-Practice/Screening-for-Perinatal-Depression?IsMobileSet=false. Accessed August 21, 2019.

American Medical Association: Improving mental health services for pregnant and postpartum mothers, policy H-420.953. Proceedings of the 2012 Annual Meeting of the American Medical Association House of Delegates, November 11, 2012. Available at: www.ama-assn.org/sites/ama-assn.org/files/corp/media-browser/public/hod/a12-resolutions_0.pdf. Accessed August 21, 2019.

American Psychiatric Association: Diagnostic and Statistical Manual of Mental Disorders, 4th Edition. Washington, DC, American Psychiatric Association, 1994

American Psychiatric Association: Diagnostic and Statistical Manual of Mental Disorders, 4th Edition, Text Revision. Washington, DC, American Psychiatric Association, 2000

American Psychiatric Association: Diagnostic and Statistical Manual of Mental Disorders, 5th Edition. Washington, DC, American Psychiatric Association, 2013

Bornmann L, Mutz R: Growth rates of modern science: a bibliometric analysis based on the number of publications and cited references. J Assoc Inf Sci Technol 66(11):2215–2222, 2015

Earls MF; Committee on Psychosocial Aspects of Child and Family Health American Academy of Pediatrics: Incorporating recognition and management of perinatal and postpartum depression into pediatric practice. Pediatrics 126(5):1032–1039, 2010 20974776

Friston KJ, Redish AD, Gordon JA: Computational nosology and precision psychiatry. Comput Psychiatr 1:2–23, 2017 29400354

Gerber AJ, Gonzalez MZ: Structural and functional brain imaging in clinical psychology, in The Oxford Handbook of Research Strategies for Clinical Psychology. Edited by Comer JS, Kendall PC. New York, Oxford University Press, 2013, pp 165–187

Gerber AJ, Kocsis JH, Milrod BL, et al: A quality-based review of randomized controlled trials of psychodynamic psychotherapy. Am J Psychiatry 168(1):19–28, 2011 20843868

Gerlach LB, Stano C, Yosef M, et al: Assessing responsiveness of health systems to drug safety warnings. Am J Geriatr Psychiatry 26(4):476–483, 2018 29066038

Grover N: FDA drops black box warning on Pfizer's anti-smoking drug. Reuters, December 16, 2016. Available at: www.reuters.com/article/us-pfizer-fda/fda-drops-black-box-warning-on-pfizers-anti-smoking-drug-idUSKBN1452JJ. Accessed August 22, 2019.

Hampton T: Early brain imaging in infants may help predict autism. JAMA 318(13):1211–1212, 2017 28973228

Haskins R, Margolis G: Show Me the Evidence: Obama's Fight for Rigor and Results in Social Policy. Washington, DC, Brookings Institution Press, 2014

Kendig S, Keats JP, Hoffman MC, et al: Consensus bundle on maternal mental health: perinatal depression and anxiety. J Obstet Gynecol Neonatal Nurs 46(2):272–281, 2017 28190757

Kupfer DJ, First MB, Regier DA: A Research Agenda for DSM-V. Washington, DC, American Psychiatric Association, 2002

Leichsenring F, Luyten P, Hilsenroth MJ, et al: Psychodynamic therapy meets evidence-based medicine: a systematic review using updated criteria. Lancet Psychiatry 2(7):648–660, 2015 26303562

Luborsky L, Singer B, Luborsky L: Comparative studies of psychotherapies. Is it true that "everyone has won and all must have prizes"? Arch Gen Psychiatry 32(8):995–1008, 1975 239666

McCabe DP, Castel AD: Seeing is believing: the effect of brain images on judgments of scientific reasoning. Cognition 107(1):343–352, 2008 17803985

O'Connor E, Rossom RC, Henninger M, et al: Primary care screening for and treatment of depression in pregnant and postpartum women: evidence report and systematic review for the U.S. Preventive Services Task Force. JAMA 315(4):388–406, 2016 26813212

Pollitt A, Cochrane G, Kirtley A, et al: Project ecosystem: mapping the global mental health research funding system. RAND Corporation, 2016. Available at: https://www.rand.org/pubs/research_reports/RR1271.html. Accessed August 22, 2019.

Psychiatric News: Lieberman, Insel issue joint statement about DSM-5 and RDoC. Psychiatric News, May 14, 2013. Available at: http://alert.psychnews.org/2013/05/lieberman-insel-issue-joint-statement.html. Accessed August 22, 2019.

Rector TS, Adabag S, Cunningham F, et al: Outcomes of citalopram dosage risk mitigation in a veteran population. Am J Psychiatry 173(9):896–902, 2016 27166093

Seligman MEP: The effectiveness of psychotherapy: the Consumer Reports study. Am Psychol 50(12):965–974, 1995 8561380

Stavrou A, Challoumas D, Dimitrakakis G: Archibald Cochrane (1909–1988): the father of evidence-based medicine. Interact Cardiovasc Thorac Surg 18(1):121–124, 2014 24140816

Thoma NC, McKay D, Gerber AJ, et al: A quality-based review of randomized controlled trials of cognitive-behavioral therapy for depression: an assessment and metaregression. Am J Psychiatry 169(1):22–30, 2012 22193528

Trivedi MH, Rush AJ, Wisniewski SR, et al; STAR*D Study Team: Evaluation of outcomes with citalopram for depression using measurement-based care in STAR*D: implications for clinical practice. Am J Psychiatry 163(1):28–40, 2006 16390886

University of Wisconsin-Madison Institute for Clinical and Translational Research. What are the T0 to T4 research classifications? Madison, University of Wisconsin, 2018. Available at: https://ictr.wisc.edu/what-are-the-t0-to-t4-research-classifications. Accessed September 8, 2019.

U.S. Food and Drug Administration: FDA Drug Safety Communication: Abnormal heart rhythms associated with high doses of Celexa (citalopram hydrobromide). Silver Spring, MD, U.S. Food and Drug Administration, March 28, 2012. Available at: www.fda.gov/drugs/drug-safety-and-availability/fda-drug-safety-communication-revised-recommendations-celexa-citalopram-hydrobromide-related. Accessed August 22, 2019.

U.S. Food and Drug Administration: FDA Drug Safety Communication: FDA revises description of mental health side effects of the stop-smoking medicines

Chantix (varenicline) and Zyban (bupropion) to reflect clinical trial findings. Silver Spring, MD, U.S. Food and Drug Administration, December 16, 2016. Available at: www.fda.gov/drugs/drug-safety-and-availability/fda-drug-safety-communication-fda-revises-description-mental-health-side-effects-stop-smoking. Accessed August 22, 2019.

Wachino V: Maternal depression screening and treatment: a critical role for Medicaid in the care of mothers and children. CMCS Informational Bulletin. Baltimore, MD, Centers for Medicare and Medicaid Services, May 11, 2016. Available at: www.medicaid.gov/federal-policy-guidance/downloads/cib051116.pdf. Accessed August 22, 2019.

Zivin K, Pfeiffer PN, Bohnert AS, et al: Evaluation of the FDA warning against prescribing citalopram at doses exceeding 40 mg. Am J Psychiatry 170(6):642–650, 2013 23640689

Zivin K, Pfeiffer PN, Bohnert AS, et al: Safety of high-dosage citalopram. Am J Psychiatry 171(1):20–22, 2014 24399424

10

Engaging the Popular Media

Daniel S. Barron, M.D., Ph.D.
Kristin S. Budde, M.D., M.P.H.
Jessica A. Gold, M.D., M.S.
Kimberly Yonkers, M.D.
Joan M. Cook, Ph.D.

Learning Objectives

By the end of this chapter, readers will be able to:

- Understand why it is important for psychiatrists to communicate scientific data via clear and concise communications for popular audiences
- Recognize storytelling as a powerful communication tool
- Describe how psychiatrists can approach media as an advocacy tool, including through the use of interviews, social media, audiovisual formats, and written publications (e.g., op-eds, articles, books)
- Identify potential barriers to engaging the popular media
- Use key writing tips to connect with a broad audience

In a 2014 article in the *New York Times*, internationally regarded columnist Nicholas Kristof observed that academics "encode their insights into turgid prose. As a double protection against public consumption, this gobbledygook is then sometimes hidden in obscure journals" (Kristof 2014). He implored scholars to find ways to disseminate scientific knowledge to a wider audience: "Don't cloister yourself like medieval monks—we need you!"

Psychiatrists and psychologists need to follow this same advice. We possess a unique view of the human mind as it relates to individuals, families, and society at large. There is much to communicate about our field that can benefit patients and their families, other practitioners, and policy makers. Whether educating about new treatments or paradigms, promoting a specific policy or concept, or sharing our clinical experiences, advocacy is an essential part of interacting with, courting, and changing public opinion. In addition, because much of our education and research is publicly funded, communicating our areas of expertise to the broader society is an essential responsibility.

Using the popular media effectively can be a powerful advocacy tool. Effective media communication strategies can ignite and stoke grassroots movements around critical issues that impact our patients. They can change cultural perceptions, galvanize popular support, and bolster critical legislation. Learning how to communicate well is critical for effective advocacy. An excellent example of the effective use of the popular media is demonstrated by physician-advocate Jeremy Kidd, whose profile is featured at the end of the chapter.

We define *media advocacy* as any topic that one wishes to persuasively communicate to the public. Such topics may be relevant to the advocate's domain of expertise (e.g., psychiatry, neuroscience, public health) or may reflect a social injustice or health inequity (e.g., access to care, mental health parity). In each case, the overarching goal is public persuasion: that the issues are important, that a policy or standard of care should be amended, or that a position (scientific, political, or social) should be supported. Advocacy's persuasive and public element separates it from standard academic communications, which are typically either declarative in nature or intended for an audience of other academicians or scholars within one's field. In this chapter, we describe different forms of media-based advocacy and outline strategies to engage these forms. We discuss several types of media advocacy (e.g., audiovisual formats, written publications, and social media) and provide examples from the psychiatry departments at Yale and Stanford universities, both of which have chosen to promote media advocacy, as models for other programs.

Why Engage the Popular Media?

Engaging the popular media is different from traditional ways in which psychiatrists and psychologists disseminate information, such as through peer-reviewed publications or formal presentations at scientific conferences. Most academics publish in scientific journals, which are not often read by the public. Even though some scholarly publication outlets also have "commentary" sections in which readers can share their opinions or advocate for a particular point or cause, the audience and tone of those sections are very different from those in publications intended to reach the lay public through popular media. Many more people, however, can be reached through the popular media than an advocate could ever hope to connect with through scientific or professional channels, and the more people an advocate can reach, the likelier it will be that change will be effected.

In a recent survey of 475 state legislators, only 27% reported that when seeking information to guide their decisions on behavioral health policy, they consulted research from universities (Purtle et al. 2018). The fact that nearly three-quarters of U.S. policy makers do not obtain their public health information from academic institutions should be shocking. These findings indicate that it is imperative for psychiatrists to branch out from traditional avenues and communicate the findings from their research and clinical work in ways that capture the public's attention and focus a spotlight on the issue.

Several mental health professionals have explained the importance of engaging the public through popular media (Friedman 2009; Pipher 2006). For example, Dr. Richard Friedman, a professor of clinical psychiatry and director of the Psychopharmacology Clinic at Weill Cornell Medicine, writes for the lay public as a regular contributor on behavior to the *New York Times*. He writes and speaks about the role of psychiatrists as experts, commentators, or educators to a broad audience. Friedman (2009) explained that the public is extremely interested in human behavior and that the *New York Times* pieces about behavior are often the most widely read and shared articles in the paper. Friedman added that whereas a typical journalist is dependent on secondhand accounts or expert opinion, psychiatrists who write for a wider audience can more directly and with authority offer their advice, opinions, and expertise. In what might be seen as a call to arms, Friedman wrote, "The fact is that if we do not take a more active role in presenting and explaining our field to the public, others will do it for us" (p. 758).

Importance of Storytelling

Live storytelling events and podcasts, such as The Moth, are part of a recent trend toward digital story sharing. Apart from providing entertainment, stories are an incredibly powerful way to share a patient story, a research implication, or a personal reflection on patient care. Our brains are hard-wired to respond to stories (Huth et al. 2016). Even if you have no desire to share a story with an audience at a live storytelling event, a basic understanding of storytelling principles can improve your advocacy endeavors. The other types of advocacy discussed in this book often involve oral communication (e.g., in legislative advocacy, as discussed in Chapter 7, advocates sometimes meet with or testify before legislators), which is usually more effective when some elements of storytelling are included. Many practitioners are more comfortable citing peer-reviewed publications, but by adding a patient or personal vignette that helps nonexperts understand and appreciate a data set, speakers can make their material more memorable and relatable.

The skills required to craft and tell a compelling story are relevant to writing, public speaking, and other forms of communication. There are many components to storytelling, and although we cannot provide an exhaustive list, we touch on a few: Stories need to generate interest. This can be done by addressing a topical issue or by explaining why the story is relevant and relatable to the reader. Articulation of conflicting views or emotions can increase relevance and interest. Character development brings a story to life. Most memorable stories involve a moment of personal realization or change, often with some element of vulnerability and honesty. Many stories include the writer in some aspect. A story may involve a patient or controversial issue, but if the storyteller is not present in the story, it will fall flat. For more storytelling tips, we recommend that readers consult *Storyworthy* by Matthew Dicks (2018).

Various Forms of Popular Media

A variety of popular media formats can be used to engage with a general audience. These include the following:

- Media interviews (print, radio, and television)
- Conventional writing (op-eds, letters to the editor, short-form and long-form articles, and books)
- Online platforms (podcasts, videos, blogs, and e-mails to subscriber lists)
- Social media

Media Interviews

The most traditional form of media involvement is interviews with journalists. Often, interviews occur when the media has questions about a research publication or a request for comment on a public initiative, such as a legislative bill or public program. In an interview, a journalist asks you questions, and you respond. The encounter can be audiotaped, visually recorded, or hand transcribed by the reporter. Reporters may also request that an expert respond to written questions. We strongly encourage readers to accept such interviews or inquiries and to prepare carefully. Consider staging a mock interview with a friend or colleague who can provide feedback about your presentation style. If you work in a large health care setting or academic institution or belong to a professional society, reach out to the communications officer. Often, these professionals can help you prepare for media interviews or for written statements about research or policy initiatives.

The following are helpful tips to keep in mind when you are asked to be part of a media-based interview:

1. Know the interviewer and their perspective, when possible.
2. Know your topic. If you are not well acquainted with the topic, do your homework and research.
3. Prepare key points (three to five maximum) that you would like to convey.
4. Practice making your key points in advance of the interview (i.e., prepare sound bites).
5. Practice ways to guide the interviewer back to the key points you want to make. This is known as a "pivot" and may be something like this: "There are many questions in this field, but what people need to know is...." Above all, practice in advance of an interview, and do not hesitate to tell the journalist if an area is outside of your expertise. Bear in mind that reporters may look for areas that are controversial, and you may say something that is taken out of context. Try to think through the possible implications of your statements as you speak to the reporter.
6. Some organizations, including academic institutions and professional societies, have communications specialists who understand media. They can provide guidance about media venues and individuals who may be fair and those who have taken statements out of context. Experts may want to contact their communications officers for help in advance of the interview.

Conventional Writing

There are several forms of written communication for the media and lay public, including op-eds, letters to the editor, short-form pieces, long-form pieces, and books.

Op-Eds

Op-eds are typically editorials, with an optimal length of 500–750 words, that define and argue for a specific position, policy, or belief. They share a common form, summarized as follows:

- *Lede:* Provide an attention-grabbing hook, often reflecting some controversy or news headline (e.g., "The opioid crisis has claimed more than 45,000 victims this year").
- *Thesis:* Describe your position as an expert in the field and explain your qualifications (e.g., "I'm a psychiatrist who treats patients with opioid use disorder").
- *Argument:* Give three to five arguments that support your position. This evidence can include research papers and/or personal experience (e.g., "Multiple clinical trials have shown that opioid replacement therapy is effective. I have seen my patients respond well to opioid replacement therapy.").
- *Preemptive antithesis:* Include a paragraph that anticipates and dispels the most likely counterargument(s). You should be familiar enough with what people will say to contradict your position to address this (e.g., "A large group of people believe that opioid replacement therapy is trading one addiction for another, but this ignores the fact that opioid replacement therapy decreases the likelihood of overdose or transmission of blood-borne illnesses").
- *Conclusion:* Restate your thesis, summarize your arguments, and provide a direction for what you wish to see happen (e.g., "We should fund more opioid replacement programs and give wider access to them"). If possible, provide a next step or action that readers can take and advise them where to find additional information on the topic.

Op-eds are meant to be read by general audiences. Thus, it is helpful to avoid medical or scientific jargon that will not be understood by a broad readership. The op-ed is often topical and addresses current news. The news cycle these days is short, and an op-ed about an event or controversy that occurred months or years ago will not be of as great interest to the media as something that occurred days ago. Finally, op-eds provide a point of view, but there will be opposing views. It is wise to anticipate counterarguments as much as possible and address them head on in the op-ed. This provides authenticity and balance and can defuse negative reactions to your argument.

Good places to send op-ed pieces are your local newspaper, magazines, or online publications. Although most media outlets are starved for content, they do not accept unsolicited material indiscriminately. Be prepared for rejection. If your piece is rejected, reach out to the media outlet and try to find out the reason for the rejection (e.g., poor timing, poor writing). It might be useful to have others read the piece and to revise it before resubmitting. A piece may need to be submitted to several venues before it is accepted. Not all venues are the same, and your piece may be suited for a specialty audience rather than a general audience.

To learn more about how to write effective op-eds, you can turn to the OpEd Project, a nonprofit organization that works with universities, foundations, corporations, and community organizations to connect thought leaders with media mentors and teaches people how to engage with the public through opinion writing (www.theopedproject.org). This organization offers seminars across the country for interested individuals. Additionally, a number of academic institutions and professional societies run seminars on writing for lay audiences, which typically include training in writing opinion pieces.

Letters to the Editor

A letter to the editor is usually written in response to a timely news topic or article. Such a letter is more likely to be accepted when it is shorter than 200 words, states your support or opposition to an issue in a concise and pithy way, and includes your experience or credentials for proffering your opinion. Unlike in an op-ed, an antithesis is not necessary in a letter to the editor because these letters tend to be very brief. For letters regarding journal articles, there may be a time frame for response to a certain publication, and authors should be aware of these and other policies when framing their letter.

Short-Form Pieces

A short-form piece is typically longer than 1,000 words and is published as a short news article. Short-form pieces differ from op-eds because they are explanatory in nature, rather than expressions of opinion. They are most effective if they provide a personal, human perspective instead of a research summary. Such a piece might begin with a personal narrative that allows the reader to empathize with or become excited about an otherwise potentially less interesting or remote topic. For example, if you want to discuss psychiatric genomics, you might begin with a story of a patient who benefited from a genetic study or who had a rare case of a particular illness. As a rule of thumb, remember that no one *needs* to read your piece, so it needs to be entertaining enough to hold the reader's interest. To achieve this goal, you could begin with a personal narrative, then explain a research or clinical complexity surrounding the issue raised in the narrative, and conclude by bringing the story back to the original narrative.

Long-Form Pieces

Long-form pieces typically involve more than 3,000 words. These are the most complex pieces to write because it is very difficult to craft a story that can keep a reader's attention for an extended period of time. Accordingly, although a short-form piece or op-ed can often be written in a single sitting, a long-form essay requires careful planning and may take weeks or even longer to complete. Long-form pieces are most engaging when they combine multiple narratives, different avenues of research, and interviews with various individuals and when each of these components explains some facet of a larger concept. The structure of longer pieces varies; the book *Draft No. 4* by John McPhee (2017) is an excellent guide to different structural forms.

Books

Book writing is another potential venue for reaching the public. There are many "pop psychology" books in print, some of which are extremely popular, as well as a number of more scholarly books that are also accessible to a lay audience. These books can be a valuable resource to patients and the general public who are trying to find out information about an illness and its treatment. The typical encounter with a physician is 10 minutes, and a person can leave the office starving for more information. For patients, a book that is accessible to the public but also medically and scientifically accurate can do much good compared with attempts at doing Internet research, which may or may not be accurate. Of course, writing a book is much harder and more time-consuming than writing other media forms, but doing so is worthwhile if the book can address a need for the general public.

Online Forms of Communication

The Internet has sparked the advent of new forms of communication that educate and inform the public. Podcasts, videos, blogs, and e-mails to subscriber lists are all ways that the Internet has innovated the dissemination of information and provided opportunities for advocating and developing grassroots support.

Podcasts

Podcasts have become an increasingly popular medium for information, particularly in medical education. In fact, studies show that trainees prefer podcasts to textbooks (Riddell et al. 2017) and enjoy them as an alternative resource or adjunct for their learning. Podcasts are also useful to medical professionals at all levels to keep current with the scientific literature and to acquire core content (Pilarski et al. 2008). Among the numerous advantages of podcasts are the ability to learn while engaging in other activities (e.g., cooking, walking), the ability to cater to learners with different study habits (Back et al. 2017; Shantikumar 2009), and perhaps even increased knowledge retention as compared with reading a book chapter (Matava et al. 2013). These same advantages apply when podcasts are used as a form of advocacy, and they can be an effective way to engage and inform the listener. For an example of how to start a podcast, see Box 10–1.

Box 10–1: How to Start a Podcast

For this example, we use the podcast Psyched! by chapter author Jessica Gold and her partner David Carreon. Ask yourself the following questions (McLean 2019):

1. *What is the purpose or theme of your podcast?* It is important to think about why you want to start a podcast and what content (that is not currently available) you want to create. Before Psyched! there were not a lot of psychiatry podcasts, so that part was easy. We decided to talk about all things psychiatry—from research to trendy practices to the current events related to psychiatry. Nothing that related to psychiatry was off limits.

2. *Who is your target audience?* This question helps you collate your material and the level at which it is presented. Some podcasts are directed at specific populations of physicians (e.g., psychiatrists, internal medicine doctors), some at physicians as a group, and some (with broader information) at the lay public. Psyched! targets both the lay public and psychiatrists in all settings of work, from community to academia. As such, we try to avoid jargon and explain the information in such a way that no prior psychiatric knowledge is needed.

Box 10–1: How to Start a Podcast *(continued)*

---

3. What is the format of your podcast?

   a. *Who is hosting?* There can be solo shows, cohosted shows, roundtable shows, and even documentary shows. Psyched! is a cohosted show simply because we felt each of us added something different (Dr. Gold is a pop culture–savvy humanities major, whereas Dr. Carreon is a mental health provider and researcher). Having cohosts with different backgrounds also contributed to the "hook."

   b. *What is the format?* Some podcasts are simply summaries of recent journal articles, some use storytelling as a medium to convey information, and others (such as Psyched!) are interviews. No matter which format is chosen, it is important to keep the format somewhat consistent so that the listeners know what to expect when tuning in.

   c. *What is the title?* The title can be creative, but keep in mind that people need to be able to search for your podcast or find your podcast when searching for their topic of interest. Psyched! was a fun, short, and easy fit that described the podcast exactly.

   d. *Do you want theme music?* Including music makes your podcast more memorable. A friend composed the catchy opening song for Psyched!

   e. *Do you want any other specific signatures across your episodes?* For Psyched! every guest is asked the same five questions at the end in a rapid round (e.g., "Who is a person dead or alive, real or fictional, that you consider your hero?" "What does psychiatry get wrong?").

Box 10–1: How to Start a Podcast *(continued)*

4. *What are the length and frequency of your podcast?* On iTunes, podcasts can vary from a few minutes to longer than an hour, and popularity does not seem to be directly related to length. However, in one study, residents preferred podcasts to be shorter than 30 minutes and were less likely to listen to podcasts that were longer than 45 minutes (McLean 2019). Therefore, Psyched! is typically under 45 minutes; if the interview goes over that time, the podcast is broken into multiple episodes. Podcasts can be weekly, biweekly, or monthly. Again, anecdotally, popularity and frequency do not seem correlated, and perhaps length and frequency decisions should be made on the basis of your internal and external resources (e.g., time and patience) for editing and producing them. One nice thing about podcasts, however, is that if you avoid mentioning dates or a specific time in your content, episodes can be "banked" and used later. In this way, content can be created in waves and is not completely dependent on your schedule. Psyched! was biweekly but shifted to monthly as our schedules became busier.

5. *What equipment and technical knowledge are needed?* To make a podcast, you need some basic equipment: microphone(s), microphone stand(s), computer(s), headphones, and a recorder. Each episode will also need some editing prior to posting (which can be done by professional sound editors or by you if you have the technical expertise) to remove any sort of mistakes or background noises such as coughing. You can also interview people who are not in the room (or even have cohosts in different places, as in the case of Psyched!), but you will need to use video conferencing and record episodes via your computer for the best sound quality.

Box 10–1: How to Start a Podcast *(continued)*

---

6. *Where will you host your podcast, and how will you get listeners?* iTunes lets you host a podcast for free; however, you should also consider making a website, creating a distribution list, and thinking of other ways to promote your episodes to obtain listeners. One suggestion is to include guests who have large social media followings, and the guests can then promote their episodes, thereby drawing listeners to your podcast. For Psyched! this technique worked particularly well with nonpsychiatrist guests who were authors, for example, or a gastroenterologist with popular press books, who focused on the interaction between the gut and the brain. Additionally, Dr. Gold had an existing relationship with the *Psychiatric Times*, and she pitched them the idea of her podcast. They previously had an unsuccessful podcast but were open to helping to make this relationship work. Having Psyched! hosted on their platform and having access to their distribution lists were seminal to our success.

7. *How much do you prepare for each episode?* Time spent preparing for interviews varies widely. For Psyched! the cohosts typically read the biographical information and current work of each guest and come up with a list of at least five questions to ask that guest. Each guest also signs a release form and sends a brief biographical statement and a headshot for use on the website.

Videos

Videos are also an increasingly popular online education form. On YouTube, the most popular video sharing site, some videos can amass millions and even billions of views. However, many other video-sharing platforms are available, including Vimeo, Metacafe, Internet Archive, and TED. If you are interested in creating a video, you can easily search the Internet and find dozens of free online videos that can provide helpful advice about how to produce your own effective online video. Common tips include using good lighting, keeping the backdrop plain, avoiding camera shake, shooting from a range of angles, and ensuring that the sound quality is clear.

Blogs

Other popular sources for information and opinions are blogs (the word *blog* is an abbreviation of *weblog*). According to the Oxford Dictionary (https://en.oxforddictionaries.com/definition/blog; accessed February 24, 2019), a blog is "a regularly updated website or web page, typically one run by an individual or small group, that is written in an informal or conversational style." Merriam Webster (www.merriam-webster.com/dictionary/blog; accessed February 24, 2019) describes a blog as either "a website that contains online personal reflections, comments, and often hyperlinks, videos, and photographs provided by the writer" or "a regular feature appearing as part of an online publication that typically relates to a particular topic and consists of articles and personal commentary by one or more authors."

Blog posts can follow the formats of traditional writing and consist entirely of written material, but they can also be highly creative endeavors that use a variety of online tools, including photographs and hyperlinks. A blog post should be brief enough to be read in one sitting, and it needs to be attention grabbing because blog readers expect a higher degree of entertainment from blogs than from other media formats.

Blog posts can be disseminated in a number of ways. You could write a post for another person's blog or for a news blog such as the *Huffington Post*, or you could start your own blog. Individuals can start a blog, for example, through one of the big outlets, such as *Psychology Today* or Ariana Huffington's relatively new *Thrive Global*. If you start your own blog, you will need to update your blog regularly in order to retain readers. You also will need to vary your approaches in order to keep the blog fresh and relevant.

E-mail Subscriber Lists

E-mail subscriber lists are mass e-mails that are regularly sent to subscribers who want to receive updates about an issue. This is an older form of online communication that is often used by groups and organizations. When e-mail first became popular in the 1990s, this form of communication was highly effective because most e-mail users opened all the e-mails they received. However, as the sheer volume of e-mails received by the average person has grown (the average American worker receives more than 120 e-mails per day), the effectiveness of this form of online advocacy communication has declined (Campaign Monitor 2019a). Today, the average e-mail open rate is 25% or less (Campaign Monitor 2019b). To improve open rates, e-mail marketing consultants recommend that writers create clear and catchy subject lines, keep the body of the e-mail short, and put links for action in the first third of the e-mail.

Social Media

Social media, such as Twitter, Instagram, and Facebook, can be key influencers of public discourse. These platforms have become an increasingly powerful way to amplify one's voice or spread ideas across a potentially broad network of people. Social media can be challenging to engage in because the amount of content a user can post is space limited for certain social media forms. In addition to sharing thoughts and ideas, social media can be used to share research, directing a broad audience to publications and useful websites. When you engage in social media, take special care to keep your personal posts separate from your professional posts. A significant drawback to social media is that sometimes these platforms spread misinformation as well as accurate information, and lay readers may not be able to tell the difference. Finally, although some social media users choose to engage with and attempt to educate "trolls," others have decided never to read the comment sections and to block chronic harassers.

Barriers to Engaging With the Media

Engaging with the popular media takes time, effort, and a different skill set from the one that psychiatrists and psychologists typically possess (Cook 2018). These skills can be learned through formal or informal instruction and require practice. Finding the time to practice these new skills can be difficult.

Some psychiatrists and psychologists may have concerns about media advocacy. They might think, "I don't want to say the wrong thing, so I better not say anything." Or they might wonder, "Would expressing this opinion impact how my patients view me?" Some might think, "This doesn't advance my academic career, so I won't take the time." Overcoming these complex, often personal obstacles can require thought and discussions with colleagues, supervisors, and friends.

Advocates should always be concerned about raising potential ethical concerns by commenting about public figures (Box 10–2) or unintentionally violating patient confidentiality by using patients' stories in such a way that the actual patients recognize themselves. Psychiatrists and psychologists need to take extra care to keep descriptions general and err on the side of obscuring revelatory details.

Another barrier that psychiatrists face is the potential for negative implicit bias toward psychiatrists by members of the general population. Psychiatrists should be aware of the frequent negative images and false stereotypes of psychiatrists that are perpetuated in the media (e.g., *New Yorker* cartoons and movies such as *One Flew Over the Cuckoo's Nest*). Some comments reflecting negative bias that the public might en-

---

Box 10–2: Ethics, Media Advocacy, and the "Goldwater Rule"

In 1964, the American quarterly publication *Fact Magazine* published a series of articles under the title "The Unconscious of a Conservative: A Special Issue on the Mind of Barry Goldwater." The editors of the magazine, Ralph Ginzburg and Warren Boroson, had polled psychiatrists, asking whether U.S. Senator Barry Goldwater was fit to be president, and they printed their findings in their magazine. The editors were subsequently sued for libel, and Goldwater won $75,000 in damages. As a result, the American Psychiatric Association's Principles of Medical Ethics (first published in 1973) state that it is unethical for psychiatrists to give a professional opinion about public figures whom they have not examined in person and from whom they have not obtained consent to discuss their mental health in public statements (American Psychiatric Association 2013). The principle is now informally known as the Goldwater rule.

---

dorse include the following: psychiatrists are elitist and withholding, psychiatrists are damaged and insane, psychiatrists want to control others by forcing them to undergo electroshock treatment or take drugs, and psychiatrists can read minds. When you engage the media for advocacy, consider how your words and actions could feed into or reinforce these or other negative stereotypes.

Examples of Media Advocacy Programs at Two University Psychiatry Departments

To address potential barriers to engaging with the popular media, we have established programs at two academic institutions: Yale University in New Haven, Connecticut, and Stanford University in Palo Alto, California.

In 2016, a group of psychiatry and neurology residents at Yale University organized a monthly writing for the public interest group. The structure was relatively simple: well-known speakers were invited every other month to teach about a media form, and then the next month, attendees shared their current ideas or drafts of works in progress. A number of ground rules were provided for the workshop portion: participants were encouraged to read their pieces slowly and clearly out loud to their colleagues. We also encouraged readers to bring hard copies for attendees. Listeners were advised to jot down notes to refer to when offering help. Notes could be passed to the reader or shared verbally. We asked listeners to resist the temptation to list "mistakes" they heard and instead asked that the critique be thoughtful, respectful, and honest and include a combination of emotional response, constructive advice, and positive reinforcement or praise. If a listener asked a question, the writer could answer or choose to think about it and follow up via e-mail or in person at a later time. Finally, if the meeting ended before everyone who wanted to read had the opportunity, we ensured that these readers would be the first name(s) on the list for the next meeting.

In our experiences, we have found that medical writers appreciate hearing both what they have communicated well and what was not coming across well. Because hearing feedback about one's writing can be painful, we encouraged bravery in sharing as well as graciousness in response. We found that arguing or disagreeing, even if a listener's response catches the writer by surprise, does not promote learning or better writing. We encouraged our writers to be careful not to "critique the critique." Responses are personal, and they are designed to be given in the spirit of being helpful. We encouraged the writer to let the point settle. This means that sometimes the best response to a listener's question or comment is simply saying thank you.

At Stanford University, we organized "Mind Over Media," a media curriculum for the psychiatry residency program that began in 2016 (Morris et al. 2018). It was initiated on the basis of the strong desire to incorporate media literacy into the residency educational structure. This program includes monthly lunchtime talks that seek to educate medical students, residents, and faculty about issues in the media related to mental health. Prior to each session, a series of articles (or videos, episodes from a television series, or video links) is sent to the residency and faculty listservs, with a "primary" article or clip selected for each session. Each e-mail also includes about five questions for attendees to think about before the session. Recent topics addressed have included the Goldwater rule, news coverage of mass shootings, public outcry over the Netflix show *13 Reasons Why*, the Logic song based on the suicide hotline number, comedy and media, and media reporting on suicide. The sessions often include guest speakers from academia, industry, and/or media outlets to facilitate discussion. Sessions have been well attended each month (30–40 people) and are among the most discussed and well-liked components of the residency curriculum.

Writing Tips for Connecting With a General Audience

A number of books and workshops are available to help academics learn to write in ways that engage the public. In *How to Write for a General Audience: A Guide for Academics Who Want to Share Their Knowledge With the World and Have Fun Doing It*, psychologist Kathleen Kendall-Tackett (2007) elaborates on what she calls the "seven deadly sins of academic writers." She identifies these as use of the passive voice, use of jargon, too many abstractions, noun pile-ups, weak voice construction, excess verbiage, and too many syllables. Her tips on how to address these potential weaknesses are extensive. Her advice includes limiting the number of nouns used in a sentence, using concrete nouns, turning nouns into verbs, reducing the quantity of words and then trying to improve the quality of words that remain, and using more simple words. Other manuals with advice on writing for a wider audience are listed in Table 10–1, with one or more tips culled from each book.

In general, we recommend these writing tips:

- Avoid the "turgid prose" described by Kristof (2014).
- Be thoughtful about the words used to frame issues. Words and phrases have the power to conjure up highly charged, evocative images, and how an idea is framed can predetermine who attends to and who shuts out your message. Framing the estate tax as a "death tax," for example, was an effective way to rally supporters, even those who were poor and would never benefit from an estate tax repeal.
- Be attentive to the negative implicit bias and general misunderstanding about the psychiatry profession; make efforts to not reinforce familiar stereotypes of psychiatrists.
- Include stories as much as possible; they will help the reader to understand and remember the advocacy issue.
- Use shorter sentences; be as clear and concise as possible.

There are many books about science communication written by professional science writers and journalists. We encourage readers to search out these books, some of which are found in the References.

TABLE 10–1. Tips from some of our favorite books on writing

Book	Tips
Bird by Bird: Some Instructions on Writing and Life (Lamott 1994)	Get started: Write one page of 300 words containing memories, dreams, or stream of consciousness about *the reason you want to write.* You don't always have to chop with the sword of truth. You can point with it too.
The Forest for the Trees: An Editor's Advice to Writers (Lerner 2000)	Write what you know. Pieces people like best are usually those that stir debate or arouse strong feeling.
Writing to Change the World (Pipher 2006)	Writing to connect is "change writing," which, like good therapy, creates the conditions that allow people to be transformed. Present yourself as a curious student rather than a smug expert. Humility is appealing.
How to Write for a General Audience: A Guide for Academics Who Want to Share Their Knowledge With the World and Have Fun Doing It (Kendall-Tackett 2007)	An academic title presents you with two distinct disadvantages: 1. Editors are concerned that you might not be able to write in an accessible level for their publication. 2. Academics often disregard deadlines. Read and review the news outlets in which you want to publish. Learn what the editor wants and the style their writers use, and follow their lead.
Only as Good as Your Word: Writing Lessons From My Favorite Literary Gurus (Shapiro 2007)	In almost all cases, editors will improve your writing. Try not to take comments personally. *No* never means *no:* It means rewrite, retitle, re-spin, add a more timely lead, and resend your writing to the hopefully nice editor at the next cubicle.
Storyworthy: Engage, Teach, Persuade, and Change Your Life Through the Power of Storytelling (Dicks 2018)	Honesty and vulnerability make for the best stories.

Conclusion

Engaging with the popular media is an important endeavor for psychiatric advocates. Doing so can help to educate the public about current psychiatric issues, such as social determinants of health, access to care, and mental health parity and can also help expand grassroots support. When psychiatric advocates effectively engage the popular media, they lay the groundwork for systemic change at all levels of care.

References

American Psychiatric Association: The Principles of Medical Ethics: With Annotations Especially Applicable to Psychiatry, 13th Edition. Arlington, VA, American Psychiatric Association, 2013

Back DA, von Malotky J, Sostmann K, et al: Superior gain in knowledge by podcasts versus text-based learning in teaching orthopedics: a randomized controlled trial. J Surg Educ 74(1):154–160, 2017 27651055

Campaign Monitor: The shocking truth about how many emails are sent. Nashville, TN, Campaign Monitor, 2019a. Available at: www.campaignmonitor.com/blog/email-marketing/2019/05/shocking-truth-about-how-many-emails-sent. Accessed December 17, 2019.

Campaign Monitor: What are the average click and read rates for email campaigns? Nashville, TN, Campaign Monitor, 2019b. Available at: www.campaign monitor.com/resources/knowledge-base/what-are-the-average-click-and-read-rates-for-email-campaigns. Accessed February 24, 2019.

Cook JM: Engaging a public audience: social justice advocacy and dissemination of trauma science. J Trauma Dissociation 19(2):131–135, 2018 28929928

Dicks M: Storyworthy: Engage, Teach, Persuade, and Change Your Life Through the Power of Storytelling. Novato, CA, New World Library, 2018

Friedman RA: The role of psychiatrists who write for popular media: experts, commentators, or educators? Am J Psychiatry 166(7):757–759, 2009 19570937

Huth AG, de Heer WA, Griffiths TL, et al: Natural speech reveals the semantic maps that tile human cerebral cortex. Nature 532(7600):453–458, 2016 19570937

Kendall-Tackett KA: How to Write for a General Audience: A Guide for Academics Who Want to Share Their Knowledge With the World and Have Fun Doing It. Washington, DC, American Psychological Association, 2007

Kristof N: Professors we need you! New York Times, February 15, 2014. Available at: /www.nytimes.com/2014/02/16/opinion/sunday/kristof-professors-we-need-you.html?mcubz=3. Accessed August 24, 2019.

Lamott A: Bird by Bird: Some Instructions on Writing and Life. New York, Anchor, 1994

Lerner B: The Forest for the Trees: An Editor's Advice to Writers. New York, Riverhead, 2000

Matava CT, Rosen D, Siu E, et al: eLearning among Canadian anesthesia residents: a survey of podcast use and content needs. BMC Med Educ 13:59, 2013 23617894

McLean M: How to start a podcast: every single step. Dundee, UK, The Podcast Host, March 21, 2019. Available at: www.thepodcasthost.com/planning/how-to-start-a-podcast/#ch-1. Accessed August 24, 2019.

McPhee J: Draft No. 4: On the Writing Process. New York, Farrar, Straus, & Giroux, 2017

Morris NP, Johansen SL, May M, et al: Media-related education in psychiatry residency programs. Acad Psychiatry 42(5):679–685, 2018 30155603

Pilarski PP, Alan Johnstone D, Pettepher CC, et al: From music to macromolecules: using rich media/podcast lecture recordings to enhance the preclinical educational experience. Med Teach 30(6):630–632, 2008 18677662

Pipher M: Writing to Change the World. New York, Riverhead, 2006

Purtle J, Dodson EA, Nelson K, et al: Legislators' sources of behavioral health research and preferences for dissemination: variations by political party. Psychiatr Serv 69(10):1105–1108, 2018 29983112

Riddell J, Swaminathan A, Lee M, et al: A survey of emergency medicine residents' use of educational podcasts. West J Emerg Med 18(2):229–234, 2017 28210357

Shantikumar S: From lecture theatre to portable media: students' perceptions of an enhanced podcast for revision. Med Teach 31(6):535–538, 2009 18937140

Shapiro S: Only as Good as Your Word: Writing Lessons From My Favorite Literary Gurus. Emeryville, CA, Seal Press, 2007

Advocacy Role Model Interview: Jeremy Kidd, M.D., M.P.H.

Advocacy Through Communication With the Public

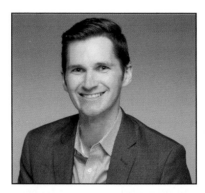

Jeremy Kidd, M.D., M.P.H.

T32 Research Fellow in Addiction Psychiatry, Columbia University; Private Practice, New York, New York

How did you come to be an advocate?

As an LGBTQ person growing up in rural Virginia, I saw a lot of anti-LGBTQ efforts going on. It was a really conservative area, and I didn't know any other gay people. By high school, I had come out as gay, but I didn't really know how to gravitate toward advocacy in that area. Instead, I got into discussions about abortion rights back then—it felt safer to talk about an issue I was less personally connected to, and it felt empowering to advocate.

In college, I joined a club called the Sexual Minority Student Alliance. I vividly remember one of the meetings, when a freshman walked in after just having been beaten up for being gay. Lots of people felt that advocacy was needed after that, so a group of friends and I formed a parallel organization called Queer Action. That's where I first learned how to be an advocate, and I continued to do advocacy work throughout college and medical training.

Could you describe the kind of advocacy work you do now?

One of the things I do is engage the media and the public. I've written letters to the editor (e.g., "Protesting Trump's Transgender Ban," www.nytimes.com/2017/07/27/opinion/protesting-trumps-transgender-ban.html) and blog posts (e.g., "The True Cost of Trump's Transgender Military Ban," www.huffpost.com/entry/the-real-cost-of-trumps-transgender-military-ban_b_59a0b426e4b0cb7715bfd58c) and given media interviews, for example. I've found this to be an effective form of advocacy because, for better or for worse, people listen to us as medical professionals.Media advocacy can be challenging for a number of reasons. For one, it can be hard to parse out when you're intentionally acting as a physician-advocate and when you're an advocate who just happens to also be a physician. In my case, I've been fortunate to be able to combine my interest in advocacy with my career as a physician because the issues I advocate for are also rooted in my professional medical opinions. That's not always true for everyone, though, so it's important to understand when you're speaking just for yourself and when you're speaking as a doctor.

Another challenging aspect of media advocacy is getting the framing right. This is about choosing the lens through which you present an idea to the media. As doctors, we're used to relying on facts and data. But that doesn't resonate with the general public. So consider what frames *will* resonate with your audience. Freedom, justice, fairness, protecting the vulnerable—these are some of the themes that you might use to achieve emotional resonance. Read lots of pieces by nonphysicians. That will help to frame your messaging.

What advice do you have for other psychiatrist-advocates?

1. One of biggest mistakes we make as physicians is thinking that we are the arbiters of truth, when in fact we are just single members of the community. As the saying goes, "Nothing about us without us." Get to know the community with whom or for whom you're advocating. Invite community members to be involved or even take the lead—they need to be part of the process.

2. Keep in mind that the results of your advocacy might come to fruition only after you've left the scene. Celebrate even small victories, knowing that incremental change can gradually re-

sult in big wins. I recently found out that an LGBTQ Resource Center campaign I started 15 years ago at my alma mater just came to fruition!

3. Don't get distracted by resistance. Change makes people nervous. When they express that, don't be too reactive. Let it motivate you. Sometimes it means you're on the right track. Integrate their criticism if it's valid and work around the resistance, without becoming overly defensive or disengaged.

4. Take care of yourself. Advocacy is hard work. Talk to your friends and fellow advocates. Support each other.

PART III
Advocacy for Special Populations

11

Advocacy for Children and Families

Debra Koss, M.D., FAACAP, DFAPA
Adam J. Sagot, D.O., FAPA

Learning Objectives

By the end of this chapter, readers will be able to:

- Identify opportunities for effective advocacy in working with, and on behalf of, child and adolescent patients and their families

- Understand strategies to navigate interactions with lawmakers at the local, state, and federal levels in advocating for children and families

- Examine opportunities for joining with stakeholders to develop grassroots advocacy efforts for child and adolescent mental health

- Identify barriers to effective advocacy for child and adolescent mental health

- Identify opportunities to expand advocacy training for psychiatrists who work with children and families

Half of all lifetime cases of mental illness begin by age 14 years, and three-quarters of cases begin by age 24 (National Institute of Mental Health 2018). One in five youth is affected by mental illness severe enough to cause significant impairment in their lives (National Institute of Mental Health 2017). Mental illness in youth is common, has an early onset, and can be disabling. However, children and adolescents often cannot advocate effectively for themselves and instead must rely on the proxy voice of others to represent their needs and to advocate on their behalf. As physicians providing health care to these patients, we must prepare ourselves well to be their advocates.

As psychiatrists, we routinely incorporate the principles of advocacy into our daily clinical practice. We advocate on behalf of children and youth in the course of routine treatment to ensure access to quality mental health care. These experiences are an integral part of our professional identity. Our advocacy efforts, however, need not be restricted to clinical practice. In fact, in order to have broader and more sustainable impact, we should seek opportunities for advocacy at the local, state, and federal levels.

In this chapter, we provide an overview of the skills necessary for effective advocacy; highlight opportunities for psychiatrists to engage in advocacy at the local, state, and federal levels, including through grassroots advocacy; examine the benefits and challenges of advocating alongside children and families; and look to the future of advocacy education and training during child psychiatry fellowship and beyond. Although much of the chapter focuses on legislative advocacy, all of the venues for advocacy described in Part II, "Practicing Advocacy"—patient-level advocacy, organizational advocacy, legislative advocacy, education as advocacy, research as advocacy, and engaging the popular media—are pertinent to advocacy for children and adolescents, and more information on these topics can be found in the respective chapters.

Also, given the nationwide shortage of child psychiatrists and the importance of advocacy for children and youth, we recognize that child psychiatrists as well as generalist psychiatrists may be involved with treating and advocating for children and families. Therefore, we have sought to include in this chapter information that pertains to all psychiatrists who work with children and families.

Psychiatrists as Advocates for Children and Families

Because mental illness in children and adolescents is common (National Institute of Mental Health 2017) and often has an early onset (National Institute of Mental Health 2018), the treatment of mental illness must involve early identification and intervention. Research has identified safe and effective treatments, yet too often families encounter barriers to care that prolong time to evaluation and interfere with initiation of treatment. When mental health treatments are blocked or delayed, children and youth experience negative outcomes, including academic failure, increased rates of substance abuse, involvement in the juvenile justice system, and suicide (National Alliance on Mental Illness 2018). In fact, suicide is now the second leading cause of death for youth ages 10–24 (National Alliance on Mental Illness 2018).

As psychiatrists who work with children and families, we have a responsibility to use our expertise and our voices to advocate on behalf of children and youth to reduce the occurrence of negative outcomes and to affirm that mental health services are an integral part of a child's overall health care. Advocacy is not only a significant part of our daily interactions on behalf of our patients but also a part of our core professional identity. We routinely advocate with school systems, child-serving agencies, and insurers, but in this time of health care reform we must also engage in legislative advocacy. Our medical training provides us with knowledge and clinical experience that can be used to inform legislators and policy makers. We can report data, translate neuroscience research, and share clinical anecdotes. With additional advocacy training, we can also expand our knowledge about the legislative process and learn strategies to more effectively engage legislators in meaningful discourse.

Moreover, it is essential that psychiatrists engage in mental health advocacy for children and adolescents because these patient populations are at a comparative disadvantage relative to other patient populations in their ability to advocate for themselves. There are a number of challenges unique to this population, from the inherent difficulty of mobilizing and organizing effective advocacy efforts for children and adolescents to the time constraints and stress levels of families and caregivers. Psychiatrists advocating for children and youth must recognize these challenges and meet them with effective action and commitment.

A commitment to advocacy may seem daunting, especially if one attempts to "do it all" or "go it alone," but advocacy need not be overwhelming or time-consuming. In an effort to increase our impact and avoid becoming fatigued, it is crucial that we use an approach that is focused and deliberate. We must develop a working knowledge of the legislative and political process in order to identify advocacy goals that are timely and attainable. At times, we may need to take the lead and organize an effort to champion the needs of children and youth. At other times, it may be more effective to add our voices to advocacy initiatives led by other stakeholders to ensure that the specific developmental needs of children and youth are considered.

Opportunities for advocacy exist on a continuum, require varying levels of competency and time, and have an impact on distinct portions of the pediatric population. The degree of our engagement in advocacy may be adjusted across time and across settings, with certain settings requiring a greater level of involvement. For instance, to advocate for an individual patient, we may speak with a school counselor on behalf of a student who has been bullied, educating school staff about the impact of bullying on the student's development and academic performance. This intervention will have a direct impact on the social and emotional needs of the student and may indirectly benefit other students as this counselor subsequently interacts with other students who are bullied. Going a step further, we may choose to advocate with school administration for policies that will address the needs of the victim, the bully, and the bystanders within the school, which involves a greater time commitment but also has the potential to positively impact more students (see the following section).

Going even further, we may choose to testify at school board hearings or run for a position on a school board, striving to have an even broader impact on the entire district through the allocation of resources that will support the implementation of evidence-based bullying prevention programs. Although serving as an elected official will require significantly more time and a specific skill set, we should not overlook opportunities for more direct involvement in local, or even state and federal, government (see section "Advocacy at the Local, State, and Federal Levels" below). Finally, grassroots advocacy is a potentially effective method of creating change at all these levels of advocacy (see section "Advocacy Through Grassroots Efforts" below). In the following sections, we use case scenarios to illustrate the principles of advocacy that can increase our efficacy and competency at the school, community agency, local, state, and federal levels, including through grassroots efforts.

Advocacy Through Schools, Child-Serving Systems, and Community Agencies

Child and adolescent psychiatrists, as well as other psychiatrists who regularly work with children and families, routinely advocate with school systems, child-serving systems such as the child welfare and juvenile justice systems, and community agencies on behalf of an individual patient as part of comprehensive treatment planning. For instance, we may advocate for modifications to an Individualized Education Program for a student with generalized anxiety disorder and school refusal. Additionally, we may be called in as consultants to assist schools in addressing an issue that pertains to the general student body, such as assessing their policies for conflict resolution and bullying prevention. Moreover, we may identify opportunities to serve as mental health advocates, championing the need for increased mental health education or school-based mental health services. In all of these cases, our knowledge of child and adolescent development and the neuroscience of mental illness guides our work. Furthermore, our knowledge of systems and our ability to navigate the different roles and responsibilities of psychiatrists when providing direct care, consulting to schools, or serving as mental health advocates also guide our decision making. The following vignette explores a scenario in which a child and adolescent psychiatrist is called in as a consultant to a school.

Case Example 1

Mr. T, the principal at a public high school, attends a monthly meeting of all county high school principals. At this meeting, he learns of an alarming trend: rates of electronic cigarette use are on the rise. School administrators are encouraged to review and update policies on cigarette use in schools to include this new electronic smoking device. Mr. T returns to his district and begins to assemble a workgroup to assist with this task. The school psychologist suggests that Mr. T contact Dr. L, a child psychiatrist who has previously treated students in the district with positive outcomes and has a reputation for being collaborative. Mr. T subsequently invites Dr. L to participate as a consultant.

Dr. L asks how he can be helpful to the workgroup. Mr. T admits that the school knows little about electronic cigarettes. Dr. L assembles some resources, including fact sheets about electronic cigarettes from the National Institute on Drug Abuse and diagrams of the adolescent brain. Dr. L makes significant contributions to the workgroup by providing factual information regarding electronic cigarette use and summarizing the impact of nicotine exposure during adolescence. These details inform the group's decisions regarding an updated school policy. Before the workgroup concludes, Dr. L is asked for any final recommendations. Dr. L advocates for a series of educational programs for educators, students, and parents about electronic cigarettes, highlighting strategies for prevention, smoking cessation, and harm reduction. The principal and school psychologist are interested and indicate they will consider the recommendation.

Psychiatrists can serve as resources within communities and are often called on as subject matter experts. In this case, Dr. L is initially contacted because of his past history of working well with the school. Dr. L is careful to understand the role he is to play as a consultant to the workgroup by asking for clarification on how he can help, and he collects resources from credible organizations to serve as teaching materials. Of note, professional organizations such as the American Psychiatric Association (APA) and the American Academy of Child and Adolescent Psychiatry (AACAP) often have educational and advocacy resources for use by members in these kinds of situations. Prior to the conclusion of the workgroup, Dr. L advocates for additional educational programming because he understands that a policy alone will not reverse the new trend in electronic cigarette use.

Advocacy at the Local, State, and Federal Levels

Opportunities exist at the local, state, and federal levels for psychiatrists to directly engage lawmakers and seek bipartisan support for policies that promote access to quality mental health care for children and youth. We offer examples in the following subsections.

Local-Level Advocacy

Getting involved in mental health advocacy at the local level, or within communities, can often feel more accessible than at the other levels, especially for psychiatrists who are entering into advocacy for the first time. We may choose to get involved in advocacy initiatives in the communities in which we live or work, where we already have personal or professional connections. These connections are valuable, and we may have a better understanding of local politics and regional child-serving agencies. On a practical level, attending community advocacy meetings may also be geographically more convenient, because they take place locally rather than at state capitals. Finally, local-level advocacy can also be impactful and rewarding, as initiatives tend to be more focused on identifying timely and attainable solutions to pressing issues.

> ## Case Example 2
>
> Dr. B is the only child and adolescent psychiatrist practicing in a rural community with limited mental health services. She has no capacity to see new patients. Dr. B frequently receives calls from families, school psychologists, and primary care providers who describe difficulty accessing mental health care. She provides information about local mental health services and referrals for psychiatric evaluation in neighboring counties but recognizes that families will likely encounter long waiting lists and transportation challenges. While Dr. B is discussing these concerns with a colleague, she learns about a newly formed coalition of mental health stakeholders who are meeting to discuss strategies to advocate for improved access to quality mental health care for children and youth across the county.

The experiences of Dr. B are not uncommon. There are approximately 9,400 child and adolescent psychiatrists in the United States, but it is estimated that more than 30,000 are needed to meet the needs of children and youth experiencing mental illness (Njoroge et al. 2016). The thought of approaching this public health crisis alone is daunting. We will be far more effective in our advocacy efforts if we share our expertise and our voices with other local stakeholders who are equally committed to improving access to care for youth in our communities.

Multiple opportunities exist to engage with coalitions in local-level advocacy, including the following:

- Hosting a children's health forum that includes providers, consumers, and legislators
- Completing inventories of local mental health resources and then distributing these inventories to the public
- Conducting community needs assessments that can lead to white papers outlining recommendations for community-based children's mental health services

Using these strategies, children's mental health coalitions can advocate for a broad range of services, such as pediatric collaborative care programs, substance use education programs, and suicide prevention programs. Psychiatrist leadership is a necessary component of these efforts to ensure that proposals for mental health system reform will be evidence based and developmentally appropriate.

State-Level Advocacy

State-level advocacy efforts have enormous potential to impact policies addressing children's mental health. The ability of experts in child and adolescent mental health to inform state policy makers is critical to the services that children and adolescents receive because many of the programs aimed at improving children's quality of life and health care are state funded. The opportunity to impact these programs must be met with resolve and creativity. The following are some of the opportunities to communicate with state legislators:

- Meeting legislators at town hall meetings or other in-district events
- Meeting with legislators in their district offices and offering to serve as a resource on children's mental health
- Inviting a legislator to visit the local children's mental health facility
- Communicating with lawmakers and their staff regarding a specific bill
- Testifying at a committee hearing
- Hosting an education day or legislative day at the state capitol

Requesting a meeting with your state legislator can serve as the first step in forming a lasting and impactful relationship. As constituents, we are empowered to request a meeting with our representatives by virtue of their obligation to their electorate. Any in-person meeting with a legislator or their staffer is considered a good meeting because the relationship formed during these meetings may lead to requests for consultation on crafting individual pieces of legislation or invitations to testify at state hearings. This relationship is also the foundation on which we can present an "ask," a request to vote for or against a piece of legislation.

In communications with policy makers, sharing data can be effective, but adding a personal story is even more memorable. Personal stories better enable policy makers to understand the perspectives specific to children and families among their electorate. For example, you might share a story about the impact of a local school-based mental health program or the impact of boarding in the local emergency department on an adolescent with a developmental disability and mental illness.

Letter-writing and e-mail campaigns (see section "Advocacy Through Grassroots Efforts" below) are additional effective strategies to reach state representatives. For example, the APA district branches and the AACAP regional organizations can request support from their respective national offices to initiate such a call to action.

Holding education days or legislative days focused on children's mental health at the state capitol are also most successfully brokered by APA district branches in collaboration with AACAP regional organizations. The resources of professional organizations such as these better enable successful scheduling and coordination. These events are effective tools to engage and inform state legislators and can provide opportunities for psychiatrists to be voices for children on a broad range of legislative topics. The events can be organized around a specific topic (e.g., the impact of marijuana on the developing brain) or a specific legislative event (e.g., the start of a new legislative session).

Federal-Level Advocacy

Mental health advocates working directly with federal legislators have been at the forefront of efforts to shape policies that are critical to improving access to care nationwide, including the Mental Health Parity and Addiction Equity Act of 2008 (P.L. 104-204) and the Patient Protection and Affordable Care Act of 2010 (P.L. 111-148). Despite these accomplishments, the need for legislative advocacy at the federal level persists. As psychiatrists working with children and families, we must remain steadfast in our efforts to ensure implementation of parity and continuation of essential health benefits. We must also be knowledgeable about programs specific to children and youth so that we can more effectively advocate for these patients.

A prime example of a successful federal advocacy effort is the Children's Health Insurance Program, or CHIP (www.healthcare.gov/medicaid-chip/childrens-health-insurance-program). This program provides essential health insurance to approximately 9 million middle- and low-income children whose families do not qualify for Medicaid and are otherwise uninsured. CHIP is administered by states according to federal requirements and is funded jointly by states and the federal government. Federal funding must be periodically renewed by Congress. The Medicare Access and CHIP Reauthorization Act of 2015 (P.L. 114-10) extended funding through September 2017.

In October 2017, when funding for CHIP had not yet been renewed, psychiatrists joined with other stakeholders to advocate for continuation of CHIP funding. Multiple strategies were used. APA and other professional organizations voiced their support for CHIP reauthorization as organizational lobbyists met with Congressional leadership. APA and AACAP also rallied the membership of both organizations to engage in a letter-writing and e-mail campaign imploring members of Congress to reauthorize CHIP. Opinion pieces and social media also were used to engage and influence the public.

In January 2018, children and families saw a crucial legislative victory when CHIP funding was secured for an additional 6 years. In February 2018, Congress also passed a budget bill that included provisions for an additional 4 years of funding for CHIP, resulting in a total of 10 years of insurance coverage for nearly 9 million youth. As mental health advocates, we were reminded of the importance of using our collective voices and of the impact of organized advocacy efforts.

Issues pertaining to children's mental health are increasingly in the national spotlight. The opioid epidemic, rates of suicide among youth, and the experiences of immigrant children are just several of the issues that must be addressed. When stakeholders organize and work together in coalitions, we can share resources to more efficiently engage lawmakers. We can break through partisan politics and build consensus as we confirm that the health of our children is a priority. Legislators recognize that coalitions represent an alliance of stakeholders constituting a significant portion of their constituency. This type of organized advocacy is compelling.

Psychiatrists interested in participating in federal advocacy efforts are invited to contact one of the many professional medical organizations or consumer advocacy organizations that champion children's mental health issues. These include, but are not limited to, APA, AACAP, the American Medical Association, the American Academy of Pediatrics, the National Alliance on Mental Illness, and the National Federation of Families for Children's Mental Health. One specific opportunity from APA is highlighted in Box 11–1.

Box 11–1: APA Congressional Advocacy Network

As mental health advocates, our efforts should not be limited to one day. We can be most impactful in our advocacy efforts if we take time to build constituent relationships with our representatives and our senators. APA has developed a specific program, the Congressional Advocacy Network (CAN), to assist with this goal. CAN advocates serve as key contacts for their members of Congress so that when an important issue arises, APA can quickly get its message to members of Congress. Psychiatrists are given tools, including policy fact sheets and talking points, and asked to set up meetings with their members of Congress. The goal is for more members of Congress to have a relationship with psychiatrists so the representatives better understand the issues facing our profession and our patients and their families.

Advocacy Through Grassroots Efforts

Grassroots advocacy refers to the actions of individuals in the general public to enact change, or to influence members of government to effect change, for a given policy or legislative action. Unlike *grasstops advocacy*, which focuses on engaging those who already have influence with or connections to policy makers, grassroots advocacy focuses on making use of "boots on the ground," such as a legislator's constituents, to engage lawmakers. Grassroots advocacy is an indispensable tool for creating change at all levels of government. For example, consider the power of an organized e-mail campaign, such as those commonly sponsored by psychiatric professional organizations, that enables hundreds of psychiatrists to contact their representatives in support of bills that positively impact mental health care (e.g., the letter-writing and e-mail campaign for CHIP reauthorization described in the previous section). Campaigns of this nature allow our collective voices to be heard with a surround-sound effect, which can make a crucial difference in attempts to effect change or compel those in power to enact change.

Individually driven advocacy efforts can face numerous challenges, chief among which is often the limitation of having only one voice. Grassroots advocacy and its potential impact encompass what is arguably the most critical component of advocacy: power in numbers. Because currently practicing child and adolescent psychiatrists, as well as psychiatrists in general, are in short supply, advocacy efforts that use our combined voices effectively are of paramount importance. When we as psychiatrists step outside our offices, we become part of the community and part of the grassroots network. Psychiatrists working with children and families in the grassroots context have the opportunity to join with community partners to advocate for system reform that ensures access to evidence-based, child-focused, family-centered treatment.

Advocating With Patients and Families

The potential for change is dramatically impacted by the involvement of patients and/or their family members as active role players in advocacy. As constituent psychiatrists, we represent a subset of the constituents to which legislators are beholden; however, there is no substitute for the impact of patients' and families' personal stories during the process, which is often profound and difficult to put into words. The impression left by a youth or parent advocate not only is memorable but also serves to educate legislators about the real-life consequences of current policies, as well as to motivate legislators and stakeholders to remain steadfast in efforts to find bipartisan support for policies that are evidence based and sustainable. As psychiatrists working with children and families, we can translate neuroscience and clinical research data in a way that makes this material accessible and relevant for legislators, and we can tell patient stories based on our professional experience. However, when psychiatrists work in coalition with other organizations that represent individuals and families affected by mental illness, this can result in even more effective advocacy. Families and youth can share compelling personal stories that serve to engage a more empathic audience. For information on ethical considerations when engaging in advocacy alongside patients and families, see Chapter 1, "What Is Advocacy, and Why Is It Important?"

Advocacy Education During Child Psychiatry Fellowship and Beyond: Where We Are and Where We Can Go

Training in health care and policy advocacy is lacking, to say the least, for physicians in general, let alone for psychiatrists and psychiatric subspecialists such as child psychiatrists. However, the need has never been greater. The current medical systems of care are rapidly growing in complexity across all fields, including those serving child and adolescent patient populations. This increased complexity requires a better-informed and more nuanced approach to health advocacy in order to promote effective change and care delivery. Medical schools have begun to address this recognized need by increasingly adopting advocacy and service-learning curricula, such as community service requirements, exposure to governmental agencies, and interactions with legislators (Croft et al. 2012; Martin and Whitehead 2013), but child and adolescent fellowships and continuing medical education courses have yet to concretely make strides toward addressing the education gap.

Child and adolescent patient populations, as noted earlier in this chapter, are at a comparative disadvantage to other populations in their dependence on proxies to advocate for change. This clear need, in combination with the gap in advocacy-based training, has already been recognized by the field of pediatrics. Pediatricians, their professional organizations, the Milestone Project initiative, and the Accreditation Council for Graduate Medical Education have taken action to adjust their training programs to incorporate modular learning requirements and more detailed language for health care and policy advocacy (Accreditation Council for Graduate Medical Education 2019b; Accreditation Council for Graduate Medical Education, American Board of Psychiatry and Neurology 2017; Lichtenstein et al. 2017). Since changes to pediatric training requirements first went into effect after 1996, a wealth of data has accumulated regarding various implementation strategies and resultant successes (Bensen et al. 2014; Delago and Gracely 2007; Goldshore et al. 2014; Schwarz et al. 2015). Much can be learned from the years of data thus gathered to inform advocacy training for child and adolescent psychiatrists.

Currently, child and adolescent fellowships have no requirements for modular learning experiences in advocacy beyond generalized recommendations that graduating trainees should be able to advocate for the prevention of disease and for quality care systems (Accreditation Council for Graduate Medical Education 2019a; Accreditation Council for Graduate Medical Education, American Board of Psychiatry and Neurology 2017). Despite the expressed desire for this training by practicing child and adolescent psychiatrists and trainees, as well as the existence of academic papers proposing advocacy training language and strategies to address the education gap (Accreditation Council for Graduate Medical Education 2019a; Dingle and Stuber 2008; Sexson 2007), there have been no significant en masse efforts for change in fellowship training. With the acknowledged need for change, where do we begin to make adjustments? The most obvious strategy would require altering training requirements for child and adolescent fellowship programs using the data and examples set by pediatric training programs over nearly two decades. Additionally, changes could be made to provide more advocacy-focused education in general psychiatry residency programs as well as advocacy-related continuing medical education courses to psychiatrists who work with children and families. More information on advocacy educational curricula, including the data to support them and potential paths forward, can be found in Chapter 8, "Education as Advocacy."

Conclusion

Psychiatrists working with children and families must take active roles in advocacy at all levels, including clinical practice; consultation to schools, community agencies, and child-serving systems; and legislative advocacy at local, state, and federal levels. Expanded advocacy training and mentorship to residents, fellows, and practicing psychiatrists is necessary to improve on our advocacy skills and thereby allow us to communicate more effectively with legislators and policy makers. With these skills, we can focus on building constituent relationships and engaging legislators on issues that are unique to children's mental health.

There are many opportunities for psychiatrists to work as individuals to advocate for children and adolescents, but working collectively is far more impactful. The benefits of organized advocacy efforts through the APA and AACAP, in collaboration with other stakeholder organizations, cannot be understated. These groups provide a wealth of resources, long-standing relationships with legislators, and educational tools that have proven effective in aiding with the implementation of advocacy-driven efforts. Ultimately, participating in organized advocacy efforts and joining children's health coalitions will amplify our voices so that we may successfully advocate for health care policies that will ensure access to evidence-based, child-focused, family-centered treatment.

References

Accreditation Council for Graduate Medical Education: Requirements for Graduate Medical Education in Child and Adolescent Psychiatry (Subspecialty of Psychiatry). Chicago, IL, Accreditation Council for Graduate Medical Education, 2019a. Available at: https://www.acgme.org/Portals/0/PFAssets/ProgramRequirements/405_ChildAdolescentPsychiatry_2019_TCC.pdf?ver=2019-03-28-161025-277. Accessed August 25, 2019.

Accreditation Council for Graduate Medical Education: Program requirements for medical education in pediatrics. Chicago, IL, Accreditation Council for Graduate Medical Education, 2019b. Available at: www.acgme.org/Specialties/Program-Requirements-and-FAQs-and-Applications/pfcatid/16/Pediatrics. Accessed August 25, 2019.

Accreditation Council for Graduate Medical Education, American Board of Psychiatry and Neurology: The Pediatric Milestones Project. Chicago, IL, Accreditation Council for Graduate Medical Education, July 2017. Available at: www.acgme.org/Portals/0/PDFs/Milestones/PediatricsMilestones.pdf. Accessed August 19, 2019.

Bensen R, Roman H, Bersamin M, et al: Legislative advocacy: evaluation of a grand rounds intervention for pediatricians. Acad Pediatr 14(2):181–185, 2014 24126045

Croft D, Jay SJ, Meslin EM, et al: Perspective: is it time for advocacy training in medical education? Acad Med 87(9):1165–1170, 2012 22836845

Delago C, Gracely E: Evaluation and comparison of a 1-month versus a 2-week community pediatrics and advocacy rotation for pediatric residents. Clin Pediatr (Phila) 46(9):821–830, 2007 17641116

Dingle AD, Stuber ML: Ethics education. Child Adolesc Psychiatr Clin N Am 17(1):187–207, xi, 2008 18036486

Goldshore MA, Solomon BS, Downs SM, et al: Residency exposures and anticipated future involvement in community settings. Acad Pediatr 14(4):341–347, 2014 24906986

Lichtenstein C, Hoffman BD, Moon RY: How do U.S. pediatric residency programs teach and evaluate community pediatrics and advocacy training? Acad Pediatr 17(5):544–549, 2017 28254496

Martin D, Whitehead C: Physician, healthy system: the challenge of training doctor-citizens. Med Teach 35(5):416–417, 2013 23444894

National Alliance on Mental Illness: Mental health by the numbers. Arlington, VA, National Alliance on Mental Illness, 2018. Available at: www.nami.org/learn-more/mental-health-by-the-numbers. Accessed August 25, 2019.

National Institute of Mental Health: Prevalence of any mental disorder among adolescents. Bethesda, MD, National Institute of Mental Health, 2017. Available at: www.nimh.nih.gov/health/statistics/mental-illness.shtml. Accessed December 12, 2019.

National Institute of Mental Health: Children and mental health. Bethesda, MD, National Institute of Mental Health, 2018. Available at: www.nimh.nih.gov/health/publications/children-and-mental-health/index.shtml. Accessed December 12, 2019.

Njoroge WF, Hostutler CA, Schwartz BS, et al: Integrated behavioral health in pediatric primary care. Curr Psychiatry Rep 18(12):106, 2016 27766533

Schwarz K, Sisk B, Schreiber J, et al: A common thread: pediatric advocacy training. Pediatrics 135(1):7–9, 2015 25535264

Sexson SB: Overview of training in the twenty-first century. Child Adolesc Psychiatr Clin N Am 16(1):1–16, vii, 2007 17141115

12

Advocacy for Older Adults

Melanie Scharrer, M.D.
Gary Epstein-Lubow, M.D.
Ilse R. Wiechers, M.D., M.P.P., M.H.S.

Learning Objectives

By the end of this chapter, readers will be able to:

- Understand the urgent need for psychiatrists to advocate for older adults, given the significant projected rise in the geriatric population coupled with geriatric mental health workforce shortages

- Identify clinical, social, and environmental factors that impact older adults' mental health, their health care delivery, and their quality of life

- Explore key health care systems issues and health policy factors that place older adults at increased risk for psychiatric syndromes and poor quality of life

- Explore opportunities to engage in advocacy for older adults

The Imperative for Advocacy for the Geriatric Population

The United States is an aging nation. Older adults represent a large portion of the U.S. population today, and the U.S. Census Bureau (2018) estimates that 1 in 5 Americans will be age 65 or older in 2030. The growing health care needs of older adults and the difficulties our current system faces in meeting those needs have been clearly laid out in multiple reports by the Institute of Medicine (2008, 2012) (the IOM was renamed the Health and Medicine Division of the National Academies of Sciences, Engineering, and Medicine in 2016).

All psychiatrists will encounter older adults in their practices, either as patients or as integral parts of other patients' lives. Specialties that have typically not engaged regularly with older adults, such as forensics (Carson and Sabol 2016), addiction (Mattson et al. 2017), and child psychiatry (Roberts et al. 2016; U.S. Census Bureau 2017) will also encounter the geriatric population with increasing frequency as the country's demographics continue to shift.

In this chapter, we follow the hypothetical case of one older adult, Ms. X, as she and her family navigate multiple systems and challenges. The situations faced by this patient—including depression, isolation, health care costs, disability, and end-of-life concerns—are typical for many older adults. At the end of each section, we provide examples of advocacy opportunities. From shower poles to voting polls, opportunities to support older adults are within reach for policy advocates who know where to look.

Case Example: Ms. X's Need for Advocacy

Ms. X is an 85-year-old Hmong woman who arrives at the local free clinic accompanied by her daughter and son-in-law. Her son-in-law states, "She stopped cooking and gardening." Her daughter shares that her mother accuses others of stealing things and now rarely leaves the apartment, although she used to be very involved with her community. Ms. X's daughter insisted on the appointment after her mother woke from another nightmare, crying and stating she wished she had died in Laos. Ms. X's daughter also reports that her mother was recently brought home by police after bystanders called in unsafe driving behaviors.

Ms. X appears anxious and frightened in the clinic. She agrees to allow her daughter and son-in-law to participate in all of the conversations with clinical staff, and she declines to be interviewed alone despite the physcian's offer to seek an interpreter (who would be difficult to locate) or use a telephone-based translation system (which would be complex for Ms. X to use because of a hearing impairment and her unfamiliarity with technology).

> ### Case Example: Ms. X's Need for Advocacy *(continued)*
>
> With her daughter and son-in-law present, Ms. X denies all symptoms of depression or anxiety and also denies any memory concerns. Ms. X denies any difficulties with activities of daily living or independent activities of daily living. However, her daughter states that because her mother began getting lost on short trips to the grocer's, she or her sisters visit daily to bring groceries. They also prepare meals, clean, and provide reassurance to their mother. Lately, Ms. X has required help changing her clothing and showering.
>
> A depression-screening questionnaire reveals moderate symptoms. A cognitive screening test conducted in English reveals moderate symptoms. Careful questioning about paranoid thoughts, hallucinations, or other psychotic symptoms shows only the concerns about "stolen" objects and the experiences of "nightmares," which clearly are reports from experiences while asleep. A visual screening test reveals significant impairments.
>
> The physician asks whether Ms. X would like to speak with a social worker to identify a health care power of attorney and sign up for Medicare and/or Medicaid, but she declines and goes home with her family.

Medicare and Medicaid

When most people think about health insurance for older adults, they think of Medicare. However, Medicaid also plays a significant role for many older Americans (Table 12–1). In recent estimates, about one-fifth of Medicare patients are dual-eligible for Medicaid (Table 12–2), representing just over about 12 million patients (Kaiser Family Foundation 2017a; Medicaid.gov 2019). For this and other reasons discussed further below, it is important to think about opportunities to advocate for policy change in both programs, working toward the goal of improving care for older adults with substance use disorders, cognitive disorders, and other mental health problems.

Patients who receive Medicare are predominantly, but not exclusively, older than age 65 (17% of recipients are patients younger than age 65 who have permanent disabilities). At least half of Medicare patients are also on a fixed, low income with minimal savings, and about

TABLE 12–1. Key eligibility and coverage provided by Medicare and Medicaid

	Description
Medicare	Federally funded and federally administered
	Eligibility: people age 65 or older, younger people with disabilities, and people with end-stage renal disease
Part A	Pays for hospitalization costs, hospice, home health, and skilled nursing for up to 100 days
Part B	Pays for physician services, laboratory and X-ray services, durable medical equipment, and outpatient and other services
Part C (Medicare Advantage Plan)	Offered by private insurance companies (e.g., an HMO or a PPO) approved by Medicare to provide Part A and Part B benefits
Part D	Assists with the cost of prescription drugs
Medicaid	Joint federal and state program
	Federal law requires coverage for low-income families, qualified pregnant women and children, and individuals receiving Supplemental Security Income
	States can have additional options for coverage
Medicaid coverage of specific interest for older adults	Covers nursing facility care beyond the 100-day limit or skilled nursing facility care that Medicare covers, prescription drugs, eyeglasses, and hearing aids

Note. HMO=health maintenance organization; PPO=preferred provider organization.

one-third have more than five chronic conditions. More than one-third of Medicare patients have impairments in at least one activity of daily living and/or report cognitive or memory impairments (Kaiser Family Foundation 2017a).

Whereas Medicare Parts A and B are federally administered, Part C's services and coverage vary across states and insurance carriers. Park et al. 2017) reported that Medicare Advantage Plans have increased co-payments for services or pharmaceuticals and decreased provider pools for poorly reimbursed services, such as substance use treatment and other mental health care, and home care services. Many patients notice the increase in cost or wait time and disenroll from the insurance, opting for a plan that better meets their individual needs (Montz

TABLE 12–2. **Characteristics of people who are dual-eligible for Medicare and Medicaid**

Sicker (>5 chronic conditions)

More hospital readmissions

Poorer (50% are below federal poverty limit)

More women

More minority patients

More patients with mental illness

More patients lacking high school diploma

More patients in nursing homes

Source.   Kaiser Family Foundation 2017a.

et al. 2016). The end result of these insurer policy decisions appears to be cost-shifting patients with lower reimbursement rates and higher costs from private Part C plans to the federal government's standard Parts A and B coverage.

Medicaid is administered by individual states, and there is high variability from state to state in the eligibility criteria and mental health and substance use service coverage. As a general rule, to be eligible for Medicaid, the households of individuals receiving Medicaid typically must meet certain income requirements, such as earning less than 200% of the federal poverty level (Medicaid.gov 2019). Medicaid is the predominant payer for long-term care, including $55 billion for nursing homes in 2015 (Kaiser Family Foundation 2017b). This means that 6 out of 10 nursing home residents have their care paid for by their state Medicaid program. Thus, policies that impact Medicaid funding have the potential to impact available funding for the majority of patients receiving long-term care.

The Centers for Medicare and Medicaid Services (CMS) collectively oversee both programs. CMS publishes its regulations in Quarterly Provider Updates. A proposed rule or proposed regulation announces CMS's intent to issue a new regulation or modify an existing regulation. CMS solicits public comments on proposed regulations, usually for at least 60 days.

Advocates can stay aware of any upcoming changes to Medicare or Medicaid policy by visiting www.cms.gov, clicking on the regulations and guidance tab, and downloading the quarterly update tab to review proposed changes. Professional organizations such as the American

Psychiatric Association and American Medical Association, among others, regularly monitor changes in CMS regulations and may notify members when public comments are being solicited. Responding to the call for public comments, either as an individual or in coordination with a professional society, is one way for psychiatrist-advocates to have an impact on policy affecting their older adult patients. Table 12–3 includes advice for responding to a call for public comments.

Social Isolation and Loneliness

Loneliness is the discrepancy between desired and actual social contacts. Poorer, sicker, and widowed or separated adults are at highest risk for loneliness. Isolation risk increases as physical or psychiatric health comorbidities increase. About one-third of all older adults report loneliness (AARP 2010).

The Older Americans Act of 1965 (P.L. 89-73) supports a range of home- and community-based services, including congregate meals and home-delivered meals (e.g., Meals on Wheels), preventive health outreach, Elder Rights, and the Senior Corp Program (SCP). Elder Rights funds Adult Protective Services and Elder Justice Initiatives, which work to protect vulnerable older Americans from fraud and abuse. The SCP coordinates and supports older volunteers, who stay active serving frail older adults and other community members. Many of these programs and other important senior programs are administered through local Area Agencies on Aging or Aging and Disability Resource Centers.

Although the Older Americans Act Reauthorization Act of 2016 (P.L. 114-144) provided an extension of funding through fiscal year 2019 and short-term extensions have provided continued funding through mid–calendar year 2020, funding beyond that time remains uncertain (U.S. Congress 2016). Over the past several decades, however, federal funding has not kept pace with the expanding population of older adults or with inflation. The Leadership Council of Aging Organizations estimates that in order for Older Americans Act funding to simply catch up with the growth in the older adult population, its appropriation would have to be increased by at least 12% each year for several years (Leadership Council of Aging Organizations 2019; National Committee to Preserve Social Security and Medicare 2018).

Opportunities for advocacy to address social isolation and loneliness start at the patient level, with the need for psychiatrists to become aware of local community resources that support older adults' social engage-

TABLE 12–3. **Tips for posting public comments on CMS regulations**

Refer to the regulation title and the Centers for Medicare and Medicaid Services (CMS) number listed at the beginning of the regulation

Indicate whether you are for or against the proposed regulation or some part of it and explain why

Use reasoning, logic, and good science to support your proposal

Include a copy of any relevant references that support your comments

ment. One useful resource is the Eldercare Locator (available at https:// eldercare.acl.gov or by calling 1-800-677-1116), which is a public service of the U.S. Administration on Aging that connects people with services for older adults and their families on the basis of zip code or city and state. Patients and families can benefit from education about the value of social engagement to support well-being. Legislative advocacy for geriatric populations should include talking with local and federal elected officials and their staff about the importance of supporting resources for older adults. This is particularly pertinent for representatives or senators serving on the House or Senate Appropriations Committees, especially the Subcommittee on Labor, Health and Human Services, Education, and Related Agencies.

Caregivers

Family and friend caregivers are a "shadow workforce, acting as geriatric case managers, medical recordkeepers, paramedics, and patient advocates to fill dangerous gaps in a system that is uncoordinated, fragmented, bureaucratic, and often depersonalized" (Bookman et al. 2007). Caregiving can be extremely time-intensive and emotionally demanding, and caregivers often have little support and also have other work and personal obligations (Table 12–4). A study of more than 5,500 caregivers of people with dementia found that 32% met criteria for depression (Covinsky et al. 2003). Caregivers of people with angry or aggressive behavioral disturbances and those who spent more time caregiving were more likely than others to experience depression (Covinsky et al. 2003).

Increasingly, some caregivers find their demands split between caring for older adults and for children or even grandchildren. Estimates suggest that up to 47% of adults ages 40–59 and 42% of Generation Xers are sandwiched between caregiving for parents age 65 or older and

TABLE 12–4. Facts about caregiving in the United States

Roughly 14.3% of all American adults are a caregiver to someone age 50 or older (39.8 million Americans)

The breakdown for recipients of caregiving is as follows:
50% parent or parent-in-law
12% spouse
23% another relative
15% nonrelated friend or neighbor

Females make up 60% of caregivers

Caregiving for a spouse/partner is particularly time-intensive (averaging 44.6 hours/week)

Only half of caregivers report feeling as if they had a choice in providing the care

Fewer than half of caregivers say they receive help from another unpaid caregiver

About one-third of caregivers report their loved one gets paid help from personal aides or housekeepers

About one-third of caregivers report no help at all—paid or unpaid

Higher-hour caregivers and those caring for a spouse receive even less help, with 57%–78% reporting no help

Six in 10 caregivers report being employed and working an average of more than 30 hours/week outside of their caregiving duties

Most caregivers report workplace issues as a result of caregiving, such as cutting back on their working hours, taking a leave of absence, and/or receiving a warning about work performance or attendance

Source. AARP 2015.

raising or financially supporting children (Parker and Patten 2013). It is unclear how many of the 1.5 million grandparents currently serving as primary caregivers for their grandchildren are also providing care for spouses or other aging family members (U.S. Census Bureau 2017).

The National Family Caregiver Support Program (funded by the Older Americans Act) helps caregivers to become more informed about available services and helps older people needing care to gain access to these services. The program also can link caregivers to individual counseling, support groups, and training to provide safer care in the home. In some instances, the program can help modify the residence or provide adaptive equipment. Unfortunately, the demand for this support far exceeds the availability of services, with a reported 40% of area aging agencies maintaining waiting lists for these services (Lewin Group 2016). Since 2009, the U.S. Administration on Aging has provided competitive grants to implement state-administered Lifespan Respite Care Programs, which are designed to help families access respite resources and afford to pay respite caregivers; currently, these programs are available in only 37 states (Administration on Aging 2016; Administration for Community Living 2019).

By advocating for caregivers, we are advocating for our older adult patients who are the recipients of that care. Family-level opportunities for advocacy should focus on connecting caregivers with local resources for support. Psychiatrist-advocates can work within their own health care organization to ensure that it provides caregiver support services for both patients and employees. On the Administration for Community Living's (ACL) website (https://acl.gov), advocates can find opportunities for public input on policies and interventions impacting older adults and their caregivers. The ACL also has e-mail updates, which can be tailored to target specific areas of advocacy interest. Psychiatrist-advocates interested in legislative advocacy can focus on discussing the National Academies of Sciences, Engineering, and Medicine (2016) caregiver policy recommendations with local, state, and federal representatives (Table 12–5).

Older Adults With Visual and Hearing Impairments

In the case example, Ms. X's visual and hearing losses compounded the challenges of her initial presentation for care. Vision is currently the leading cause of age-related disability. Worldwide, 285 million people are visually impaired, and much of this disability is preventable. Acquired vision loss has severe personal, social, and economic consequences, extending beyond the patient to family members and caregivers (International Federation on Ageing 2013). Although Medicare covers corrective vision surgeries, such as artificial lens replacement in cataracts, corrective lenses are covered only after the surgery has been completed, not before. Additionally, visual screening and ophthalmologic exams are not covered for all recipients but rather are limited to those with diabetes, glaucoma, or macular degeneration (Medicare.gov 2019).

Although data show that the prevalence of hearing loss in the United States continues to increase with age, hearing aids are not covered un-

TABLE 12–5. National Academies of Sciences, Engineering, and Medicine caregiver policy recommendations

In 2016, the National Academies of Sciences, Engineering, and Medicine reviewed the role of family caregivers in aging and published the following recommendations:

- Develop, test, and implement effective mechanisms within Medicare, Medicaid, and the U.S. Department of Veterans Affairs to ensure that family caregivers are routinely identified and that their needs are assessed and supported in the delivery of health care and long-term services and supports

- Direct the Centers for Medicare and Medicaid Services to develop, test, and implement provider payment reforms that motivate clinicians to engage family caregivers in delivery processes across all modes of payment and models of care

- Strengthen the training and capacity of health care and social service providers to recognize and engage family caregivers and to provide evidence-based supports, including referrals to services in the community

- Increase funding for programs that provide explicit supportive services for family caregivers to facilitate the development, dissemination, and implementation of evidence-based caregiver intervention programs

- State governments that do not have caregiver support programs should implement them

- Explore, evaluate, and, as warranted, adopt federal policies that provide economic support for working caregivers

- Expand the data collection infrastructures within the U.S. Departments of Health and Human Services, Labor, and Veterans Affairs to facilitate monitoring, tracking, and reporting on the experience of family caregivers

- Establish a public-private, multi-stakeholder innovation fund for research and innovation to accelerate the pace of change in addressing the needs of caregiving families

- Launch a multi-agency research program sufficiently robust to evaluate caregiver interventions in real-world health care and community settings, across diverse conditions and populations, and with respect to a broad array of outcomes

Source. National Academies of Sciences, Engineering, and Medicine 2016.

der traditional Medicare plans. Research shows worsening delirium and dementia outcomes for patients with uncorrected hearing or visual impairments, and some advocates have argued that it is time to revisit the U.S. Preventive Services Task Force recommendations for the screening of older adults (du Feu and Fergusson 2003; Whitson and Lin 2014).

Psychiatrist-advocates for older adults can engage in patient-level advocacy by educating patients and their caregivers on the health and safety risks of untreated sensory impairments and by regularly screening for sensory impairment among patients. At an organizational level, advocates can work to encourage standardized screening for sensory impairment and address barriers to correcting impairments, especially in inpatient care settings, in which the organization has greater control over policies, resources, and services directly provided to patients. Legislative advocacy can focus on educating state and federal officials about the importance of supporting primary prevention, standardized screening, and early intervention to address sensory impairments.

Driving and Older Adults

Although many older adults continue to drive safely in their communities, some hesitate to limit or discontinue driving even in the face of worsening disability. Ms. X became lost in a familiar area before her family intervened to limit her driving. For older adults who do not have access to reliable public transportation or who lack the physical and cognitive capacity to successfully navigate public transportation, options can be limited.

Individual states have different policies for how frequently licenses may be renewed, whether they must be renewed in person, and when visual testing occurs. Eighteen states have relatively short renewal periods and require more frequent vision screening for older drivers; 16 states and the District of Columbia do not allow license renewal by mail for older drivers; the District of Columbia requires a physician's approval for drivers age 70 and older to renew their licenses; and Illinois requires applicants age 75 and older to take a road test at every renewal (Insurance Institute for Highway Safety, Highway Loss Data Institute 2019). For older adults who no longer drive, the Federal Transit Administration's Section 5310 Program and Title III B of the Older Americans Act are important sources of funding for accompanied ride programs and some medical transport (National Aging and Disability Transportation Center 2018).

Patient-level advocacy in this area includes psychiatrists regularly asking older patients and their caregivers about driving safety during clinical evaluations. Advocates should be aware of state laws and institutional policies when it comes to licensing and physician roles in reporting potentially impaired drivers. Depending on your state, there may be opportunities for state-level advocacy to improve existing age-related driving laws and regulations. Legislative advocacy can focus on maintaining and expanding access to transportation for older adults who no longer drive.

Stigma and Suicide in Older Adults

Case Example: Ms. X's Emergency, Treatment, and Release

Within a week of Ms. X's initial visit, she is taken to the emergency department (ED) by emergency medical services after she tried to harm her daughter at home with a kitchen knife. The ED evaluation is completed with an interpreter, and it is clear that Ms. X is reporting current active thoughts that are paranoid and suicidal. This is explained to her family, and Ms. X is involuntarily hospitalized on a psychiatric unit.

During the first overnight on the psychiatric unit, Ms. X has a fall that results in a hip fracture, and she is transferred to the orthopedic service. In the surgical setting, Ms. X tries to get out of bed and leave the hospital. The orthopedic team consults the hospital's consultation-liaison psychiatry service for a decisional capacity evaluation and for recommendations on management of psychiatric symptoms.

The psychiatry consultant assesses Ms. X and determines that she has delirium and lacks capacity at the current time to make most medical decisions. Ms. X's daughter is provided with education, including strategies to help Ms. X feel safe in the hospital setting. Over time and with attentive pain management and judicious use of opioids, the delirium slowly clears, the paranoia and suicidal thoughts resolve, and Ms. X is discharged to the care of her daughter at home, with recommendations for in-home physical and occupational therapy and home health support from a visiting nurse.

> ### Case Example: Ms. X's Emergency, Treatment, and Release *(continued)*
>
> In contrast, Ms. S, a geriatric patient across the hall from Ms. X, receives the same discharge instructions following hip fracture repair. She and her husband have supplemental insurance and health savings accounts that somewhat offset the high cost of health care. In addition to having Social Security retirement benefits, both Ms. S and her husband draw on pensions. As white American citizens, Mr. and Ms. S were able to obtain federal housing loans to buy property that has appreciated in value during the course of their lifetimes. To increase accessibility, the couple renovate their home and invest in adaptive technology and assistive devices. This reduces the risk of accidents and helps the couple remain as independent as possible.

According to the Suicide Prevention Resource Center (2017), "older adults are not inclined to seek mental health services due to social, cultural, and financial reasons." Older adults are less likely to access mental health services for many reasons, including general stigma about mental illness; fear of others' perceptions regarding their loss of mental capacity; worries about limitations on their right to own a firearm, drive a car, or continue working; and worry about involuntary admission to a psychiatric hospital. Because of stigma and stoicism, older adults are less likely than younger individuals to call a traditional suicide hotline, and most would not identify their problem as a "crisis" (Institute on Aging 2019).

Even for skilled clinicians, depression can be difficult to detect when patients have multiple chronic conditions. Depression may be assumed to be a natural part of aging, leading to underdiagnosis and undertreatment. Currently, mental health services are rarely integrated into non–mental health settings, including aging services. Increasing access to mental health care and screening at more common points of care for older adults could reduce the burden of unrecognized, untreated mental illness. Preventing suicide means meeting older adults where they are, rather than expecting them to go to mental health clinicians for assistance.

Shifting the focus of examination from illness to wellness may also improve identification of older adults at risk. One example of this shift of focus is the Institute on Aging's 24-hour phone line for older adults; since 1973, the Friendship Line (1-800-971-0061) has provided support for older adults, including outreach calls to check on well-being.

Trained volunteers offer support and assess for grief, loneliness, and suicidal thoughts in their conversations with older adults (Institute on Aging 2019).

Older adults have a higher rate of suicide than the national average. Specifically, Asian women over age 65 have the highest rate of older female suicides (Duldulao et al. 2009), and white males over age 85 have a markedly higher suicide rate, about four times higher than the national average (Canetto 2015). Table 12–6 lists some facts about older adults and suicide.

Because depressed older adults who complete suicide do so with a firearm 67% of the time (Administration on Aging, Substance Abuse and Mental Health Services Administration 2012), asking older adult patients and their families about firearm safety and storage is an essential part of the health assessment and is the first step in advocating for older adult safety. Most states have very minimal laws regarding mental health and firearm ownership. As of January 1, 2020, 18 states have passed and implemented "red flag" gun laws allowing a court order to temporarily seize guns from someone who exhibits dangerous behavior (Segers 2019). Older adults with neurocognitive impairments exhibit worse judgment and less impulse control. Patients with delirium can present with paranoia, increasing risks to family and friends if firearms are accessible.

Advocates for older adults can work within their local communities or organizations to implement screening programs for depression in local senior centers, aging and disability resource centers, and primary care offices. Education as advocacy is important because training all staff within organizations that serve older adults to recognize signs and symptoms of depression and other mental health and cognitive problems will result in increased access to much-needed help. Increasing the awareness among health care colleagues about the high risk for suicide in older adult populations can also help save lives.

Legal and Ethical Considerations in Geriatric Mental Health Advocacy

Once a patient is determined to have lost decision-making capacity, procedures vary from state to state as to how surrogate decision makers are appointed or activated. The state of residence and any advance directives completed by the patient determine which decisions the surrogates

TABLE 12–6. Older adults and suicide

Older adults who attempt suicide

- Use deadly methods more frequently (67% use firearms)
- Plan attempts more carefully
- Are discovered and rescued less frequently
- Are less likely to recover from an attempt

Source. Administration on Aging, Substance Abuse and Mental Health Services Administration 2012; Suicide Prevention Resource Center 2017.

are allowed to make for the patient. Difficulties can arise when incapacitated relatives move closer to their caregivers and, in so doing, cross state lines. Advance directives prepared in one state may not be accepted in another state. Guardians' ability to consent to some mental health or medical treatments varies by state as well. Consultation-liaison psychiatrists are often involved in helping work through some of these challenging decisional capacity situations, especially when patients are receiving inpatient medical or surgical care (for more information, see Chapter 18, "Advocacy for Patients in Medical Settings").

Vulnerable older adults have been victimized by both court-appointed and familial guardians (Teaster et al. 2004). Data suggest that 1 in 10 older adults (approximately 5 million Americans) have been exposed to some sort of abuse (Acierno et al. 2010). Vulnerable older adults are also at risk of self-neglect. Abuse and neglect compromise older adults' independence and dignity, threatening their physical safety and financial security.

In 2010, Congress passed the Elder Justice Act as part of the Patient Protection and Affordable Care Act of 2010 (P.L. No 111-148), the first piece of comprehensive legislative authority designed to address and combat abuse, neglect, and exploitation of older adults. Adult protective services provides local and federal advocacy for older adults. The Administration for Community Living, the Older Americans Act, and the National Center on Elder Abuse fund, organize, and train investigative teams. Different states have different mandatory reporting laws for vulnerable adults.

Effective advocates for older adults are always mindful of patient-level advocacy that includes asking specific, targeted questions to identify potential physical, sexual, or financial abuse. This questioning can be challenging, given that this population may face physical, emotional, and cognitive barriers to reporting. A strong patient-level advocate also ensures that patients and caregivers are educated and aware of resources related to advance directive planning. Knowing your state's mandatory reporting laws and who should be notified of a vulnerable adult in a potentially abusive situation is also necessary for good patient-level advocacy.

Social Determinants of Health

Social determinants of health represent the conditions in which people are born, live, and age, and they are the primary factors affecting health inequities. Socioeconomic status is a significant social determinant of health. Low-income older adults are more likely to face hardships such as food insecurity, medication cutbacks, skipped meals, or difficulty paying bills (Levy 2015). More than 25 million Americans age 60 and older are economically insecure, living at or below 250% of the federal poverty level (National Council on Aging 2016).

Social Security remains the primary source of retirement income for most older Americans, accounting for $4 out of every $5 of income for older people with low to moderate incomes (AARP 2012). Social Security tends to benefit married one-earner couples more than single workers or married couples with substantial dual incomes (Liebman 2001). Supplemental Security Income (SSI), which is separate from Social Security retirement benefits, pays monthly benefits to people with limited income and resources who are disabled, blind, or age 65 or older. SSI is available for U.S. citizens or nationals and to people in one of seven categories of "qualified aliens" (see list at www.ssa.gov/ssi/spotlights/spot-non-citizens.htm). For most seniors, the average additional benefit SSI provides is approximately $459/month (www.payingforseniorcare.com/longtermcare/resources/supplemental_security_income.html). For refugees and immigrants, including Ms. X, SSI can be quite difficult to obtain. Many clinicians are unaware of the assistance they can offer their patients in accessing SSI, such as recommending the support of an interpreter or the waiving of the SSI interview altogether for those with more substantial impairments. Even if psychiatrists are aware of the help they could offer, many clinic resources are stretched too thin to provide the support needed to complete the paperwork.

Understanding your older adult patients' socioeconomic status and existing sources of income is vital for successful coordination of care. Advocates can work within their organization to lobby for the resources needed to support patients with SSI applications. Advocates can support efforts at all levels that aim to reduce income inequality and decrease disparities in the social determinants of health. Being aware of any proposed changes to Social Security policies at the federal level is also important for advocates of older adults because this program provides the bulk of financial support for most older Americans. Advocates can also support antidiscrimination laws and work to fight mandatory retirement ages in an effort to help combat ageism.

Although Social Security and SSI benefits remain vital to most older adults, an increasing percentage of older adults are delaying retirement (Johnson 2018). This is likely due to a combined effect of economic insecurity and improved health in old age. It is important to recognize that older adults who continue to work likely face ageism in the workplace, and this can add to stress levels. The World Health Organization (2019) defines *ageism* as "the stereotyping and discrimination against individuals or groups on the basis of their age...including prejudicial attitudes, discriminatory practices, or institutional policies and practices that perpetuate stereotypical beliefs."

Aging in Place

Patients and their families can promote healthy aging at home by adapting their homes to prevent falls and increase accessibility. Local, state, and national programs are available that can support families financially as they make these changes. Ultimately, keeping older adults at home, and injury free, prevents unnecessary hospitalizations or placements at supportive facilities. Psychiatrists working with older adults should screen for safe home environments and encourage intervention when it appears that patients cannot meet their needs in their current environment. Psychiatrists can recognize the individual and community benefits of aging in place. Successful aging in place is not limited to the home. Advocates for older adults can urge community leaders to take steps to create dementia-friendly communities, which can help individuals with cognitive impairments and their caregivers remain active in their neighborhoods. Dementia-friendly communities are villages, towns, cities, or counties that are informed, safe, and respectful of individuals with dementia and their families and caregivers and provide supportive options that help improve quality of life (Dementia Friendly America 2018).

Case Example: Continued Advocacy for Ms. X

Unfortunately, Ms. X is unable to follow the hospital team's discharge recommendations because of a combination of cultural and financial barriers. She is taken back to the ED, rehospitalized, and then transferred to a local skilled nursing facility.

> ### Case Example: Continued Advocacy for Ms. X (continued)
>
> Shortly after being admitted to the facility, Ms. X begins to lose weight. She refuses to eat any of the facility's food. Her family brings food that is familiar, but her appetite has waned significantly. Psychiatric consultation is ordered, but a workforce shortage contributes to a delay in face-to-face assessment. Because of cultural barriers and other factors, Ms. X has difficulty engaging in the skilled rehabilitation, and because of decreased mobility, she develops a pressure ulcer.
>
> The pressure ulcer results in cellulitis, and reduced mobility plus aspiration then lead to pneumonia. Ms. X is rehospitalized, and during this stay, her family arranges care around the clock. She requires placement in the intensive care unit; it is explained to Ms. X and her family that the multiple comorbidities and frailty suggest she may die soon. While this information is sinking in, Ms. X becomes delirious again and consistently states her wish to die at home with traditional treatments.
>
> Because Ms. X has no legal health care proxy, the medical team must spend extra time reengaging psychiatry consultation and speaking with multiple family members. Ultimately, with the help of palliative care, Ms. X is discharged to her home, with family supporting her 24 hours a day. A shaman is contacted, but Ms. X dies before the traditional soul-calling ceremony can be performed. The shaman reassures the family that she will be at peace with the completion of funeral rites.

Many Hands Make Light(er) Work?

Geriatric mental health care workforce shortages are another major contributor to poor outcomes, long waits, and difficulties accessing treatment in a timely and equitable fashion. According to a report by the Institute of Medicine (2012), the U.S. health care system is not prepared to deal with the current mental health and substance use problems facing older adults and is even less prepared to face the increasing needs that the expanding aging population will present.

The scope of the workforce deficit in geriatric psychiatry is daunting in view of the aging demographics. The IOM's 2012 report concludes,

"The breadth and magnitude of inadequate workforce training and personnel shortages have grown to such proportions, that no single approach, nor a few isolated changes in disparate federal agencies or programs, can adequately address the issue. Overcoming these challenges will require focused and coordinated action by all" (Institute of Medicine 2012, p. 285). To meet current needs and prepare for the future, the IOM recommended a series of interventions that focused on coordinating federal efforts to develop and strengthen the workforce, building capacity, conducting additional needed research, funding training and loan-forgiveness programs, and requiring geriatric mental health and substance use competencies for all levels of personnel who care for older adults (Institute of Medicine 2012).

Sadly, many of the IOM's recommendations remain unaddressed today, and this situation provides ripe opportunities for psychiatrists to advocate for older adults by addressing the shortages in geriatric mental health care. Psychiatrist-advocates working in clinical educator roles can advocate within their academic organizations for inclusion of geriatric mental health and substance use competencies in curricula for all manner of health care trainees. One potential legislative advocacy target is medical school loan-forgiveness legislation, ensuring that any legislation regarding forgiveness of loans for medical school or mental health training has broad and inclusive language that includes in its eligibility requirements psychiatrists who complete geriatric subspecialty training.

End-of-Life Care

Addressing end-of-life care issues is an inevitable part of providing care to older adults. Although these issues are not unique to this population, they certainly are more common. Ensuring that patients receive high-quality, person-centered, and family-oriented care at the end of life is paramount. Many opportunities for advocacy exist for psychiatrist-advocates in this area, as highlighted by the recommendations of the IOM report *Dying in America* (Table 12–7). (Institute of Medicine 2014).

There are great opportunities to use education as advocacy with end-of-life care issues because many health care providers as well as patients and their caregivers are poorly informed. Of particular importance is patient- and family-level advocacy that encourages people to develop advance care planning. Understanding the wishes of older adults when they still have the capacity to decide how they wish to be cared for alleviates substantial burden and guilt for loved ones down the road. It also facilitates the speed with which transitions in care at the end of life can take place.

TABLE 12–7. **Key end-of-life recommendations from the Institute of Medicine**

All insurers should cover the provision of comprehensive care for individuals with advanced serious illness who are nearing the end of life

Professional societies should develop standards, and insurers should integrate these standards into assessments, care plans, and the reporting of health care quality

Educational institutions, accrediting boards, and regulatory agencies should establish the appropriate training, certification, and/or licensure requirements to strengthen the palliative care knowledge of clinicians who may encounter patients near the end of life

The government should require insurers to finance medical and social services, consistent with patient goals at the end of life, and should require reporting on quality measures, outcomes, and costs for this care

Community stakeholders should educate members about the care of people with advanced serious illness and encourage advance care planning and informed choice based on individuals' needs and values

Source.   DeStefano and Stith Butler 2014; Institute of Medicine 2014.

Conclusion

The older adult population is growing, and the impacts their needs will have on our health care system in coming years will be profound. Understanding the myriad of policies and health system factors that impact the quality of care received by older adults provides physicians with many avenues for advocacy. However, solutions will not be simple. Older adult patients have complex care needs, and fixing the system to support those needs is also a complex task. As a psychiatrist-advocate working in this space, you will need tenacity and creativity to keep things moving forward, but your persistence will be rewarded. Improvements in care for older adults with substance use and other mental health disorders will create huge positive impacts for patients, communities, and society.

References

AARP: Loneliness in Older Adults: A National Survey of Adults 45+. Washington, DC, AARP, September 2010. Available at: https://assets.aarp.org/rgcenter/general/loneliness_2010.pdf. Accessed August 26, 2019.

AARP: Sources of income for older Americans. Washington, DC, AARP, 2012. Available at: www.aarp.org/content/dam/aarp/research/public_policy_

institute/econ_sec/2013/sources-of-income-for-older-americans-2012-fs-AARP-ppi-econ-sec.pdf. Accessed August 26, 2019.

AARP: Caregiving in the U.S.. 2015 Report. Washington, DC, AARP, June 2015. Available at: www.aarp.org/content/dam/aarp/ppi/2015/caregiving-in-the-united-states-2015-report-revised.pdf. Accessed August 26, 2019.

Acierno R, Hernandez MA, Amstadter AB, et al: Prevalence and correlates of emotional, physical, sexual, and financial abuse and potential neglect in the United States: the National Elder Mistreatment Study. Am J Public Health 100(2):292–297, 2010 20019303

Administration for Community Living: Lifespan Respite Care Program. Washington, DC, Administration for Community Living, 2019. Available at: https://acl.gov/programs/support-caregivers/lifespan-respite-care-program. Accessed August 26, 2019.

Administration on Aging: Older Americans 2016: Key Indicators of Well-Being. Washington, DC, Administration on Aging, 2016. Available at: https://agingstats.gov/docs/LatestReport/Older-Americans-2016-Key-Indicators-of-WellBeing.pdf. Accessed August 26, 2019.

Administration on Aging, Substance Abuse and Mental Health Services Administration: Older Americans behavioral health issue brief 4: preventing suicide in older adults. Washington, DC, Administration on Aging, 2012. Available at: www.sprc.org/sites/default/files/migrate/library/OABH_IssueBrief4PreventingSuicide.pdf. Accessed August 26, 2019.

Bookman A, Harrington M, Pass L, et al: Family Caregiver Handbook: Finding Elder Care Resources in Massachusetts. Cambridge, Massachusetts Institute of Technology, 2007

Canetto SS: Suicide: why are older men so vulnerable? Men and Masculinities 20(1):49–70, 2015

Carson A, Sabol W: Aging of the state prison population, 1993–2013. Bureau of Justice Statistics Special Report. Washington, DC, Office of Justice Programs, U.S. Department of Justice, May 2016. Available at: www.bjs.gov/content/pub/pdf/aspp9313.pdf. Accessed August 26, 2019.

Covinsky KE, Newcomer R, Fox P, et al: Patient and caregiver characteristics associated with depression in caregivers of patients with dementia. J Gen Intern Med 18(12):1006–1014, 2003

Dementia Friendly America: What is DFA? Washington, DC, Dementia Friendly America Network, 2018. Available at www.dfamerica.org/what-is-dfa. Accessed December 29, 2019.

DeStefano L, Stith Butler A: Dying in America: improving quality and honoring individual preferences near the end of life. Washington, DC, National Academies of Sciences, Engineering, and Medicine, September 17, 2014. Available at: http://nationalacademies.org/HMD/Reports/2014/Dying-In-America-Improving-Quality-and-Honoring-Individual-Preferences-Near-the-End-of-Life.aspx. Accessed August 26, 2019.

du Feu M, Fergusson K: Sensory impairment and mental health. Advances in Psychiatric Treatment 9(2):95–103, 2003

Duldulao AA, Takeuchi DT, Hong S: Correlates of suicidal behaviors among Asian Americans. Arch Suicide Res 13(3):277–290, 2009 19591001

Institute of Medicine: Retooling for an Aging America: Building the Health Care Workforce. Washington, DC, National Academies Press, 2008

Institute of Medicine: The Mental Health and Substance Use Workforce for Older Adults: In Whose Hands? Washington, DC, National Academies Press, 2012

Institute of Medicine: Dying in America: Improving Quality and Honoring Individual Preferences Near the End of Life: Brief Report. Washington, DC, National Academies Press, 2014

Institute on Aging: Friendship line. San Francisco, CA, Institute on Aging, 2019. Available at: www.ioaging.org/services/all-inclusive-health-care/friendship-line. Accessed August 26, 2019.

Insurance Institute for Highway Safety, Highway Loss Data Institute: Older drivers: license renewal procedures. Arlington, VA, Insurance Institute for Highway Safety, 2019. Available at: www.iihs.org/topics/older-drivers#driver-license-renewal. Accessed August 26, 2019.

International Federation on Ageing: The high cost of low vision: the evidence on ageing and the loss of sight. Toronto, ON, Canada, International Federation on Ageing 2013. Available at: www.ifa-fiv.org/wp-content/uploads/2013/02/The-High-Cost-of-Low-Vision-The-Evidence-on-Ageing-and-the-Loss-of-Sight.pdf. Accessed August 26, 2019.

Johnson R: Delayed retirement and the growth in income inequality at older ages. Washington, DC, Urban Institute, February 1, 2018. Available at: www.urban.org/research/publication/delayed-retirement-and-growth-income-inequality-older-ages. Accessed August 26, 2019.

Kaiser Family Foundation: An overview of Medicare. Washington, DC, Kaiser Family Foundation, February 13, 2017a. Available at: www.kff.org/medicare/issue-brief/an-overview-of-medicare. Accessed August 26, 2019.

Kaiser Family Foundation: Medicaid's role in nursing home care. Washington, DC, Kaiser Family Foundation, June 20, 2017b. Available at: www.kff.org/infographic/medicaids-role-in-nursing-home-care. Accessed August 26, 2019.

Leadership Council of Aging Organizations: LCAO supports increased funding for OAA programs. Washington, DC, Leadership Council of Aging Organizations, 2019. Available at: www.lcao.org/files/2019/08/LCAO-letter-to-Senate-Appropriations-Committee-and-Subcommittee-on-Labor-HHS-and-Education-and-Subcommittee-on-Transportation-Housing-re-2020-funding-for-aging-services.pdf. Accessed December 19, 2019.

Levy H: Income, poverty, and material hardship among older Americans. RSF 1(1):55–77, 2015 27857982

Lewin Group: Process evaluation of the Older Americans Act Title III-E National Family Caregiver Support Program: final report. Falls Church, VA, Lewin Group, March 2016. Available at: www.acl.gov/sites/default/files/programs/2017-02/NFCSP_Final_Report-update.pdf. Accessed August 26, 2019.

Liebman JB: Redistribution in the current U.S. Social Security system (NBER Working Paper No 8625). Cambridge, MA, National Bureau of Economic Research, December 2001. Available at www.nber.org/papers/w8625. Accessed August 26, 2019.

Mattson M, Lipari RN, Hays C, et al: A day in the life of older adults: substance use facts, in The CBHSQ Report. Rockville, MD, Substance Abuse and Mental Health Services Administration, 2017. Available at: www.ncbi.nlm.nih.gov/books/NBK436750. Accessed Decemer 19, 2019.

Medicaid.gov: Seniors and Medicare and Medicaid enrollees. Baltimore, MD, Centers for Medicare and Medicaid Services, 2019. Available at: www.medicaid.gov/medicaid/eligibility/medicaid-enrollees/index.html. Accessed June 25, 2019.

Medicare.gov: Eye exams. Baltimore, MD, Centers for Medicare and Medicaid Services, 2019. Available at: www.medicare.gov/coverage/eye-exams. Accessed August 26, 2019.

Montz E, Layton T, Busch AB, et al: Risk-adjustment simulation: plans may have incentives to distort mental health and substance use coverage. Health Aff (Millwood) 35(6):1022–1028, 2016 27269018

National Academies of Sciences, Engineering, and Medicine: Families Caring for an Aging America. Washington, DC, National Academies Press, 2016.

National Aging and Disability Transportation Center: Older adults & transportation: unique issues related to older adults and transportation. Washington, DC, National Aging and Disability Transportation Center, 2018. Available at: www.nadtc.org/about/transportation-aging-disability/unique-issues-related-to-older-adults-and-transportation. Accessed December 19, 2019.

National Committee to Preserve Social Security and Medicare: Fiscal year 2018 omnibus appropriations bill includes increased funding for several programs crucial to seniors. Washington, DC, National Committee to Preserve Social Security and Medicare, March 23, 2018. Available at: www.ncpssm.org/documents/social-security-policy-papers/fiscal-year-2018-omnibus-appropriations-bill-includes-increased-funding-several-programs-crucial-seniors. Accessed August 26, 2019.

National Council on Aging: Economic security fact sheet. Arlington, VA, National Council on Aging, 2016. Available at: https://d2mkcg26uvg1cz.cloudfront.net/wp-content/uploads/NCOA-Economic-Security.pdf. Accessed August 26, 2019.

Park S, Basu A, Coe N, Khalil F: Service-level selection: strategic risk selection in Medicare Advantage in response to risk adjustment. NBER Working Paper No 24038. Cambridge, MA, National Bureau of Economic Research, November 2017. Available at: www.nber.org/papers/w24038. Accessed December 16, 2019.

Parker K, Patten E: The Sandwich Generation: rising financial burdens for middle-aged Americans. Washington, DC, Pew Research Center, 2013. Available at: www.pewsocialtrends.org/2013/01/30/the-sandwich-generation. Accessed September 13, 2019.

Roberts A, Ongunwoke S, Blakeslee L, et al: The population 65 years and older in the United States. American Community Survey Reports 2018:ACS–A38, 2016

Segers G: What are "red flag" laws, and which states have implemented them? CBS News, August 9, 2019. Available at: www.cbsnews.com/news/what-are-red-flag-laws-and-which-states-have-implemented-them. Accessed November 4, 2019.

Suicide Prevention Resource Center: Older adults. Waltham, MA, Suicide Prevention Resource Center, September 2017. Available at: www.sprc.org/sites/default/files/spark-talk/JoAnne%20Sirey_keypoints%28REV%29.pdf. Accessed August 26, 2019.

Teaster PB, Dugar T, Mendiondo M, et al: The 2004 survey of Adult Protective Services: abuse of vulnerable adults 18 years of age and older. Alhambra, CA, National Center on Elder Abuse, 2004. Available at: www.napsa-now.org/wp-content/uploads/2012/09/2-14-06-FINAL-60+REPORT.pdf. Accessed August 26, 2019.

U.S. Census Bureau: Grandparents still work to support grandchildren. 2015 American Community Survey. Suitland, MD, U.S. Census Bureau, July 12, 2017. Available at: www.census.gov/library/visualizations/2017/comm/grandparents-support-grandchildren.html. Accessed August 26, 2019.

U.S. Census Bureau: Older people projected to outnumber children for first time in U.S. history. Suitland, MD, U.S. Census Bureau, 2018. Available at: www.census.gov/newsroom/press-releases/2018/cb18-41-population-projections.html. Accessed August 26, 2019.

U.S. Congress: Older Americans Act Reauthorization Act of 2016, Pub. L. No. 144-144. Washington, DC, 114th Congress, 2016. Available at: www.congress.gov/114/plaws/publ144/PLAW-114publ144.pdf. Accessed December 29, 2019.

Whitson HE, Lin FR: Hearing and vision care for older adults: sensing a need to update Medicare policy. JAMA 312(17):1739–1740, 2014 25369486

World Health Organization: Frequently asked questions: ageism. Geneva, Switzerland, World Health Organization, 2019. Available at: www.who.int/ageing/features/faq-ageism/en. Accessed August 26, 2019.

13

Advocacy for LGBTQ Patients

Eric Yarbrough, M.D.

Learning Objectives

By the end of this chapter, readers will be able to:

- Understand the spectrum of sexual orientation and gender identity
- Understand the complex history of LGBTQ people and psychiatry
- Understand basic affirming approaches when working with LGBTQ people
- Understand the impact that society and laws can have on the LGBTQ population

Advocating may be the most important and impactful intervention that a psychiatrist can do for patients who are part of the lesbian, gay, bisexual, transgender, and queer/questioning (LGBTQ) population. By advocating for medications or specialized therapies, as well as for equal rights, respect, and validation, psychiatrists can significantly impact the mental health of a community that continues to face discrimination from many fronts (Pandya 2014). In this chapter, LGBTQ is used as an inclusive term to represent the full spectrum of gender and sexual diversity.

The ability to sit with a patient and normalize their experience without pathologizing aspects of their identity can provide fertile ground for healing. As clinicians, we typically provide evaluation, diagnosis, and treatment to the patients who come to see us. For LGBTQ people, how-ever, it is often the *absence* of a diagnosis regarding diverse identities that can provide the necessary intervention to improve their overall well-being.

This is not to say that LGBTQ people are not in need of psychiatric in-tervention. They generally suffer from the same symptoms as the larger non-LGBTQ population; in fact, they have higher rates of depression, anx-iety, substance use, and suicidal ideation (Levounis et al. 2012). Notably, these higher rates have largely been attributed to the impact of minority stress—being LGBTQ in a non-LGBTQ world (Meyer 2015).

Approaching therapy with LGBTQ patients requires exploring how having a minority identity has impacted them in various aspects of their lives. For example, LGBTQ people frequently experience struggles within their own mind in the form of internalized homophobia and transphobia (see section "Advocating With LGBTQ Patients" below). Furthermore, LGBTQ patients need our advocacy in their struggles for civil rights and access to care and against stigma within their families as well as in religious communities, hospital systems, and other facilities. Finally, these patients need our advocacy at the local, state, federal, and global levels to promote psychotherapeutic approaches that help them and to halt the practice of interventions that harm.

History of LGBTQ People and Psychiatry

LGBTQ people have existed as long as humankind has existed. Evidence of diverse sexual orientations and gender identities is scattered throughout history (Stern 2009). For significant portions of modern history, however, being LGBTQ has been pathologized and criminal-ized, forcing LGBTQ people to live in hiding and keep their identities se-cret. It is only in the past 100 years that an LGBTQ movement has formed, enabling LGBTQ people to emerge safely and reveal their iden-tities without fear of ridicule, incarceration, institutionalization, or even death.

LGBTQ people have a complicated history with psychiatry. From the beginnings of modern psychiatric thought, early psychiatric leaders, such as Sigmund Freud, struggled with whether or not to pathologize di-verse sexual orientations; individuals who fell outside the norm were of-ten thought to be deviant or to possess arrested development (Freud 1923). For the sexual minority (gay, lesbian, and bisexual) portion of the LGBTQ population, it took the pioneering research of Evelyn Hooker

(1957) and advocacy on the part of sexual minority psychiatrists within the American Psychiatric Association—who formed the Caucus of Gay, Lesbian, and Bisexual Members of the American Psychiatric Association in 1973 and then the Association of Gay and Lesbian Psychiatrists in 1985 (Association of Gay and Lesbian Psychiatrists 2019)—to change the categorization of homosexuality as a pathology.

During the American Psychiatric Association's annual meeting in 1972, a brave gay psychiatrist named John Fryer was accompanied by Barbara Gittings and Frank Hamany in a symposium called "Psychiatry: Friend or Foe to the Homosexual? A Dialogue." For this symposium, Dr. Fryer put on a mask, a wig, and padding and disguised his voice out of fear of being censured and fired as a gay psychiatrist. He publicly stated, "I am a psychiatrist, and I am a homosexual" (Clendinen 2003). It was a significant moment in the history of psychiatry and for all sexual minority people because this event helped to spur the American Psychiatric Association's 1973 removal of homosexuality from the list of mental illnesses in the second edition of the *Diagnostic and Statistical Manual of Mental Disorders* (DSM-II; Drescher 2015) and the World Health Organization's removal of homosexuality from its list of diseases in 1990 (Cochran et al. 2014).

Transgender and gender-nonbinary people have only recently been able to see similar classification changes. In DSM-5 (American Psychiatric Association 2013), the diagnosis of gender identity disorder was changed to gender dysphoria (Drescher 2010). This name change sparked significant controversy between two opposing factions within the DSM-5 work group on sexual and gender identity disorders: in an effort to decrease the stigma of gender diversity, one faction advocated for the removal of any diagnostic code from DSM-5, whereas the other faction advocated to keep a diagnostic label in order to maintain access to medical care, which requires diagnostic codes for third-party payment purposes. After spirited advocacy by both sides, the two factions agreed to removal of the word "disorder" and settled on the new diagnosis of gender dysphoria (Drescher 2013). Keeping a diagnostic code has enabled payment by insurers for hormone therapy and other gender-affirming surgical procedures for transgender patients. The hope is that gender dysphoria, which continues to pathologize gender diversity (in contrast, no diagnosis for religious dysphoria or racial dysphoria exists), will eventually be removed from DSM. However, before this occurs, a new third-party payment structure needs to be in place to allow for continued and equal access to gender-affirming medical care.

In some parts of the world, LGBTQ people are now being given the rights to legally marry, raise a family, live out of the closet in society, and receive medical care without discrimination. This is only a recent phenomenon, however, and in many parts of the world, even in the United States, disparities still exist. We are still situated, historically speaking, in the middle of culture wars that continue to debate and define what is within the realm of human experience versus what is pathology. It is on the side of acceptance and validation that the psychiatrist can play a significant role in these battles.

LGBTQ Overview

To advocate for LGBTQ people, one must first understand what the acronym means and how the different identities of the LGBTQ rainbow intersect. The word *queer* is sometimes used as an umbrella term for all LGBTQ people. This is a derogatory term that has been reclaimed by the community as a name that many diverse people use to define themselves.

Sexual orientation is the attraction that a person has toward a particular sex or gender. This attraction can be to the same sex, to the opposite sex, to both sexes, or to neither sex. People used to be classified as either straight or gay. Alfred Kinsey helped the general public understand that there is actually a range of sexual desires, which may or may not line up with romantic desires or even sexual acts (Kinsey et al. 1948/2010).

Straight   Gay

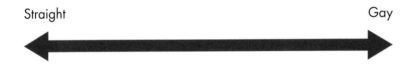

The spectrum of sexual orientation is now known to be multilayered, and every person can have a range of feelings and desires outside of the gay/straight dichotomy. It is probably better to consider that people may be attracted to varying levels of femininity and masculinity. This can include a lack of attraction to both.

Gender also is starting to be understood on a spectrum. *Sex* is something that is defined by a person's genitalia at birth, but *gender* resides in the mind and can exist in a multitude of diverse ways. An informed way to think about gender is not to split it into male or female but to consider instead "how male" and "how female" each person expresses themselves. These definitions are largely culturally defined, and there are variations in what is considered masculine and feminine. There can be different levels of maleness or femaleness within one person. There can also be an absence of both (Yarbrough 2018).

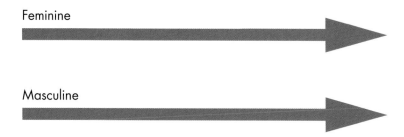

Gender expression, or how someone presents to the outside world, is external. Gender identity, or how a person views themselves, resides within the mind. These need not align with sex, which is defined by the person's genitalia. All of these are also different from sexual orientation (Figure 13–1). These distinctions can be confusing. The simplest way to understand gender and sexuality is that they are individualistic in nature and that we should approach each patient as a unique combination of all these factors. As part of this approach, you can ask patients about their preferred pronouns. Some patients might go by the pronouns he and him or she and her; nonbinary patients may prefer pronouns such as they and them or ze and zir.

Advocating With LGBTQ Patients

The internal struggle of growing up different is a universal experience with LGBTQ people. Some spend the better part of their lives trying to find families and communities that will accept them for who they are. Society has bombarded generations of LGBTQ people with the message that they are abnormal, not wanted, deviant, and even sick. Unless LGBTQ children grow up in an environment that provides support and validation, they may succumb to the experience of many LGBTQ people and experience isolation during their most formative years. This sad but common experience is thought to be one of the reasons for the continued health disparities within the LGBTQ population.

Everyone digests negative messages about diverse groups, and the LGBTQ population is no different. When LGBTQ people accept incorrect and/or harmful information about themselves and then believe that in-

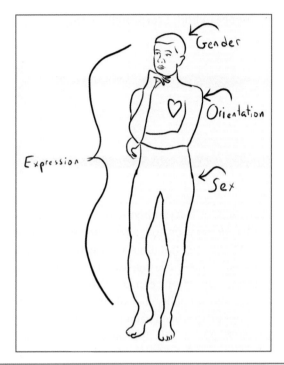

FIGURE 13–1. **Sex, sexual orientation, gender, and gender expression should be thought of as separate characteristics.**

Source. Yarbrough E: *Transgender Mental Health.* Washington, DC, American Psychiatric Association Publishing, 2018, p. 26. Copyright © American Psychiatric Association Publishing, 2018. Used with permission.

formation, this can be described as internalized homophobia and/or internalized transphobia (Drescher 2001). Regardless of how supportive the environment or a particular community is toward them, LGBTQ people still absorb negative information from individuals, groups, and the media. LGBTQ-affirming psychiatrists generally accept that these negative messages over time are at least partly, if not mostly, responsible for the increased levels of suicidal ideation, suicide attempts, anxiety, depression, and substance abuse in the LGBTQ population.

Advocating for LGBTQ people starts with the individual. Psychiatrists are trained to work one on one with patients; this work may include providing various forms of psychotherapy. LGBTQ people require gay-affirming and gender-affirming therapy stances. That is to say, therapeutic interventions should start with the stance that diverse sexual orientations and gender identities are part of the human condition and not a pathology or mental illness. Whatever problems or symptoms a patient may be reporting, it is important that the psychiatrist inform the patient that the process of treatment will help discover and support who they are without attempts to change their identity.

Many LGBTQ people are afraid that psychiatric treatment may force them to change their gender and/or sexual identities because, in many states, clinicians practice conversion therapy. *Conversion therapy* is a dangerously misleading term for a practice that attempts to correct or convert an LGBTQ person's identity to "normal." Conversion therapy attempts to change a person's sexual orientation to heterosexual or their gender identity to cisgender (i.e., back to the sex they were assigned at birth). Outcomes with conversion therapy are poor and can lead to worsening of psychiatric symptoms and even suicide (Schroeder and Shidlo 2002). Patients may need to be reassured that conversion therapy is unethical and, in some states, unlawful and will not be part of their treatment.

Case Example: Conversion Therapy

Adam is an 18-year-old cisgender male who grew up in Utah in a very religious household and who started to realize around the time of puberty that he might be different from his peers. He became more and more aware of his attraction to boys. His parents noticed and sent him to a therapist to attempt to convert his sexual orientation to straight. After a year of therapy, Adam felt increasingly depressed and became suicidal. He decided that he couldn't live in his current situation anymore and would rather either run away or kill himself. He chose the former.

Adam made it to Seattle and lived in a youth shelter. He bonded with other youth there and continued to pursue his education. He is now in college and doing well academically, but he is suffering from depressive symptoms secondary to the social struggles he has endured over the last 5 years.

Adam comes to your office because his friends have convinced him to get help. He reports classic symptoms of depression and is hesitant to disclose his sexual orientation to you. He is worried that you, like the previous therapist, will pathologize him and attempt to "cure" him of his sexual diversity.

With patients like Adam, psychiatrists should inform patients that the goal of therapy is to help them understand who they are and to support them. Psychiatrists need to provide basic psychoeducation around the current understanding of gender and sexuality and to teach LGBTQ patients about internalized homophobia and internalized transphobia. Patients may incorrectly believe that their gender and/or sexual diversity is pathological. Psychiatrists should also be mindful that some LGBTQ people might blame their symptoms on their LGBTQ status. These individuals might believe that if they were not gay or transgender, for instance, they might not have problems with depression, with school, or with work. Their symptoms, however, might be better explained by minority stress. Transgender people, for example, might end up homeless because their families are not accepting of their gender identity, and the emotional strains of isolation and poverty can bring on symptoms of depression. The key is to understand that in many cases, the symptoms are likely caused by society's response to gender-diverse people and not a result of being gender diverse in and of itself. This is the essence of advocacy with the LGBTQ individual.

Patients have grown up with ideas of what their lives might look like in the future. For example, they might have long wanted to get married and have children. Although it may seem obvious to a psychiatrist, LGBTQ patients might not realize that these same dreams are still available to them. Psychiatrists can provide hope and reassurance that a patient's gender or sexual identity will not arrest these lifelong goals. On the other hand, it is also important for psychiatrists to validate that patients have an open road of possibilities beyond what they imagine. It is always the patient who will ultimately decide the direction their life will take.

It is our duty as psychiatrists to provide validation to our patients with diverse sexual orientations and gender identities and to be a part of the supportive and nurturing environment many have not had access to. By experiencing a corrective emotional experience, LGBTQ patients can begin to heal from the unjust scars that have been left on them by the larger invalidating world.

Advocating With Relationships

Internalized homophobia and internalized transphobia frequently surface when psychiatrists work with couples. Although relationships in general come with their own sets of stressors, LGBTQ people might be quick to think their sexual or gender identity is to blame for any relational problems. Many straight couples deal with problems in their relationships, too, but they rarely blame their heterosexuality for these problems. LGBTQ people, however, sometimes blame their identities as a contributing factor. When working with couples, psychiatrists need to be ready to provide psychoeducation and to guide their patients through the murky waters of relationships.

Heterosexual relationships are widely portrayed and endorsed in modern society, and heterosexual people have relationship role models in the form of family members and media portrayals of how a relationship or marriage is supposed to look. Having these examples provides validation to the straight couple that they are experiencing a common human condition and provides reassurance during their times of struggle. LGBTQ people typically do not have access to these same models of behavior. When problems occur in an LGBTQ relationship, there are few references to turn to in order to gauge whether their struggles are reason for concern. Psychiatrists must be careful not to blame the patients' sexual or gender identity as the root cause of conflict in relationships. Paying attention to all of the possible conflicts—the internal conflict, the relationship conflict, and also the larger-world conflict—makes the process of working with LGBTQ couples challenging.

Advocating With Families

Psychiatrists may need to advocate for their LGBTQ patients when it comes to familial relationships. Some families will connect their loved one to psychiatric treatment in the hopes that the loved one will be "cured" of their "homosexual tendencies" or gender diversity. Psychiatrists must remember that the primary relationship of concern is with the patient, not the family, and that navigating family dynamics can be difficult. Parents, in particular, might not be ready to accept the idea that their child is gay, bisexual, or transgender. They might blame their marriage or the child or come up with a host of other factors that have caused the "problem" of diversity.

Providing psychoeducation to families in this situation requires some understanding of motivational interviewing. The psychiatrist needs to assess whether the family is at all ready to consider that the patient might be different and to identify where the family is on the acceptance spectrum. The psychiatrist might need to gently provide information or outside resources to family members and to help educate the family about diversity and acceptance. Parents might need to grieve the loss of the child they had envisioned. Although their dreams of what the future might look like will need to shift, family members can be reassured that their child will be best served when that person's differences are seen as strengths. Organizations such as the Parents and Friends of

Lesbians and Gays (https://pflag.org) can help families better understand and support their LGBTQ loved ones.

Case Example: Support for the Family

Daniel is a 5-year-old boy who is brought to your office by his parents because he is displaying gender-atypical behavior. Daniel likes to keep his hair long and wear female clothing and has friends who are mostly female. When you ask Daniel if he identifies as a boy or a girl, he says he thinks he is a girl, but people keep telling him he is a boy and should act like a boy.

Daniel's parents have heard about transgender people. They are upset because they are worried that if Daniel turns out to be transgender, he will have a difficult life because people won't accept him and he is likely to be bullied. They also are dealing with the realization that their son won't grow up to be the son they thought. They were dreaming that he would have children and carry on the family name (he was named after his father). Daniel's parents had fantasized about how his life would unfold, and his potential gender change would upset their plans.

In addition to providing support to Daniel, you realize that his parents need support as well. Although Daniel is fortunate to have open-minded and supportive parents, his parents still have core beliefs and ideals that may affect Daniel. They might communicate to him in some way their disappointment with his gender identity, which could lead to internal conflicts for Daniel and perhaps even result in symptoms of mental illness down the road.

One of the main ways in which families can help their children of different sexual orientations or gender identities is to be supportive and accepting. Many parents believe they need to do something proactive and help their children "figure out" who they really are. However, identifying a person's gender identity and sexual orientation takes time and may occur over many years. Parents and families of LGBTQ people need to practice listening more than providing advice. Telling a child that they are LGBTQ will not help them with this process. But normalizing LGBTQ people and correcting any misconceptions or feelings of stigma that a child might have can be helpful.

Advocating With Other Clinicians

Patients are rarely treated by only one clinician and are likely to interact with a host of other providers with varying degrees of LGBTQ knowledge. When working with LGBTQ people, it is often necessary for psychiatrists to advocate for their patients with other clinicians. For example, a psychiatrist and a primary care clinician might both be treating a gender-diverse patient when the patient reports wanting to start hormone treatment. Although the primary care clinician may not feel comfortable providing hormones to a transgender patient, the psychiatrist can advocate for the patient by speaking to the primary care clinician and discussing any concerns. The psychiatrist can also refer the primary care clinician to organizations such as the World Professional Association for Transgender Health (WPATH; www.wpath.org), which provides guidelines and suggests medical follow-up when prescribing hormones. In this way, a provider who previously was not comfortable prescribing hormones might become an advocate and provider for transgender people. Taking the time to teach other clinicians about such concepts as minority stress, internalized homophobia and transphobia, and basic gender-affirming practices is part of our duty as psychiatrists.

Advocating with other clinicians also involves information sharing on behalf of patients. For example, a lesbian-identified woman might not feel comfortable sharing her sexual experiences with a primary care clinician, particularly if office visits are brief. A psychiatrist, however, might have more insight into an individual patient's sexual health risk factors due to sexual orientation, identity, or practices. A patient's sexual orientation or gender identity will not dictate their sexual practices; rather, a medical interview should determine sexual health risks by identifying the specifics around which body parts are being used and how they are used. Psychiatrists need to provide both the requisite time and a safe environment for discussion of these sexual practices. With the patient's permission, the psychiatrist can contact the patient's primary care clinician to discuss the ways in which the patient's sexual identity and behavior might affect the need for care and screening.

Advocating With Hospitals

Hospital systems can be slower to change than individual providers when it comes to policies and procedures involving treatment of LGBTQ individuals. Transgender people in particular may avoid going to hospitals to seek care because the environment exacerbates their psychiatric symptoms. Transgender individuals who go to an emergency department for evaluation might experience hostility and discrimination from the staff because of their gender identity. These patients might be misgendered (referred to by the wrong pronoun) or called the wrong name. Some staff might even refuse to work with these patients altogether on the basis of personal views.

Some inpatient clinicians might also be quick to blame a person's LGBTQ identity as the reason for hospitalization. They might claim that a person's sexual orientation is causing lability or that prescribed hormones are causing psychotic symptoms. As clinicians who are in a place to advocate for LGBTQ people, psychiatrists should approach these situations with facts and attempt to educate other clinicians on standards of care. At an organizational level, psychiatrists can advocate for hospital-wide programs to educate clinicians about caring for LGBTQ patients and work with hospital administration to implement procedures based on best practices around the treatment of LGBTQ people.

Advocating Around Religion

Religion can be a deeply personal and meaningful aspect of patients' lives. It can serve as a source of comfort and reassurance and give people a sense of belonging to something larger than themselves. Many religions teach unity, acceptance, and peace—but not necessarily for LGBTQ individuals. Some of the world's most prominent religions condemn homosexuality, and some even consider that homosexuality should be punishable by death.

Some LGBTQ patients struggle with religious perspectives about their gender and sexual diversity and fear that they are somehow "ill" or "flawed." Faith leaders and members may either support these beliefs or challenge them. For instance, it is quite difficult for patients to disagree with their priest if he tells them they are evil for being homosexual and have no future with God. For us as psychiatrists, toeing the line between supporting a patient's faith and providing education on what we know about gender and sexual diversity may be challenging, depending on the patient's sexual/gender identity and religious beliefs. We need to be sensitive and help patients understand that LGBTQ people represent a diverse expression of the human condition and are not mentally ill. At the same time, we should refrain from making assumptions about how patients identify. Labeling a person with a gender or sexual identity is not helpful; instead, we should facilitate the patient's self-exploration and identification. Patients will often experience some level of ambivalence, especially if their identity conflicts with their religion, and we, as psychiatrists, should be prepared to sit with them through these processes.

Advocating With Public Facilities

Public places such as homeless shelters and prisons can be dangerous for LGBTQ people, and in particular for the transgender population. The placement of prisoners is typically up to the management of the facility. The majority of public facilities split up people based on sex, meaning that the gender marker on a person's identification card will dictate whether they are assigned to a male or female section.

Some transgender people may look either masculine or feminine on the basis of social standards. A woman of trans experience—that is, a person assigned male at birth but who identifies as female—may look very feminine according to societal norms but be placed in a male prison because of being labeled as male on their identification card. Appearing feminine but being surrounded by men in a prison environment can be highly stressful and unsafe for the individual.

Although it may seem that the rules of public facilities are out of the hands of psychiatrists, these facilities often look to psychiatrists for guidance. A psychiatrist should communicate with these facilities and advocate for patients' safety. Patients should be asked in which environment they would feel most comfortable and safe. Patients also should have access to the same treatment that others receive. A transgender man, for example, may need access to feminine hygiene products, and staff should be educated about this need. These are just a few of the ways in which a psychiatrist can advocate for safety and encourage facilities to think more broadly when working with gender-diverse people. Communicating clearly and looking at each case on an individual basis will lead to the best outcomes for all involved.

Advocating for Gender-Affirming Medical Care

When working with transgender people, psychiatrists are still actively debating what treatment is acceptable and necessary for symptoms of gender dysphoria. However, access to hormones and surgery has been shown to lead to better mental health outcomes and is supported by the American Psychiatric Association (Drescher and Haller 2012).

Underscoring the unmet need for gender-affirming medical care among transgender people, only a limited number of psychiatric providers are knowledgeable about gender-affirming treatments, and even fewer surgeons are trained to do gender-affirming procedures effectively. In an effort to educate more clinicians, WPATH publishes clinical guidelines on how to work with and evaluate gender-diverse patients (World Professional Association for Transgender Health 2012). The WPATH criteria have been changing as knowledge and understanding about transgender people have grown. In the past, transgender people were required to live as the opposite gender to prove their transgender identity before they could receive hormones or gender-affirming procedures. Now, WPATH has moved toward an informed consent model, in which it is the job of the clinician not to question a person's transgender identity but to make sure that they understand the risks and benefits of medications or procedures before having them.

As psychiatrists, we are in a difficult position of being, in many cases, the gatekeepers to gender-affirming hormone treatment and surgeries. We are often asked to assess a patient's gender identity and say whether the patient is ready for surgery—for example, by writing a letter of support prior to gender-affirming procedures. This situation has hurt the relationship between psychiatrists and transgender people. Our goal should be to assess a person's capacity to make a decision about what is best for them. Transgender people have a growing number of treatment options available to them, and psychiatrists can advocate for their patients by understanding these treatment options and discussing with patients what might be best for them. Beyond the individual patient level, advocacy may include supporting the removal of unnecessary and burdensome barriers to care, such as policies requiring letters of support from mental health providers prior to gender-affirming surgeries.

Some clinicians still think that gender-diverse patients are mentally ill and that gender dysphoria should be treated as a psychosis. Having conversations with these clinicians on behalf of our patients is a necessary role for psychiatrists. In addition, helping our patients get access to gender-affirming procedures may be more helpful than any medication or therapy we could provide.

Advocating in the Larger World

Psychiatrists are in a unique and privileged position to be able to advocate not only for patients but also for individuals in the larger world when it comes to gender and sexual diversity. By removing homosexuality as a disorder from DSM in 1973, members of the American Psychiatric Association communicated to the larger world that they believed homosexuality was a normal human variant. This stance by psychiatrists laid the groundwork for the civil rights legislation that followed, leading to marriage equality in the United States today. However, these civil rights are continuously being challenged. At the time of this writing, for example, gender diversity remains a point of controversy, with continuing debate concerning transgender people in the military and public bathrooms.

Psychiatrists can help protect and strengthen the civil rights of LGBTQ people by educating U.S. lawmakers and the public about gender and sexual diversity. Furthermore, in some countries, homosexuality is a crime punishable by death. Psychiatrists can advocate by connecting with clinicians and government leaders in these nations in order to provide education about gender and sexual diversity. These efforts not only might help the mental health of LGBTQ people, but also could save lives.

One example of an ongoing advocacy effort for LGBTQ people in the larger world is the movement to ban conversion therapy. Major professional organizations, including the American Psychiatric Association, the American Psychological Association, and the American Academy of Child and Adolescent Psychiatry, have repudiated the practice of conversion therapy. In 2015, the Obama administration issued a statement calling for an end to conversion therapies, although this White House edict ended after the election of a new federal administration in 2016. So far, many states, including California, Connecticut, Delaware, Hawaii, Illinois, Maryland, Massachusetts, Nevada, New Hampshire, New Jersey, New Mexico, New York, Oregon, Rhode Island, Vermont, and Washington, have successfully banned the practice of conversion therapy. Continued legislative advocacy by psychiatrists is needed to ensure that this ban extends throughout all 50 U.S. states and U.S. territories. In addition, this ban has raised novel issues for state regulatory agencies, ethics committees, and licensing boards (Drescher et al. 2016), which are grappling with how to sanction practitioners of conversion therapy. Psychiatrist-advocates can work to educate these governing bodies and the public about the harmful effects of conversion therapies.

Conclusion

Advocacy is an integral part of the clinical work of a psychiatrist. LGBTQ patients are in need of people who will advocate for them and validate their experience. Psychiatrists are in a unique position to understand psychopathology and identify what is within the realm of human experience. Diversity of gender and sexual orientation is becoming more understood as existing on a spectrum rather than as a dichotomy. There are as many expressions of the human condition as there are people to express them. When we work with patients, we must look at their entire life experience and attempt to identify places where we can make a difference. Sometimes that involves psychotherapy or medication on the level of the individual patient and systems or legislative advocacy in the larger world. Making a difference also might involve simply telling individuals that they matter, that you see them, and that they are who they are without a need for change.

References

American Psychiatric Association: Diagnostic and Statistical Manual of Mental Disorders, 5th Edition. Arlington, VA, American Psychiatric Association, 2013

Association of Gay and Lesbian Psychiatrists: AGLP history. Philadelphia, PA, Association of Gay and Lesbian Psychiatrists, 2019. Available at: www.aglp.org/pages/AGLPHistory.php. Accessed August 28, 2019.

Clendinen D: Dr. John Fryer, 65, psychiatrist who said in 1972 he was gay. March 5, 2003. Available at: www.nytimes.com/2003/03/05/us/dr-john-fryer-65-psychiatrist-who-said-in-1972-he-was-gay.html. Accessed August 28, 2019.

Cochran SD, Drescher J, Kismodi E, et al: Proposed declassification of disease categories related to sexual orientation in the International Statistical Classification of Diseases and Related Health Problems (ICD-11). Bull World Health Organ 92(9):672–679, 2014 25378758

Drescher J: Psychoanalytic Therapy and the Gay Man. Hillsdale, NJ, Analytic Press, 2001

Drescher J: Queer diagnoses: parallels and contrasts in the history of homosexuality, gender variance, and the diagnostic and statistical manual. Arch Sex Behav 39(2):427–460, 2010 19838785

Drescher J: Controversies in gender diagnosis. LGBT Health 1(1):10–14, 2013 26789504

Drescher J: Out of DSM: depathologizing homosexuality. Behav Sci (Basel) 5(4):565–575, 2015 26690228

Drescher J, Haller E: Position Statement on Access to Care for Transgender and Gender Variant Individuals. Washington, DC, American Psychiatric Association, 2012

Drescher J, Schwartz A, CasoyF, et al: The growing regulation of conversion therapy. J Med Regul 102(2):7–12, 2016 26789504

Freud S: Certain neurotic mechanisms in jealousy, paranoia, and homosexuality. Int Rev Psychoanal 4:1–10, 1923

Hooker E: The Adjustment of the Male Overt Homosexual. Glendale, CA, Society of Projective Techniques and Rorschach Institute, 1957

Kinsey A, Pomeroy W, Martin C: Sexual Behavior in the Human Male (1948). Bronx, NY, Ishi Press International, 2010

Levounis P, Drescher J, Barber M (eds): The LGBT Casebook. Washington, DC, American Psychiatric Publishing, 2012

Meyer I: Resilience in the study of minority stress and health of sexual and gender minorities. Psychology of Sexual Orientation and Gender Diversity 2(3):209–213, 2015

Pandya A: Mental health as an advocacy priority in the lesbian, gay, bisexual, and transgender communities. J Psychiatr Pract 20(3):225–227, 2014 24847996

Schroeder M, Shidlo A: Ethical issues in sexual orientation conversion therapies: an empirical study of consumers. Journal of Gay and Lesbian Psychotherapy 5(3–4):131–166, 2002

Stern K: Queers in History. Dallas, TX, BenBella, 2009

World Professional Association for Transgender Health: Standards of Care, Version 7. East Dundee, IL, World Professional Association for Transgender Health, 2012. Available at www.wpath.org/media/cms/Documents/ SOC%20v7/Standards%20of%20Care_V7%20Full%20Book_English.pdf. Retrieved December 19, 2019.

Yarbrough E: Transgender Mental Health. Washington, DC, American Psychiatric Association Publishing, 2018

14

Advocacy for Immigrants, Refugees, and Their Families

Jennifer Severe, M.D.
Michelle B. Riba, M.D., M.S.
Allan Tasman, M.D., DFAPA, FRCP

Learning Objectives

By the end of this chapter, readers will be able to:

- Understand how immigration status is a social determinant of mental health
- Recognize how foreign-born populations are impacted by implicit bias
- List five or more advocacy actions that reflect an appreciation of cultural competency
- Understand how advocacy through mental health services can help foreign-born patients
- Understand the need for a curriculum on immigration literacy in training programs

The foreign-born population is on an upward trajectory, approximating 1 in 7 residents in 2017 (Figure 14–1) compared with 1 in 11 in

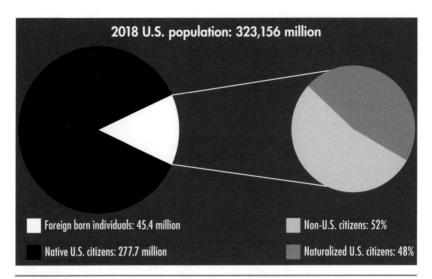

FIGURE 14–1. **U.S. foreign-born population.**
Data manually extracted and calculated by Jennifer Severe, M.D., from the U.S.
Census Bureau Population Survey 2018 Report.
Source. U.S. Census Bureau: Table 1.1.: Population by sex, age, nativity, and U.S.
citizenship status: 2018, in Foreign Born: 2018 Current Population Survey Detailed
Tables. Suitland, MD, U.S. Census Bureau, 2019. Available at: www.census.gov/
data/tables/2018/demo/foreign-born/cps-2018.html. Accessed December 15,
2019.

1997 (Pimienti and Polkey 2019; Schmidley and Gibson 1999), and is
expected to reach 1 in 6 by 2060, with a more racially diverse cohort
(Vespa et al. 2018). This population comprises every individual on U.S.
soil who is not a U.S. citizen at birth, including naturalized U.S. citizens,
lawful permanent migrants or green card holders, temporary migrants
such as students, humanitarian migrants such as refugees, and unlawful
migrants (Pimienti and Polkey 2019; U.S. Census Bureau 2019). Contemporary immigration continues to generate contentious debates that
transcend the problem of illegal migrants and affect the entire foreign-
born population, from naturalized U.S. citizens to temporary workers
(Fussell 2014: Hirschman 2014; Zamora-Kapoor et al. 2017).

Advocating for this population is inherently complex and daunting
for the simple reason that doing so challenges the biased views of inclusion and exclusion woven into the American social, economic, and political fabric. On such slippery advocacy ground, psychiatrists need to be
cognizant of and to separate themselves from their own personal views
and biases in service of advocacy actions truly rooted in the promotion
of the mental health and well-being of their patients. Although advocacy

competency may not be a natural extension of psychiatrists' training and expertise (Clifford 2014; Kirmayer et al. 2018a), we believe that psychiatrists are already engaged in crucial advocacy actions without identifying their actions as such. Advocacy transpires through actions that range from calling an interpreter line during a psychiatric assessment to helping foreign-born patients navigate the complex health care system.

Immigration: A Social Determinant of Mental Health

Mental health is shaped throughout the life course by factors and forces that affect the environments in which an individual is born, grows, lives, works, and ages (Allen et al. 2014; Andermann 2016; World Health Organization and Calouste Gulbenkian Foundation 2014). These factors and forces are referred to as the social determinants of mental health, and they include social status, education, food, economic stability, employment, and housing. Immigration status stands as an equally powerful factor as these other correlates at influencing the mental health trajectory of the foreign-born patient (Castañeda et al. 2015). Immigration status is a complex demographic variable that is ever-changing, except for individuals who arrived via naturalization (Bureau of Consular Affairs 2019; U.S. Census Bureau 2019) (Figure 14–2).

Beyond the demographic nature of immigration status, the underlying psychological mechanism exerts both positive and negative effects on an individual's mental health and well-being. According to a risk and protective factors paradigm, lack of community integration, fear of apprehension and deportation, perceived discrimination, acculturative stress, and family separation are psychological correlates of immigration status for depression, anxiety, and substance-related disorder, whereas social networking, aspirations to employment and economic opportunities, and family cohesion raise hope and reduce psychosocial stresses (Leong et al. 2013; Patler and Laster Pirtle 2018; Perreira and Pedroza 2019).

Evidence of this paradigm is demonstrated by the Deferred Action for Childhood Arrivals (DACA) program, a U.S. immigration policy that provides a status that protects eligible unlawful migrants from deportation and grants temporary work permits (Patler and Laster Pirtle 2018; Venkataramani et al. 2017). Although the program is not a pathway to citizenship, a recent quasi-experimental study showed that participation in the DACA program dropped by nearly 40% the odds of reporting mental suffering on the six-item Kessler Psychological Distress Scale, which encompasses symptoms of feeling nervous, restless, depressed,

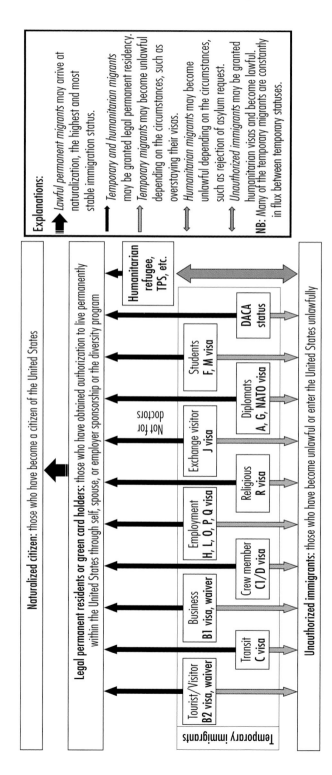

FIGURE 14–2.   The five categories of non-immigrant and immigrant U.S. statuses.

Abbreviations.   DACA=Deferred Action for Childhood Arrivals; NATO=North Atlantic Treaty Organization; TPS=temporary protected status.
Source.   Bureau of Consular Affairs: Directory of Visa Categories. Washington, D.C., U.S. Department of State, 2019. Available at: https://travel.state.gov/content/travel/en/us-visas/visa-information-resources/all-visa-categories.html. Accessed July 1, 2019.

hopeless, worthless, and that everything was an effort (Venkataramani et al. 2017). Another study demonstrated that reports of psychological wellness were predicted by DACA status (Patler and Laster Pirtle 2018).

Immigration status and history have important implications for psychiatric care. They are the fundamental elements of the foreign-born individual's sense of belonging and perceived experiences with discrimination, marginalization, threats to family, education, employment, and health care services (Kirmayer et al. 2018b; Lommel and Chen 2016; Patler and Laster Pirtle 2018). Considering these factors, we encourage psychiatrists to carefully explore not only patients' symptoms during their assessments but also the patients' narratives around immigration issues. Building and maintaining trust while assuring individuals of confidentiality remain crucial throughout such sensitive inquiries.

Overcoming Implicit Bias

It is of clinical and policy value for agents of advocacy and social justice to remain cognizant of the power and pervasiveness of implicit bias. Implicit biases are the assumptions we harbor over the course of a lifetime and that cause us to understand, experience, and react toward others on the basis of such characteristics as race, ethnicity, gender, socioeconomic status, age, and appearance (FitzGerald and Hurst 2017; Hall et al. 2015). Implicit bias affects the judgment of health care professionals and policy makers as much as it affects the judgment of the wider population (FitzGerald and Hurst 2017; Hall et al. 2015). It is known to contaminate the therapeutic milieu and advocacy efforts in ways that perpetuate health care disparities for certain ethnic and racial groups (FitzGerald and Hurst 2017; Hall et al. 2015; Schroeder 2017). Although the problem of implicit bias does not impact only the foreign-born patient, the vulnerability of foreign-born patients and the heterogeneity of their narratives and cultures make them susceptible to misconstrued views, beliefs, and assumptions (Mayell 2017; Rousseau et al. 2017; Schroeder 2017).

Addressing implicit bias starts by our acknowledging and reflecting on our own bias. Of equal importance is the need for formalized and longitudinal implicit bias training beginning early in medical training when it is likely to be more effective. We have at our disposal substantial scientific research on the issue as well as published evidence-based strategies to address stereotypes, prejudice, and discrimination in our environment and for health policy recommendations (Burgess et al. 2017; King and Jones 2016; Mayell 2017; Schroeder 2017). In Figure 14–3, we summarize under the acronym IMPACT those strategies that are found to be largely beneficial at individual, institutional, and system levels. Private

I	Increase self-awareness and awareness in your environment about implicit bias
M	Monitor and manage the influence of bidirectional implicit bias
P	Promote mindfulness and empathy-related techniques
A	Aim for structured evaluations and evidence-based treatment
C	Cultivate a culture of diversity, equity, and inclusion in your environment
T	Train on implicit bias through experiential learning and share lessons learned

FIGURE 14–3.   Advocacy efforts for overcoming implicit biases.

and public entities, such as the judicial system, have also joined the movement of implementing dialogues and trainings around implicit bias, empowering both service providers and users (Mayell 2017; Schroeder 2017). In immigration courts, such undertaking has proven to be invaluable in legal proceedings for judges, lawyers, and asylum seekers (Mayell 2017). We encourage psychiatrists to capitalize on existing efforts and resources in their institutions and to develop partnerships across disciplines for greater impact and sustainability in their advocacy activities.

Embracing Cultural Competency

Cultural competency has become central to psychiatry training, practice, and research, with the aim of reducing health care disparities for immigrant and ethnic minority patients and improving their access to care (Aggarwal et al. 2016; Butler et al. 2016). Cultural competency involves proficiency in intercultural communication and patient-provider relationship as well as sophistication in culturally appropriate diagnosis and treatment (Aggarwal et al. 2016; Butler et al. 2016). The literature is scarce on the interface between advocacy and cultural competency or the impact of one on the other. Nevertheless, since the advent of cultural competency, psychiatrists have gained a better understanding of the visible and invisible barriers to mental health service use and have given themselves permission to go beyond conventional psychiatric care to surmount those barriers (Aggarwal et al. 2016; Derr 2016; Nassar-McMillan 2014).

These barriers consist of gender, English proficiency, health literacy, cost, health insurance, alternative treatment, and transportation, as well as stigma, attitudes, norms, bias, and discrimination.

More attention is now given to the diverse nature of the foreign-born patient's socioeconomic background, cultural traditions, acculturative abilities, experiences with discrimination and marginalization, and inherent physical and mental health characteristics (Aggarwal et al. 2016; Jackson et al. 2007). Health care providers have come to learn that foreign-born patients may prioritize informal mental health support from religious leaders, folk practitioners, family, and friends and delay timely contact with mental health professionals (Derr 2016). It is crucial for psychiatrists to understand the nuances in the care they provide and to foster a welcoming environment while remaining culturally humble, sensitive, and curious. In the following list, we provide a set of advocacy actions anchored in cultural competency strategies for psychiatrists to consider (Derr 2016; Lewis-Fernández et al. 2016; Nassar-McMillan 2014; Slade 2017):

- Communicate effectively, using the help of a skilled interpreter as needed
- Engage in informed and shared decision-making
- Ensure comprehensive, culturally sensitive interviews touching multiple facets such as strengths, values, and perceived prejudice
- Consider evidence-based screenings, such as the DSM-5 Cultural Formulation Interview (Díaz et al. 2017), Harvard Trauma Questionnaire (Berthold et al. 2019), and Patient Health Questionnaire–9 (Muñoz-Navarro et al. 2017)
- Explore experiences with the migration process, including premigration and postmigration
- Search for potential hidden social challenges, such as food insecurity or illiteracy
- Adhere to evidence-based practice
- Be culturally curious and open-minded to traditional treatments that derive from a patient's cultural/ethnic history
- Empower patients and their families through psychoeducation
- Welcome the patient's support system in the treatment and advocacy interventions
- Understand patient's ties with the community, including local ethnic groups
- Make human rights and social justice principles a focus throughout treatment

Advocacy Through Mental Health Services

Community Mental Health Care

The migration process and acculturative stress (the stress of creating a new life and assimilating into a new culture in a foreign country) have varying impacts on the mental health and quality of life of foreign-born individuals (Derr 2016; Nap et al. 2015). However, foreign-born patients use mental health services at lower rates than the rest of the population despite equal or greater need for them, and timely access to care remains a major public health challenge (Bauldry and Szaflarski 2017; Chan et al. 1996; Derr 2016; Jackson et al. 2007; Lee and Matejkowski 2012). For guidance on advocacy actions that are rooted in community mental health and expected to positively impact access (Cerully et al. 2016; Frost et al. 2017; Salami et al. 2019; Sutton et al. 2016; Woodhead et al. 2017), see Table 14–1.

The care-seeking paradigm of foreign-born patients varies greatly on the basis of their immigration status, which determines their legality on U.S. soil and eligibility for health care coverage, medical visits, prescriptions, transportation to clinics, and more (Centers for Medicare and Medicaid Services 2017; National Immigration Law Center 2014; U.S. Census Bureau 2018) (see Table 14–2). However, access to care does not equate with use of that care because many may be afraid to fully engage with treatment out of concern that it might impact their immigration status. Unlawful migrants cite restrictions on their immigration status, lack of funding, and lack of knowledge of other sources of care as major reasons for favoring care in emergency departments rather than community clinics (Chan et al. 1996).

At a community and organizational level, we suggest that psychiatrists aim for advocacy interventions that promote mental health as a human right; emphasize prevention, early diagnosis, and treatment; and reduce the financial burden of health care (see Table 14–1). Psychiatrists serving on local, national, and international organizations have the vantage point to scale up conversations on immigration issues. For instance, the Council on International Psychiatry at the American Psychiatric Association plays a pivotal role in educating psychiatrists through position and action statements, curriculum development, and active engagement in immigration-related advocacy. At a state level, we recommend that psychiatrists review their states' elected officials' involvement in particular mental health–related activities to leverage opportunities stemming from mutual interests.

In addition to taking the conventional steps in treatment termination, Ms. V's psychiatrist may want to be proactive by 1) exploring and

> ### Case Example: Advocating for a Patient Facing Change in Immigration Status
>
> Ms. V is being treated for depression, which has finally improved after multiple medication trials. Her 10-year employment-based immigration visa is ending soon, with potential consequences on her socioeconomic status, family unit, employment, health insurance coverage, and, more importantly her psychiatric care and well-being. She has only a few months in which to return to her home country or face deportation. What does this mean for continuation of care? What preemptive steps could her psychiatrist take?

helping her process possible underlying psychological distress linked to the termination of her status; 2) educating her on the benefits of safety net clinics in case she runs out of insurance coverage (see Table 14–1); 3) discussing ways to transfer her care to providers or health care facilities in her home country; 4) reviewing psychotropic drugs on the formulary in the destination country and adjusting treatment if possible; and 5) involving care management for more guidance, support, and possible referral to appropriate social or legal services. This is by no means an exhaustive list of actions that could be accomplished.

Health Care Coverage

Foreign-born individuals are twice as likely as U.S. citizens to have no health insurance coverage (16.8% vs. 7.5%; U.S. Census Bureau 2018). The gap is larger for unlawful migrants. Unlawful nonelderly adults are four times as likely as nonelderly U.S. citizen adults to lack health insurance coverage (40% vs. 10%), and unlawful children are nearly five times as likely as U.S. citizen children to have no coverage (23% vs. 5%) (Kaiser Family Foundation 2019a). Foreign-born nationals who arrived at naturalization and those who have domiciled in the United States for longer than 19 years tend to have health insurance coverage, mainly private insurance (U.S. Census Bureau 2018). Naturalized and native U.S. citizens have substantially higher rates of employer-sponsored health insurance coverage than do the rest of the foreign-born population (Buchmueller et al. 2007). Approaching such disparity issues requires an understanding of the health care coverage for the foreign-born patient population (Table 14–2) (Burke and Kean 2019; Centers for Medicare and Medicaid Services 2017; National Immigration Law Center 2014).

TABLE 14–1. **Advocacy actions anchored in community mental health care**

Advocacy themes	Community interventions
Stigma reduction	Scale up stigma-reduction activities through engagement with the general public as well as private, federal, and state entities
Mental illness prevention	Enhance collaboration across sectors in mental illness prevention and treatment outside traditional settings, such as by expanding to religious organizations, schools, and local ethnic societies
Outpatient care	Scale up and prioritize ambulatory care over inpatient psychiatric care as much as possible
Connection with care	Inform patients about safety net hospitals and clinics, which have the legal mandate to provide care regardless of patients' immigration status or ability to pay; these include federally qualified health centers, federally qualified health center look-alikes, rural health centers, community health centers, and disproportionate share hospitals
Connection with support	Enlist social workers, patient navigators, peer supporters, and cultural brokers for assistance
Recovery	Promote recovery-oriented treatment and interventions
Psychoeducation	Empower patients through psychoeducation, information, and connection with key services such as legal counseling
Partnership	Partner with local social service agencies that are able to assist with specific social challenges, such as sex trafficking or refugee resettlement

Medicaid remains the single largest payer for mental health services. Its administratively complex health plans for such services vary mainly on the basis of states' options to carve in or carve out behavioral health benefits and states' adoption or refusal of Medicaid expansion through the Patient Protection and Affordable Care Act of 2010 (ACA; P.L. 111-148). It is useful to know whether one's state Medicaid program has taken steps to keep behavioral health services under the same roof with physical health plans (carve in) or has delegated some or all behavioral health services to a private entity, such as a managed care organization, or a governmental entity (carve out) (Giord et al. 2017). By 2019, 37

TABLE 14–2. Overview of government and private insurance coverage for the foreign-born population

Type of insurance	Managed or overseen by	Criteria for coverage	5-year U.S. residence required?	Specific characteristics
Medicaid (nonemergency and emergency) in states with *no* Medicaid expansion	State and federal government	*Must be* U.S.-born citizen or naturalized citizen *or* Lawful permanent migrant (green card holder) *or* Humanitarian migrant *And must* Have a family (with children) *or* Be living with a disability or HIV *or* Have a low income (amount varies by state)	No Yes, except children and pregnant women No	Unlawful migrants can benefit *only* from emergency Medicaid in the face of an emergency

TABLE 14–2. Overview of government and private insurance coverage for the foreign-born population *(continued)*

Type of insurance	Managed or overseen by	Criteria for coverage	5-year U.S. residence required?	Specific characteristics
Children's Health Insurance Program	State	Lawful children younger than age 19	No	States can choose to include more children and pregnant women from other lawful migrant categories
		Pregnant women	No	
		Income less than 200%–300% FPL	No	
		Some Medicaid lawful migrant categories	No	

TABLE 14–2. Overview of government and private insurance coverage for the foreign-born population (continued)

Type of insurance	Managed or overseen by	Criteria for coverage	5-year U.S. residence required?	Specific characteristics
Affordable Care Act	Private health insurance marketplace State Federal	All lawful migrants, including • Lawful permanent migrants not meeting the Medicaid 5-year residence period • Childless lawful migrants • Lawful migrants who did not qualify for Medicare Part A • Lawful migrants with or without disability or HIV No income limit (offered on a sliding scale)	No	Premium subsidies are available for those meeting these requirements: 1. Income between 100% and 400% of the FPL in states with *no* Medicaid expansion (for income less than 100%, the gap is left at the discretion of the state to fill) 2. Income between 139% and 400% of the FPL in states *with* Medicaid expansion (for income less than 139%, states provide Medicaid coverage for all)
Medicare Part A (hospital coverage)	Federal	Naturalized and lawful permanent migrants older than age 65 years Those who worked for at least 40 quarters (about 10 years)	Yes for lawful permanent migrants	Anyone who meets the criteria is eligible to *obtain* this coverage

TABLE 14–2. Overview of government and private insurance coverage for the foreign-born population *(continued)*

Type of insurance	Managed or overseen by	Criteria for coverage	5-year U.S. residence required?	Specific characteristics
Medicare Parts B and D (outpatient and prescription coverage)	Federal	Naturalized and lawful permanent migrants older than age 65 years	Yes for lawful permanent migrants	Anyone who meets the criteria is eligible to *purchase* this coverage
Private insurance	Private	All categories of lawful migrants	NA	Private insurance can be used to augment student health insurance, which may not cover much
Student health insurance	Private	Migrant students	NA	Private insurance can be used to augment student health insurance, which may not cover much
Travel insurance	Private	Migrant visitors, tourists, scholars, missionaries, or business travelers	NA	Private insurance can be used to augment student health insurance, which may not cover much

Note. FPL=federal poverty line; NA=not applicable.

states had adopted Medicaid expansion, and 9 states were currently with Medicaid behavioral health carve-outs (Kaiser Family Foundation 2019b; OPEN MINDS 2019).

The ACA significantly changed the health insurance landscape since its inception in 2010 (Borelli et al. 2016). The number of uninsured individuals is believed to have been reduced from 18% in 2013 to 11.9% in 2015 (Borelli et al. 2016). However, the future is uncertain for this version of the ACA, and many of the improvements from the ACA witnessed by uninsured people may be lost with future health care legislation. The ACA largely benefited lawfully present foreign-born patients by expanding Medicaid, offering premium subsidies and lower copayments, and reinforcing safety net clinics. The ACA also allowed more enrollment of lawfully present foreign-born patients, including low-income childless foreign-born adults who did not qualify before the extension because of their childless status. Moreover, the ACA permitted lawful permanent migrants (green card holders) to access Medicaid and Medicare Part A in a timely manner without waiting for the 5-year residency period in the United States that Medicaid normally requires. In essence, states that have expanded Medicaid have better coverage for lawfully present foreign-born patients than do states that have not chosen to expand. (For a comprehensive overview of health care coverage, see Table 14–2.)

> ### Case Example: Advocacy for a Patient Who Might Be Deported
>
> Ms. Q is an undocumented immigrant and mother of two who has bipolar disorder. Ms. Q started to deteriorate and has become floridly manic, but her sister is reluctant to bring her to the local emergency room because of heightened fear of profiling and deportation from the hospital. Ms. Q's sister finally decides to bring her to the emergency room but choose not to provide much information about her sister to the hospital staff and health providers, which limits the evaluations.

Ms. Q will qualify for emergency Medicaid (EM) if her psychiatric team can prove that she meets EM criteria—mainly that her acute mental health condition, if left untreated, could put her life in peril. Once stable, Ms. Q will no longer be eligible for EM and should consider a safety net clinic (see Table 14–1). Because of her unlawful status, Ms. Q does not qualify for private insurance and Medicaid, even in states that have expanded Medicaid with ACA.

U.S. Immigration and Customs Enforcement (ICE) and Customs and Border Protection (CBP) are two federal agencies in charge of immigration enforcement (CLASP 2018), and their activities create fear and emotional distress in both documented and undocumented immigrants (Hacker et al. 2011). Health care providers also witness and fear the negative effects of ICE activities on their immigrant patients (Hacker et al. 2012). Both ICE and CBP have issued memoranda that consider health care facilities to be "sensitive locations" exempt from immigration enforcement actions (CLASP 2018). Such agreements should be respected as long as they are in effect. Psychiatrists can advocate for new legislation and policy changes that will allow vulnerable patients like Ms. Q to access care without fear. This is one of the best examples that promoting human rights promotes and protects mental health.

Essentials in Immigration Literacy

As the U.S. foreign-born population grows (Pimienti and Polkey 2019) and personalized preventive care becomes the focus of health care quality, utilization, and expenditures (Al-Hachim 2017; Musich et al. 2016), psychiatrists are showing a genuine interest in caring for these individuals and understanding how to address their unique mental health issues (Hausmann-Stabile and Guarnaccia 2015). The psychiatric assessment can be complicated and may require special skills, knowledge, and training (Hausmann-Stabile and Guarnaccia 2015). Immigration literacy remains a poorly explored domain with multiple uncharted areas of training. Immigration-literate psychiatrists would be expected to be comfortable with what to ask, assess, and consider as an assessment unfolds (Hausmann-Stabile and Guarnaccia 2015). One common area of concern, for example, is refugee mental health. Some psychiatry training programs offer specific competency training that equips residents with the necessary tools to appropriately conduct pro bono psychological assessments for people seeking asylum (Patel and Sreshta 2017). As of this writing, however, we are aware of no immigration literacy curricula. We deeply hope that such a curriculum is in the making and will be revealed soon. Topics discussed in the following subsection and the content of the chapter overall could be taken into consideration in developing such an immigration literacy curriculum.

Immigration-Related Topics

Even without immigration literacy training, psychiatrists can still make substantial contributions to an individual's well-being through a single encounter. Psychiatrists can use the assessment as the main advocacy tool and build on recommendations provided in this chapter to explore immigration-related issues and solutions within a therapeutic framework. Psychiatrists may also want to consider the following recommendations for an efficient encounter:

- Manage expectations, ensure transparency, and confirm understanding on both sides
- Avoid making promises
- Accept your limits for issues that go beyond your capacity as a health care provider
- Remain humble, sensitive, and curious
- Engage a multidisciplinary team; the role of care managers remains vital
- Consult with a mentor or colleague familiar with the issue under consideration and/or pursue legal counsel within or outside your organization (e.g., Office of International Affairs, nonprofit groups, or local embassies)
- Expect to testify in a courtroom or to have documentations subpoenaed at any time

We end this subsection with a list of important immigration-related advocacy issues that have a damaging impact on patients' health and that represent significant hurdles to surmount without proper guidance. For each of the issues listed, we encourage psychiatrists to start their advocacy actions in their immediate surroundings, where they are likely to have the most meaningful impact for their patients, and then to expand their voice to targeted audiences in private, state, and federal entities as well as to the general public. Common practical steps include gathering with others around shared advocacy interests, educating stakeholders, writing letters or op-ed pieces, communicating with local elected officials, and promulgating patients' stories.

- **Family separation or reunification:** The negative and lifelong impact of family separation on both children and parents is well studied (Miller et al. 2018).

  What can you do? Advocacy interventions should start by elucidating family structures and roles; facilitating decision-making through distress reduction; and linking with organizations, advocacy groups, legal resources, and other available supports, which in turn need our help for mental health services for their clients and staff (Kohrt et al. 2018).

- **Human rights violations:** Affected populations include victims of human trafficking, forced marriages, and female genital mutilation or cutting; vulnerable children and battered spouses; and children and parents exposed to trauma premigration or during the migration process (U.S. Citizen and Immigration Services 2019a).

  What can you do? Go to the U.S. Citizen and Immigration Services (USCIS) website (www.uscis.gov/humanitarian) to familiarize yourself with a comprehensive list of human rights violations. Ensure patient safety, address underlying psychological distress, and point your patients to the list of humanitarian visa programs specifically designed by USCIS (U.S. Citizen and Immigration Services 2019a).

- **International students:** International students with mental illness may see their student visas jeopardized by days of absence from classes, as stated by USCIS (U.S. Citizen and Immigration Services 2019b).

  What can you do? A leave of absence or reduced course load can be granted to international students in need of treatment and a period of convalescence (e.g., University of Southern California Office of International Services 2019a, 2019b). The psychiatrist's note should specify whether the student should remain in the United States or return to the home country to receive treatment and/or recover.

- **Mental health–based inadmissibility grounds:** USCIS reserves the right to refuse adjusting immigration status or granting visas to applicants who have current physical or mental disorders with either 1) associated harmful behavior or past physical or mental disorders or 2) associated harmful behavior that is likely to recur or lead to other harmful behavior (Hong et al. 2017; U.S. Citizen and Immigration Services 2019c). This is also true for applicants with current substance use disorders or controlled substance–induced disorders (U.S. Citizen and Immigration Services 2019d). If the USCIS-designated doctor checks the Class A Condition box on USCIS Form I-693, the applicant is inadmissible (U.S. Citizen and Immigration Services 2019c, 2019d). In exceptional cases, USCIS may seek a case review from the Centers for Disease Control and Prevention.

  What can you do? Address underlying psychological distress. Encourage patients to seek legal guidance and to consider applying for a waiver of inadmissibility.

- **Mental disability and naturalization process:** Certain patients are unable to satisfy the English and civics requirements for U.S. citizenship because of a physical or developmental disability or mental impairment.

  What can you do? Address underlying psychological distress. A licensed psychiatrist can complete the Medical Certification for Disability Exceptions form (USCIS Form N-648) and certify, under penalty of perjury, that the patient's health condition precludes their ability to meet the English and/or civic requirements (U.S. Citizen and Immigration Services 2019e).

- **Discharge of undocumented migrants:** Hospitals have repatriated immigrant patients back to their home countries because of lack of an appropriate disposition plan for discharge (Wei et al. 2016). This practice, which seems to have involved mostly undocumented immigrant patients, also occurs when patients have long-term medical needs for which no reimbursement is available (Kuczewski 2012).

  What can you do? Ensure that shared decision-making is occurring (Kuczewski 2012; Slade 2017). Psychiatrists may want to familiarize themselves with the health care landscape of the receiving country and adjust a patient's treatment plan accordingly. Interagency cooperation usually occurs in an informal manner and without established protocols; effective cooperation relies on trust and interdependence of resources (Yetzi et al. 2017). The local consulate of the country in question should be involved in the process (Wei et al. 2016; Yetzi et al. 2017).

Asylum Proceedings

Another immigration-related topic that deserves a chapter of its own is asylum proceedings. We outline here a few key facts that are valuable for psychiatrist advocates. *Refugees* and *asylees* are two different terms that are often used interchangeably. *Refugees* are people crossing national borders to seek safety; they are outside the United States. *Asylees* are already in the United States and are referred to as *asylum seekers* for as long as their claims and applications as refugees are pending (Humberg 2018).

In order to be granted asylum, an individual needs to show 1) a reasonable fear 2) of future persecution 3) on account of race, religion, national origin, political opinion, or membership in a social group. The road to asylum from the country of origin to the United States is filled with hurdles, and asylum applicants have to satisfy an exceedingly high burden of proof of well-founded fear of persecution (Humberg 2018;

Patel and Sreshta 2017). The rates of mental illness—especially post-traumatic stress disorder—are known to be high among asylum seekers. However, the asylum psychiatric interviews are not primarily therapeutic (Humberg 2018; Moran 2013; Patel and Sreshta 2017); rather, the interviews are intended to elicit traumatic history and experiences to shape a narrative, and this can be distressful for asylum seekers. Psychiatric narratives are powerful and increase the applicants' odds of being granted asylum. The court relies to some degree on psychiatrists' evaluation and diagnosis to support individuals' claims. Lack of credibility is the main reason for asylum refusal (Humberg 2018).

Anecdotally, a platform of collaboration between medical, law, and social work schools has been shown to synergistically elevate the quality of interventions for those taking part in the psychological evaluation of asylum seekers (Moran 2013). As a physician-advocate, you should talk to your institution to understand existing collaborations with other parties or to lay the groundwork for advocacy collaboration with stakeholders.

Conclusion

Foreign-born patients need more and better advocates. In an era during which contentious debates on immigration and health care reform are in full swing, psychiatrists are called on to ensure the welfare of this population, familiarize themselves with available resources, and create momentum for advocacy actions truly rooted in the promotion of health interests. This chapter lays out in broad strokes basic principles to keep in mind, practical recommendations to consider, and avenues for training to ponder. We hope that after reading this chapter, psychiatrists will understand that by restricting themselves to a narrow view of clinical practice, they risk losing the vitality and urgency of advocating at an individual, community, or system level to arrive at definite solutions. We expect that the current generation of psychiatrists will tackle this undertaking and then share lessons learned with future generations to ensure sustainability.

References

Aggarwal NK, Cedeño K, Guarnaccia P, et al: The meanings of cultural competence in mental health: an exploratory focus group study with patients, clinicians, and administrators. Springerplus 5:384, 2016 27065092

Al-Hachim SG: Barriers to preventive healthcare for immigrants in Michigan. Minneapolis, MN, Walden Dissertations and Doctoral Studies Collection, Walden University, December 2017

Allen J, Balfour R, Bell R, Marmot M: Social determinants of mental health. Int Rev Psychiatry 26(4):392–407, 2014 25137105

Andermann A; CLEAR Collaboration: Taking action on the social determinants of health in clinical practice: a framework for health professionals. CMAJ 188(17–18):E474–E483, 2016 27503870

Bauldry S, Szaflarski M: Immigrant-based disparities in mental health care utilization. Socius Jan:3, 2017 28845455

Berthold SM, Mollica RF, Silove D, et al: The HTQ-5: revision of the Harvard Trauma Questionnaire for measuring torture, trauma and DSM-5 PTSD symptoms in refugee populations. Eur J Public Health 29(3):468–474, 2019 30561573

Borelli MC, Bujanda M, Maier K: The Affordable Care Act insurance reforms: where are we now, and what's next? Clin Diabetes 34(1):58–64, 2016 26807011

Buchmueller TC, Lo Sasso AT, Lurie I, Dolfin S: Immigrants and employer-sponsored health insurance. Health Serv Res 42(1 Pt 1):286–310, 2007 17355593

Bureau of Consular Affairs: Directory of visa categories. Washington, DC, U.S. Department of State, 2019. Available at: https://travel.state.gov/content/travel/en/us-visas/visa-information-resources/all-visa-categories.html.html. Accessed July 1, 2019.

Burgess DJ, Beach MC, Saha S: Mindfulness practice: a promising approach to reducing the effects of clinician implicit bias on patients. Patient Educ Couns 100(2):372–376, 2017 27665499

Burke G, Kean N: Older immigrants and Medicare. Issue Brief. Washington, DC, Justice in Aging, April 2019.

Butler M, McCreedy E, Schwer N, et al: Improving cultural competence to reduce health disparities. Comparative Effectiveness Reviews No 170. Rockville, MD, Agency for Healthcare Research and Quality, March 2016

Castañeda H, Holmes SM, Madrigal DS, et al: Immigration as a social determinant of health. Annu Rev Public Health 36:375–392, 2015 25494053

Centers for Medicare and Medicaid Services: Serving special populations: immigrants. Fast facts for agents and brokers. Baltimore, MD, Centers for Medicare and Medicaid Services, 2017. Available at: www.cms.gov/CCIIO/Programs-and-Initiatives/Health-Insurance-Marketplaces/Downloads/Immigration-Fact-Sheet.pdf. Accessed July 2, 2019.

Cerully JL, Collins RL, Wong EC, et al: Effects of stigma and discrimination reduction trainings conducted under the California Mental Health Services Authority: an evaluation of Disability Rights California and Mental Health America of California trainings. Rand Health Q 5(3):5, 2016 28083402

Chan TC, Krishel SJ, Bramwell KJ, Clark RF: Survey of illegal immigrants seen in an emergency department. West J Med 164(3):212–216, 1996 8775931

CLASP: The Department of Homeland Security's "sensitive locations" policies: protecting immigrant families, advancing our future. Washington, DC, CLASP, 2018. Available at: www.clasp.org/sites/default/files/publications/2018/06/2018_sensitivelocationsdetailed.pdf. Accessed December 16, 2019.

Clifford JC: Patient advocacy. CMAJ 186(2):138, 2014

Derr AS: Mental health service use among immigrants in the United States: a systematic review. Psychiatr Serv 67(3):265–274, 2016 26695493

Díaz E, Añez LM, Silva M, et al: Using the Cultural Formulation Interview to build culturally sensitive services. Psychiatr Serv 68(2):112–114, 2017 27799018

FitzGerald C, Hurst S: Implicit bias in healthcare professionals: a systematic review. BMC Med Ethics 18(1):19, 2017 28249596

Frost BG, Tirupati S, Johnston S, et al: An integrated recovery-oriented model (IRM) for mental health services: evolution and challenges. BMC Psychiatry 17(1):22, 2017 28095811

Fussell E: Warmth of the welcome: attitudes toward immigrants and immigration policy. Annu Rev Sociol 40:479–498, 2014 26966338

Giord K, Ellis E, Edwards BC, et al: Medicaid moving ahead in uncertain times: results from a 50-state Medicaid budget survey for state fiscal years 2017 and 2018. San Francisco, CA, Henry J Kaiser Family Foundation and Health Management Associates, October 2017

Hacker K, Chu J, Leung C, et al: The impact of Immigration and Customs Enforcement on immigrant health: perceptions of immigrants in Everett, Massachusetts, USA. Soc Sci Med 73(4), 586–594, 2011 21778008

Hacker K, Chu J, Arsenault L, Marlin RP: Provider's perspectives on the impact of Immigration and Customs Enforcement (ICE) activity on immigrant health. J Health Care Poor Underserved 23(2):651–665, 2012 22643614

Hall WJ, Chapman MV, Lee KM, et al: Implicit racial/ethnic bias among health care professionals and its influence on health care outcomes: a systematic review. Am J Public Health 105(12):e60–e76, 2015 26469668

Hausmann-Stabile C, Guarnaccia PJ: Clinical encounters with immigrants: what matters for U.S. psychiatrists. Focus Am Psychiatr Publ 13(4):409–418, 2015 27330456

Hirschman C: Immigration to the United States: recent trends and future prospects. Malays J Econ Studies 51(1):69–85, 2014 25620887

Hong MK, Varghese RE, Jindal C, Efird JT: Refugee policy implications of U.S. immigration medical screenings: a new era of inadmissibility on health-related grounds. Int J Environ Res Public Health 14(10):1107, 2017 28946650

Humberg J: Trauma and the paradox of asylum seekers' credibility. Master's thesis, Human Rights Studies Master of Arts Program Graduate School of Arts and Sciences. New York, Columbia University, January 2018

Jackson JS, Neighbors HW, Torres M, et al: Use of mental health services and subjective satisfaction with treatment among Black Caribbean immigrants: results from the National Survey of American Life. Am J Public Health 97(1):60–67, 2007 17138907

Kaiser Family Foundation: Uninsured rates among nonelderly adults and children by immigration status, 2007, in Health Coverage of Immigrants. San Francisco, CA, Kaiser Family Foundation, 2019a. Available at: www.kff.org/disparities-policy/fact-sheet/health-coverage-of-immigrants. Accessed July 3, 2019.

Kaiser Family Foundation: Status of Medicaid expansion decision. San Francisco, CA, Kaiser Family Foundation, November 15, 2019. Available at: www.kff.org/health-reform/state-indicator/state-activity-around-expanding-medicaid-under-the-affordable-care-act/?currentTimeframe=0&sortModel=%7B%22colId%22:%22Location%22,%22sort%22:%22asc%22%7D. Accessed December 16, 2019.

King E, Jones K: Why subtle bias is so often worse than blatant discrimination. Harv Bus Rev July 13, 2016

Kirmayer LJ, Kronick R, Rousseau C: Advocacy as key to structural competency in psychiatry. JAMA Psychiatry 75(2):119–120, 2018a 29261839

Kirmayer LJ, Sockalingam S, Fung KP, et al: International medical graduates in psychiatry: cultural issues in training and continuing professional development. Can J Psychiatry 63(4):258–280, 2018b 29630854

Kohrt BA, Lu FG, Wu EY, et al; Culture and Mental Health Services: Caring for families separated by changing immigration policies and enforcement: a cultural psychiatry perspective. Psychiatr Serv 69(12):1200–1203, 2018 30122136

Kuczewski M: Can medical repatriation be ethical? Establishing best practices. Am J Bioeth 12(9):1–5, 2012 22881842

Lee S, Matejkowski J: Mental health service utilization among noncitizens in the United States: findings from the National Latino and Asian American Study. Adm Policy Ment Health 39(5):406–418, 2012 21755392

Leong F, Park YS, Kalibatseva Z: Disentangling immigrant status in mental health: psychological protective and risk factors among Latino and Asian American immigrants. Am J Orthopsychiatry 83(2 Pt 3):361–371, 2013 23889027

Lewis-Fernández R, Aggarwal NK, Hinton L (eds): DSM-5® Handbook on the Cultural Formulation Interview. Arlington, VA, American Psychiatric Association Publishing, 2016

Lommel LL, Chen JL: The relationship between self-rated health and acculturation in Hispanic and Asian adult immigrants: a systematic review. J Immigr Minor Health 18(2):468–478, 2016 25894534

Mayell DS: Applying implicit bias scholarship to real-world issues: an immigration toolkit, in Race and Ethnicity: Views From Inside the Unconscious Mind. State of the Science: Implicit Bias Review 2017 Edition. Edited by Staats C, Capatosto K, Tenney L, Mamo S. Columbus, Kirwan Institute for the Study of Race and Ethnicity, Ohio State University, pp 16–17

Miller A, Hess JM, Bybee D, Goodkind JR: Understanding the mental health consequences of family separation for refugees: implications for policy and practice. Am J Orthopsychiatry 88(1):26–37, 2018 28617002

Moran M: Psychiatrists have role in assessing candidates for asylum. Psychiatr News 48(12):13, 2013

Muñoz-Navarro R, Cano-Vindel A, Medrano LA, et al: Utility of the PHQ-9 to identify major depressive disorder in adult patients in Spanish primary care centres. BMC Psychiatry 17(1):291, 2017 28793892

Musich S, Wang S, Hawkins K, Klemes A: The impact of personalized preventive care on health care quality, utilization, and expenditures. Popul Health Manag 19(6):389–397, 2016 26871762

Nap A, van Loon A, Peen J, et al: The influence of acculturation on mental health and specialized mental healthcare for non-western migrants. Int J Soc Psychiatry 61(6):530–538, 2015 25488952

Nassar-McMillan SC: A framework for cultural competence, advocacy, and social justice: applications for global multiculturalism and diversity. Int J Educ Vocat Guid 14(1):103–118, 2014

National Immigration Law Center: Immigrants and the Affordable Care Act (ACA). Los Angeles, CA, National Immigration Law Center, 2014. Available at: www.nilc.org/wp-content/uploads/2015/11/Immigrants-and-the-ACA-2014-01.pdf. Accessed July 1, 2019.

OPEN MINDS: Nine states with behavioral health carve-outs to CMOs remain: OPEN MINDS releases annual analysis on state Medicaid behavioral health carve-outs. Gettysburg, PA, OPEN MINDS, February 22, 2019. Available at: www.openminds.com/press/nine-states-with-behavioral-health-carve-outs-to-cmos-remainopen-minds-releases-annual-analysis-on-state-medicaid-behavioral-health-carve-outs. Accessed December 16, 2019.

Patel NA, Sreshta N: The role of psychiatrists in the growing migrant and refugee crises. Am J Psychiatry Residents J 12(7)6–8, 2017

Patler C, Laster Pirtle W: From undocumented to lawfully present: do changes to legal status impact psychological wellbeing among Latino immigrant young adults? Soc Sci Med 199:39–48, 2018 28318760

Perreira KM, Pedroza JM: Policy of exclusion: implications for the health of immigrants and their children. Annu Rev Public Health 40:147–166, 2019 30601722

Pimienti M, Polkey C: Snapshot of U.S. Immigration. Washington, DC, National Conference of State Legislatures. March 29, 2019. Available at: www.ncsl.org/research/immigration/snapshot-of-u-s-immigration-2017.aspx#7. Accessed July 1, 2019.

Rousseau C, Oulhote Y, Ruiz-Casares M, et al: Encouraging understanding or increasing prejudices: a cross-sectional survey of institutional influence on health personnel attitudes about refugee claimants' access to health care. PLoS One 12(2):e0170910, 2017 28196129

Salami B, Salma J, Hegadoren K: Access and utilization of mental health services for immigrants and refugees: perspectives of immigrant service providers. Int J Ment Health Nurs 28(1):152–161, 2019 29984880

Schmidley AD, Gibson C: Profile of the foreign-born population in the United States: 1997. U.S. Census Bureau Current Population Rep Ser P23-195. Washington, DC, U.S. Government Printing Office, 1999

Schroeder JL: The vulnerability of asylum adjudications to subconscious cultural biases: demanding American narrative norms. Boston Univ Law Rev 97:315–347, 2017

Slade M: Implementing shared decision making in routine mental health care. World Psychiatry 16(2):146–153, 2017 28498575

Sutton JP, Washington RE, Fingar KR, Elixhauser A: Characteristics of safety-net hospitals, 2014. Statistical Brief 213. Rockville, MD, Healthcare Cost and Utilization Project, 2016

University of Southern California Office of International Services: Leave of absence. Los Angeles, University of Southern California, 2019a. https://ois.usc.edu/students/maintainingstudentstatus/leaveofabsence. Accessed July 2, 2019.

University of Southern California Office of International Services: Reduced course load. Los Angeles, University of Southern California, 2019b. https://ois.usc.edu/students/maintainingstudentstatus/reducedcourseload. Accessed July 2, 2019.

U.S. Census Bureau: HI-09. Health insurance coverage status by nativity, citizenship, and duration of residence (total universe). Suitland, MD, United States Census Bureau, 2018. Available at: www.census.gov/data/tables/time-series/demo/income-poverty/cps-hi/hi-09.html. Accessed July 3 2019.

U.S. Census Bureau: About foreign born. Suitland, MD, U.S. Census Bureau, May 8, 2019. Available at: www.census.gov/topics/population/foreign-born/about.html#par_textimage. Accessed December 16, 2019.

U.S. Citizen and Immigration Services: Humanitarian. Washington, DC, U.S. Citizen and Immigration Services, 2019a. Available at: www.uscis.gov/humanitarian. Accessed December 17, 2019.

U.S. Citizen and Immigration Services: Students and exchange visitors. Washington, DC, U.S. Citizen and Immigration Services, 2019b. Available at: www.uscis.gov/working-united-states/students-and-exchange-visitors. Accessed December 17, 2019.

U.S. Citizen and Immigration Services: Physical or mental disorder with associated harmful behavior, in U.S. Citizen and Immigration Services Policy Manual, Vol 8, Admissibility: Part B—Health-Related Grounds of Inadmissibility. Washington, DC, U.S. Citizen and Immigration Services, 2019c

U.S. Citizen and Immigration Services: Drug abuse or drug addiction, in U.S. Citizen and Immigration Services Policy Manual, Vol 8, Admissibility: Part B—Health-Related Grounds of Inadmissibility. Washington, DC, U.S. Citizen and Immigration Services, 2019d

U.S. Citizen and Immigration Services: Medical disability exception form N-648), in U.S. Citizen and Immigration Services Policy Manual, Vol 12, Citizenship and Naturalization: Part E—English and Civics Testing and Exceptions. Washington, DC, U.S. Citizen and Immigration Services, 2019e

Venkataramani AS, Shah SJ, O'Brien R, et al: Health consequences of the US Deferred Action for Childhood Arrivals (DACA) immigration programme: a quasi-experimental study. Lancet Public Health 2(4):e175–e181, 2017 29253449

Vespa J, Armstrong DM, Medina L: Demographic turning points for the United States: population projections for 2020 to 2060. Current Population Rep P25-1144, Suitland, MD, U.S. Census Bureau, 2018

Wei W, Lubarsky K, Han B: Undocumented immigrants in psychiatric wards. Am J Psychiatry Residents J 11(2):10–11 2016

Woodhead C, Khondoker M, Lomas R, Raine R: Impact of co-located welfare advice in healthcare settings: prospective quasi-experimental controlled study. Br J Psychiatry 211(6):388–395, 2017 29051176

World Health Organization; Calouste Gulbenkian Foundation: Social Determinants of Mental Health. Geneva, World Health Organization, 2014

Yetzi RM, Ietza BC, René LF, César IX: Health services provision for migrants repatriated through Tijuana, Baja California: inter-agency cooperation and response capacity. Frontera Norte 29(57):107–130, 2017

Zamora-Kapoor A, Moreno Fuentes J, Schain M: Race and ethnicity in context: international migration, political mobilization, and the welfare state. Ethn Racial Stud 40(3):353–368, 2017 30546173

Advocacy for People With Substance Use Disorders

Myra Mathis, M.D.
Ayana Jordan, M.D., Ph.D.
Bachaar Arnaout, M.D.

Learning Objectives

By the end of this chapter, readers will be able to:

- Appreciate the unique medical, psychiatric, social, and economic sequelae of unhealthy substance use

- Identify three types of advocacy for people with substance use disorders (PWSUD): destigmatization, remedicalization, and decriminalization

- Learn about past successes, proposed current solutions, and future directions in advocating for PWSUD

- Appreciate several advocacy implementation strategies based on practical case scenarios

According to a report on the National Survey on Drug Use and Health (Substance Abuse and Mental Health Services Administration 2018), in 2017 approximately 20.7 million people ages 12 and older—about 1 in 13 Americans—needed treatment for substance use. Among those who needed substance use treatment, only 12.2% received treatment at a specialty facility during the previous year. Long considered the number one health problem in the United States, unhealthy substance use and addiction that go untreated result in significant medical, psychiatric, social, and economic sequelae (Robert Wood Johnson Foundation 2001). Unfortunately, antiquated models of addiction that formulate it as a moral and criminal problem have shaped policy and popular perceptions for decades. Such frameworks have resulted in practices that lag behind current scientific evidence, while simultaneously stigmatizing and criminalizing individuals with addiction. Health advocacy is crucial in influencing public discourse and informing policies that address unhealthy substance use and addiction as one of the nation's primary public health crises, with the goal of promoting prevention strategies and decreasing barriers to accessing treatment. In this chapter focusing on advocacy for people with substance use disorders (PWSUD), we highlight the need for various advocacy efforts and review past successes, current proposed solutions, and future directions, organized along three types of advocacy: destigmatization, remedicalization, and decriminalization.

Need for Varied Advocacy Efforts

Physicians and PWSUD as Advocates

Physician leadership in advocacy efforts for PWSUD is critical to the continued shift of public discourse toward more accurate models for understanding, preventing, and treating addiction. Political campaigns of the 1970s–1990s put law enforcement agencies at the center of public policies addressing substance use, resulting in increased policing efforts and harsher sentences as the solution for what is now widely acknowledged as a public health crisis (Shatterproof 2019). To ensure that the next wave of public policy related to addiction promotes responses that reflect clinical and medical knowledge, physicians must be at the forefront of advocacy initiatives.

When thinking about physician leadership in advocacy for PWSUD, it is necessary to acknowledge widespread concern regarding physician culpability in the current opioid epidemic (Kunz 2019). Such complicity has been viewed as an abdication of moral authority, and physicians cannot respond by retreating from public discourse. Instead, the medical community must acknowledge its role in the current crisis and change the narrative by being at the forefront of efforts that advocate for systems change at the local, state, and national levels, thereby promoting the destigmatization, remedicalization, and decriminalization of addiction.

The medical community alone cannot change the discourse regarding unhealthy substance use and addiction. As individuals with lived experience, PWSUD share narratives that speak to the challenges in accessing care and the human cost of untreated addiction. Conversations taking place in town halls, at city council meetings, and before state and national legislative bodies need the complement of personal accounts and medical evidence, moving policy makers toward action and ensuring that such actions are in keeping with current clinical best practices. In addition to these face-to-face interactions, clinical and narrative expertise can be mobilized through various forms of media, targeting larger audiences and influencing public perceptions in a way that reduces stigma and creates an impetus for social change. Additionally, engaging PWSUD in advocacy efforts directly counters the narrative of disempowerment that too often frames their interactions within the health care system and in society more broadly. Complementing the process of recovery by advocating for oneself and others empowers PWSUD by increasing a sense of self-efficacy and promotes seeking help.

Advocacy Needs According to Type of Substance Use Disorder

Advocacy needs vary according to the type of substance use disorder (SUD) because each type has unique medical, psychiatric, social, and economic sequelae. A brief summary of special considerations follows.

Alcohol Use Disorder

In 2017, approximately 14.5 million people ages 12 and older, representing 5.3% of the U.S. population, had alcohol use disorder (Substance Abuse and Mental Health Services Administration 2018). With its significant medical sequelae, alcohol use is the third leading cause of preventable death in the United States, following tobacco use and poor diet/physical inactivity (Mokdad et al. 2004). Of the nearly 89,000 deaths attributable to alcohol each year, more than half are due to acute causes, such as motor vehicle and other accidents, and the rest are the results of chronically mediated medical conditions, such as pancreatitis and liver disease (Centers for Disease Control and Prevention 2013). Advocacy is needed both to increase public awareness of the chronic health impact of unhealthy alcohol use and to promote evidence-based policy interventions, which include increasing prices, restricting availability, and limiting promotions and advertising (Walley et al. 2019). Physicians can also advocate for and implement harm reduction strategies, which will be discussed later in this chapter (see the subsection "Remedicalization").

Cannabis Use Disorder

At the time of this chapter's writing, 10 states have fully legalized marijuana, and another 34 have made it partially legal by approving it for medical use (DISA Global Solutions 2019). As public opinion and policy shift toward legalization, the number of marijuana users in the United States continues to rise (Substance Abuse and Mental Health Services Administration 2018). Health advocacy is needed to ensure that the public is informed of the medical and psychiatric health risks associated with cannabis and that policies are implemented to minimize those risks. Similar to what has been done in the alcohol and tobacco industries, attention must be given to limiting promotions and advertisements that target adolescents.

Cocaine Use Disorder

Approximately 966,000 people ages 12 and older had a cocaine use disorder in 2017 (Substance Abuse and Mental Health Services Administration 2018). Overdose deaths involving cocaine have more than tripled in the past two decades, increasing from about 3,800 in 1999 to almost 14,000 in 2017 (Centers for Disease Control and Prevention 2018). Much of the increase in cocaine-involved overdose deaths has been attributed to use in combination with opioids or other narcotics (Centers for Disease Control and Prevention 2018). Special considerations must be provided regarding decriminalization—removing criminal penalties for personal possession of all narcotics—given the disparities in criminal charges for various forms of cocaine. Possession of crack cocaine has been associated with harsher sentences, resulting in disproportionate criminalization in urban communities of color (Kurtzleban 2010).

Stimulant Use Disorder (Including Methamphetamine)

In 2017, an estimated 572,000 people ages 12 and older had a stimulant use disorder in the past year (Substance Abuse and Mental Health Services Administration 2018). With stimulants, as with cocaine, there is an increased risk of overdose when taken in combination with opioids. Stimulant-involved overdose deaths have increased twentyfold from 500 in 1999 to more than 10,000 in 2017, due in large part to this dangerous combination (Centers for Disease Control and Prevention 2018). Because rates of methamphetamine use are higher in rural communities, special consideration should be given to improving access to substance use treatment in rural counties. Harm reduction strategies being considered for stimulant use include drug checking to decrease harm from use of contaminated stimulants that may contain fentanyl or other synthetic opioids (Walley et al. 2019).

Sedative-Hypnotic Use Disorder

Overdose deaths involving sedative-hypnotic use have also increased in the past 20 years, with benzodiazepine-related deaths increasing tenfold from 1,100 in 1999 to more than 11,000 in 2017 (Centers for Disease Control and Prevention 2018). Again, this increase is in large part due to combination with opioids. Other health consequences of unhealthy sedative-hypnotic use include risk of withdrawal, falls, and cognitive impairment. As with other prescribed medications, sedative-hypnotics are at risk for diversion. Advocacy in support of policies aimed at reducing supply, such as state prescription monitoring systems, is necessary in addressing unhealthy use of sedative-hypnotics.

Opioid Use Disorder (Including Heroin and Prescription Opioids)

The current opioid epidemic has captured the nation's attention, with its impact being highlighted through media, film, literature, and politics, as communities across the country are devastated by the crisis. In the 1990s and early 2000s, prescription opioids flooded the market as a result of targeted efforts by pharmaceutical companies to increase the prescription of long-term opioids for pain management (Lyapustina and Alexander 2015). Although many states have passed laws to regulate health care providers' ability to prescribe opioids, annual death rates continue to rise (CO*RE 2018) (Figure 15–1). Between 2010 and 2015, the quantity of opioids prescribed nationally fell by 19%, yet the overdose rate rose by 25% (Szalavitz 2018c).

There is an ongoing need for physician leadership in advocating for policies to address the opioid crisis and ensuring that proposed interventions are based in evidence. Policies are needed to continue expanding access to opioid agonist therapies (i.e., buprenorphine and methadone). Harm reduction strategies, including needle exchange, sites for supervised

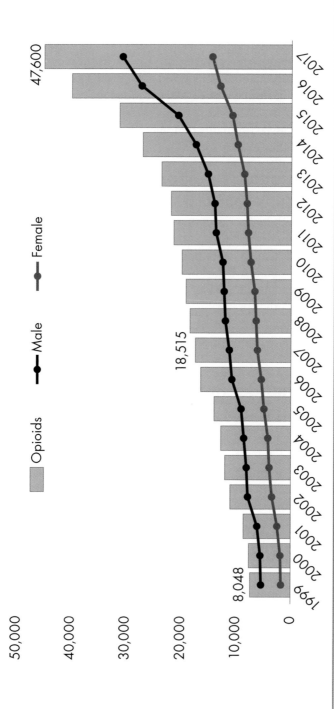

FIGURE 15–1.   National drug overdose deaths involving any opioid, number among all ages, by gender, 1999–2017.

Source.   Reprinted from National Center for Health Statistics: Multiple cause of death 1999–2017 on CDC WONDER online database, in Overdose Death Rates, Figure 3. Bethesda, MD, National Institute on Drug Abuse, January 2019. Available at: www.drugabuse.gov/related-topics/trends-statistics/overdose-death-rates. Accessed August 28, 2019.

injection, and naloxone for overdose prevention, reduce the morbidity and mortality associated with opioid use. The need for solutions to the opioid crisis has contributed to reframing popular opinion regarding substance use and demands that the medical community take action. It is a critical time in which advocates have increased opportunities to promote the destigmatization, remedicalization, and decriminalization of SUDs.

Advocacy Needs in Rural Versus Urban Settings

The public health impact of SUDs and the availability of treatment resources can vary on the basis of population density, resulting in differing advocacy needs in rural versus urban settings. Rural settings have fewer substance use treatment facilities and are rated lower in terms of certain quality measures, including access to highly educated counselors, presence of a physician, and availability of wraparound services (Bond Edmond et al. 2015). As of 2015, rural overdose death rates outpaced rates in urban settings (Mack et al. 2017). Because of the lack of opioid treatment programs in rural settings, advocacy efforts are needed to continue expanding access to opioid agonist treatment and the use of telemedicine. In contrast, urban communities are impacted by different structural factors, including higher rates of criminalization, with drug diversion programs being used at lower rates. Table 15–1 summarizes differing SUD treatment characteristics and needs in rural and urban settings (Substance Abuse and Mental Health Services Administration 2012).

Advocacy Needs for Underrepresented Minority Groups

Although patterns and types of substance use vary across racial and ethnic groups, rates of use are generally the same across all demographics. However, the effects of stigmatization and criminalization have disproportionately impacted underrepresented minorities and have led to health disparities in substance use treatment (Lagisetty et al. 2019). Responses to previous addiction crises in black and Latino communities were mediated through the judicial system, resulting in heavy policing, increased rates of incarceration, and higher sentencing in the absence of medical treatment. Advocacy efforts are needed to ensure that treatment resources are being directed toward communities of color and that treatment is provided in a culturally informed manner. Additionally, implementation of drug policies should include racial impact assessments to reduce the harm caused by criminalization of minority com-

TABLE 15–1. **Differing substance use disorder treatment characteristics and needs in rural and urban settings**

Rural treatment admissions are more likely than urban treatment admissions to:	Urban treatment admissions are more likely than rural treatment admissions to:
Be non-Hispanic white	Be non-Hispanic black
Be American Indian or Alaska Native	Be Hispanic
Report full-time employment source	Not be in the labor force
Have wage/salary as primary income	Report not having a primary source of income
Be referred to substance abuse treatment through the criminal justice system	Be self- or individually referred to treatment
Report no past month use of their primary substance of abuse	Engage in daily use of their primary substance of abuse
Report primary alcohol abuse	Report primary cocaine abuse
Report primary abuse of non-heroin opiates	Report primary heroin abuse
Be age 18–25	Be age 18 or older at first use

Source.   Substance Abuse and Mental Health Services Administration: The TEDS Report: A Comparison of Rural and Urban Substance Abuse Treatment Admissions. July 31, 2012. Available at: https://www.samhsa.gov/sites/default/files/teds-short-report043-urban-rural-admissions-2012.pdf. Accessed August 30, 2019.

munities (James and Jordan 2018). Special considerations must also be given to the availability of treatment service to American Indian, Alaskan Native, and Native Hawaiian communities, with advocacy efforts aimed at developing the human and infrastructural resources needed to provide quality, evidence-based treatment (Novins et al. 2011).

Examples and Proposed Solutions

In this section, we review past successes, current proposed solutions, and future directions, organized along three types of advocacy: destigmatization, remedicalization, and decriminalization. Although we discuss these aspects of advocacy individually, we hope readers will note that the corresponding areas of disempowerment for PWSUD do not operate in silos. The effects of stigmatization, demedicalization, and criminalization are not mediated independently, and advocacy efforts within each domain have impacts across all three.

Destigmatization

Stigma has been defined as a mark of disgrace associated with a particular circumstance, quality, or person (Lexico 2019). This "mark of disgrace" has been assigned to PWSUD and many types of addiction through popular adherence to the concept that PWSUD have flawed characters. Many consider that a return to substance use, despite significant medical, psychiatric, social, and economic consequences, is due to a moral failing. The stigmatized formulation of addiction as a moral problem affects individuals' self-perceptions (Wakeman and Rich 2018).

Past Solutions

An important advancement in destigmatizing addiction occurred through updates to DSM-5 (American Psychiatric Association 2013), which adopted less stigmatizing terminology in the diagnosis of substance-related and addictive disorders. Diagnostic categories were updated, employing the term *substance use disorders* rather than *substance abuse* and *substance dependence*. DSM-5 also removed legal consequences as a part of the diagnostic criteria, focusing on the medical, physiological, psychological, and social impacts of substance use (Saitz et al. 2019). The adoption of nonstigmatizing language in the diagnoses themselves sets the tone for a more rational discussion of addiction in clinical settings.

Current Proposed Solutions and Future Directions

Language used in clinical environments can perpetuate or mitigate stigma imposed on PWSUD; therefore, physicians must take the lead in addressing stigmatizing language and advocating for a culture of recovery. Destigmatization in clinical settings includes the use of nonstigmatizing language in the written and verbal communications that take place between physicians and PWSUD, physicians and clinical staff, and physicians and their colleagues across specialties. The use of nonstigmatizing language not only acts as a model for members of the treatment team but

TABLE 15–2. Examples of stigmatizing versus nonstigmatizing language

	Terms to avoid	Preferred terminology
Urine toxicology screen	Dirty	Positive
	Clean	Negative
		Detected
		Not detected
Descriptions of patients	Addict	Patient with a substance use disorder
	Alcoholic	
	Drunk	Patient with alcohol use disorder
	Junkie	
	Crackhead	Patient with opiate use disorder
	Abuser	
		Patient with cocaine use disorder

Source.   Saitz et al. 2019.

also affects providers' perceptions of PWSUD. This concept has been highlighted in the literature: Kelly and Westerhoff (2010) demonstrated that clinicians who were assigned a clinical vignette in which the patient was described as a "substance abuser" rather than someone with a "substance use disorder" were more likely to view the patient as personally responsible for their substance use and to agree that more punitive measures should be taken. These findings suggest that stigmatizing language not only informs perceptions but also can impact treatment decisions. Table 15–2 provides examples of stigmatizing versus nonstigmatizing language that can be used when communicating with patients, families, staff, and peers.

Efforts to destigmatize addiction and PWSUD must extend beyond the clinical setting and into the public domain. In addition to writing op-eds and participating in other forms of media outreach, physicians and PWSUD can further decrease stigma by educating lay audiences at community centers, schools, and places of worship. There is also an important role for the physician in advocating for policy change at each level of government. Currently, we see how framing addiction as a public health crisis results in resources being allocated toward research and treatment. As nonstigmatized and remedicalized language becomes commonplace in the media and public discourse, we hope that policy will continue to shift away from punitive responses toward substance use and toward more comprehensive medical and social interventions.

Case Example: Stigmatizing Language About Mr. E

Mr. E is a 57-year-old Latino male with a history of coronary artery disease and cocaine use who presents to the emergency department with chest pain. An electrocardiogram reveals nonspecific ST segment changes. Initial troponin is elevated to 0.45 ng/mL, and the urine toxicology is positive for cocaine and benzodiazepines. Mr. E is admitted to the hospital to rule out myocardial infarction. While on the cardiology observation floor, he becomes agitated, pulls off the telemetry monitoring pads, and demands to be discharged. The psychiatry department is called to determine whether the patient has capacity to leave against medical advice.

The medicine intern's admission note recounts the above history and reports that the patient "is a cocaine abuser" and "a frequent flyer who often demands to leave AMA." Nursing notes report that the patient had "a dirty urine" on admission, which is his third one this month. On arrival to the unit, the psychiatry resident speaks with a member of the nursing staff, who states, "That man is a pain! Every time he comes here, he leaves AMA and goes right back to that stuff. He just can't stay clean! I wonder if he's just trying to avoid jail time—they say he's got so many possession charges, ya know?"

In the room, Mr. E is pacing back and forth. He says to the resident, "Are you gonna let me outta here? These people don't know how to help me!" He proceeds to tell the resident that he overheard staff members saying they couldn't believe he was back again. He didn't feel like the team was listening to him and felt he was being judged. He said, "Every time I come here, they just treat me like an addict. I'm not a junkie. I don't even do heroin, but they treat us all the same." After a complete evaluation, Mr. E was found to have capacity to leave AMA and was discharged from the hospital.

In this case example, there were multiple instances when medical providers could have used less stigmatizing language to describe the patient and his SUD. Substitution of terms such as *clean, dirty,* and *abuser* with nonstigmatizing language may have changed both the patient's experience and the providers' perceptions of Mr. E and his presentation. The use of nonstigmatizing language reinforces a nonjudgmental stance, which is necessary for mitigating the effects of stigma and facilitating engagement in care.

Remedicalization

Demedicalization of substance use can be traced back to the prohibition era of the early 1900s, which coincided with emerging moral formulations of addiction in the medical literature (Kunz and White 2019). Although advances in the medical understanding of substance use were brought forth throughout the twentieth century, it was imaging studies published in the early 2000s demonstrating neurobiological changes occurring as a result of addiction that helped to reestablish the medical basis for these disorders (Volkow et al. 2004).

Unhealthy substance use is now considered one of the most pressing public health crises in the United States. Discussion of substance use as a public health issue represents a shift away from moralization as a frame for understanding and responding to addiction (Robert Wood Johnson Foundation 2001); by conceptualizing addiction within a medical framework, the response to substance use is mediated through improving access to treatment and promotion of policies that reduce the morbidity and mortality associated with substance use. Physician advocacy in this area can set the course for policies that impact treatment delivery to PWSUD and can create an avenue for empowering PWSUD to better engage with and effectively navigate through the health care system.

Past Solutions

Remedicalization of addiction was effectively signed into law with the passage of the Mental Health Parity and Addiction Equity Act of 2008 (MHPAEA; Centers for Medicare and Medicaid Services 2019). As an example of successful legislative advocacy, MHPAEA requires insurance companies to cover mental health and addiction services equitably with respect to other health conditions. Additionally, it has been shown that increasing access to health care increases access to addiction treatment. Specifically, states that expanded Medicaid under the Patient Protection and Affordable Care Act of 2010 (P.L. No 111-148) saw an increase in the number of people accessing addiction treatment (Beronio et al. 2014). Unfortunately, advocacy is still needed in the enforcement of MHPAEA to ensure access to care for PWSUD; studies suggest that people in need of mental health services are less likely to have access to care and more likely to be charged more for mental health treatment than for primary care services (Dangor 2019).

Advocacy efforts to regulate the tobacco industry represent an example of successful medicalization of a specific SUD leading to improved public health outcomes. Concerted efforts by local, state, and national public health agencies informed the general public and policy makers about the public health impact of cigarette smoking and tobacco use. Advocates promoted policies that regulated the tobacco industry through increasing prices, increasing taxes, and banning promotions and advertisements that targeted children and adolescents. As a result, there has been a steady decline in the prevalence of tobacco use over the past 50 years (Wang et al. 2018).

Current Proposed Solutions

Increase access to addiction treatment. Remedicalization of addiction includes advocating for expanded access to evidence-based treatments. In particular, access to life-saving treatments for opioid use disorder must be expanded in order to combat the opioid epidemic. Efforts are under way to increase access to opioid agonist therapy (i.e., methadone and buprenorphine) by advocating for policies that 1) increase the number of opioid treatment centers, 2) increase the number of buprenorphine prescribers, and 3) decrease the regulatory burden to become a buprenorphine prescriber. Importantly, as of December 2018, the 8-hour medication-assisted treatment training required to receive an X-license waiver to prescribe buprenorphine is available for free online through the Providers Clinical Support System (PCSS) website (Providers Clinical Support System 2019). The effort by some physicians, academicians, and policy leaders to totally eliminate the need for X-license waiver training is gaining traction on various social media platforms (#XtheXlicense). Physicians are also advocating for changes within local health systems to provide immediate access to buprenorphine in emergency departments without requiring a negative urine toxicology screen. Policies that promote access to opioid agonist treatment while individuals are incarcerated are another important area of advocacy with life-saving implications, given that individuals released from prison have decreased opioid tolerance and are at higher risk for overdose.

Harm reduction. Harm reduction is a pragmatic, person-centered public health approach that seeks to reduce harm to individuals and communities by emphasizing the measurement of health, social, and economic outcomes over the measurement of substance consumption (Stancliff et al. 2015). Features of harm reduction include the following (Walley et al. 2019):

- Reducing the acute risks of harm (e.g., overdose education, take-home naloxone rescue kits, needle exchange programs, drug checking, supervised drug consumption venues)

- Reducing complications of risk (e.g., preexposure HIV prophylaxis, postexposure HIV prophylaxis, managed alcohol programs, housing first programs)
- Reducing harm by reducing use (e.g., access to opioid agonist or antagonist medication, heroin treatment, managed alcohol programs)
- Reducing harm by engaging in care (e.g., needle exchange programs, access to opioid agonist or antagonist medications, housing first programs)

The Prevention Point Philadelphia (https://ppponline.org) needle exchange program is an example of a harm reduction program that minimizes the acute risk of substance use (death) by engaging individuals in care. Individuals who engage with this program also can be initiated on buprenorphine and receive a variety of medical and nonmedical services.

Future Directions

Moving forward, ongoing advocacy is needed to improve access to addiction treatment. Although parity laws have been passed, patients still face barriers when trying to get insurance companies to cover addiction services (Dangor 2019; Szalavitz 2018a). Advocacy efforts by physicians and PWSUD are needed to ensure that patients get access to the services that are guaranteed to them by law. Additionally, as was demonstrated by Medicaid expansion, universal access to quality health care is a promising policy solution that can expand access to substance use treatment (Andrews et al. 2019).

Case Example: Use of Harm Reduction Strategies for Mr. E

Six months after he was found to have capacity to leave the hospital, Mr. E returns to the emergency department following an overdose reversal with naloxone. Mr. E reports that he was visiting a friend, Ms. D, on the other side of town and purchased cocaine from a new dealer. He remembers snorting a few lines of cocaine, then waking up in the ambulance. He was told by the emergency medical technicians that a friend of Mr. E's administered naloxone when she noticed that he was slumped over and nodding out. The urine toxicology report is positive for benzodiazepines, cocaine, and a synthetic opioid. Review of the state prescription monitoring system reveals that Mr. E received 100 tablets of lorazepam from four different providers in the last month.

> ## Case Example: Use of Harm Reduction Strategies for Mr. E *(continued)*
>
> Mr. E is thankful that Ms. D had a naloxone kit available and could recognize the signs of an overdose. He is also frightened by what happened and wants to get addiction treatment for cocaine and benzodiazepine use disorders. Although he is unemployed, he was enrolled in Medicaid during a previous hospital visit. Mr. E is placed on a waiting list for a treatment facility nearby that accepts Medicaid, but he must wait 6 weeks before a spot becomes available.

In this case example, Mr. E had an unintentional overdose involving benzodiazepines and cocaine that was likely contaminated with a synthetic opioid. His friend Ms. D had received education in recognizing the signs of an overdose and was provided a take-home naloxone overdose reversal kit, which she was able to use to help Mr. E. This case illustrates the importance of harm reduction strategies in reducing acute risk of harm and the need for expanded access to substance use treatment. Additionally, it demonstrates the importance of advocating for policies that reduce the supply of prescribed narcotics and the need for more mechanisms to follow patient supply of controlled substances through systems such as state prescription drug monitoring programs (PDMPs). However, it is important to note that more research must be done to fully understand whether state PDMPs cause more harm than good for PWSUD because there is often undue scrutiny placed on this population (Carr 2016).

Decriminalization

Criminalization of addiction in the United States has a long history, dating back to the prohibition era of the early 1900s and escalating with the "War on Drugs" in the 1970s. A generous interpretation of policies that criminalize addiction is that they intend to deter individuals from use by enforcing laws against use. Inherent in this practice is the notion that returning to substance use despite consequences is a choice and not a symptom. Therefore, criminalization relies on stigma as a premise of its implementation, and punitive responses to PWSUD reinforce it. People of color, specifically black and nonwhite Latinos, are disproportionately stigmatized and criminalized by these policies, with racism and xenophobia shaping the development of U.S. drug policy since the early 1900s (Szalavitz 2018b). Criminalization resulted in increased rates of incarceration, harsher sentences, and less access to necessary addiction treatment for these populations.

Criminalization of SUDs comes at a high financial and human cost. In 2010, law enforcement costs for marijuana alone totaled $3.6 billion, with a low estimate of $750 being spent per arrest (Bradford 2013). From 2001 to 2010, about 8.2 million marijuana arrests were made, with blacks being 3.73 times more likely to be arrested than whites (American Civil Liberties Union 2019). These figures estimate cost to the states but do not account for cost to the individual in terms of time, lost potential days of work, and disruption in daily life that has varied downstream effects.

Past and Current Proposed Solutions

Past and ongoing efforts to decriminalize addiction include the expansion of drug diversion programs. For example, the Law Enforcement Assisted Diversion (LEAD) programs (www.leadbureau.org) allow police officers discretionary authority to divert individuals to community-based harm reduction interventions for violations driven by unmet behavioral health needs. This diversion allows individuals to avoid the normal legal system cycle, including booking, detention, prosecution, conviction, and incarceration. Instead, referrals are made to a trauma-informed intensive case management service that includes services such as transitional housing and/or drug treatment. Through the LEAD National Support Bureau, municipalities can receive technical support and guidance in establishing their local LEAD programs. Although care must be given to mitigate implicit bias in this system, local municipalities have been successful in diverting individuals away from incarceration, with one Seattle-based LEAD program reporting that its participants are 58% less likely to be arrested.

Future Directions

Many advocates point to Portugal as an example of the future for drug policy in the United States (Kristoff 2017). In 2001, Portugal fully decriminalized all drugs and began treating addiction as a medical issue rather than a legal concern. Rates of overdose deaths decreased by 85% because decriminalization came with a resultant expansion in access to evidence-based treatment (Kristoff 2017). This sweeping policy change reflects the principle that instead of operating independently of one another, destigmatization, remedicalization, and decriminalization are interdependent processes, each of which is necessary to improve population health in relation to addiction.

> ### Case Example: Advocacy's Impact on Mr. E
>
> Four weeks before Mr. E's bed is available in the substance use treatment program, he is approached by police officers after a call was made that he was loitering in front of a convenience mart. He tells the officers that he has recently experienced homelessness and is awaiting a bed in a treatment facility. His city just started a LEAD program, and the officers refer him for intensive case management services. As a result, he is connected to transitional housing and assigned a caseworker who is able to advocate for moving his substance use treatment admission date up by 2 weeks.

Conclusion

Stigmatization, demedicalization, and criminalization result in disempowerment of PWSUD and create barriers to accessing needed care. Physicians and PWSUD have a role in reversing these processes by engaging in multifaceted advocacy efforts that influence public opinion and promote policy change on the local, state, and national levels. As explained in this chapter, previous and current advocacy efforts have resulted in improved public health outcomes. Ongoing conversations taking place in community centers, places of worship, city halls, and legislative chambers are needed to continue reshaping the national discourse. These public discussions are critical in reforming public policy to provide more equitable access to evidence-based treatments for addiction in the United States.

Online Resources

Medication Assisted Treatment Waiver Training

Providers Clinical Support System: Waiver Training for Physicians. https://pcssnow.org/medication-assisted-treatment/waiver-training-for-physicians. Accessed September 28, 2019.

Overdose Prevention

Harm Reduction Coalition: Overdose Prevention. Available at: https://harmreduction.org/issues/overdose-prevention/. Accessed September 28, 2019.

Prescribe to Prevent: https://prescribetoprevent.org. Accessed September 28, 2019.

Substance Abuse and Mental Health Services Administration: Opioid Overdose Prevention Toolkit. Available at: https://store.samhsa.gov/system/files/sma18-4742.pdf. Accessed December 29, 2019.

References

American Civil Liberties Union: Marijuana arrests by the numbers. New York, American Civil Liberties Union, 2019. Available at: www.aclu.org/gallery/marijuana-arrests-numbers. Accessed August 29, 2019.

American Psychiatric Association: Diagnostic and Statistical Manual of Mental Disorders, 5th Edition. Arlington, VA, American Psychiatric Association, 2013

Andrews CM, Pollack HA, Abraham AJ, et al: Medicaid coverage in substance use disorder treatment after the Affordable Care Act. J Subst Abuse Treat 102:1–7, 2019 31202283

Beronio K, Glied S, Frank R: How the Affordable Care Act and Mental Health Parity and Addiction Equity Act greatly expand coverage of behavioral health care. J Behav Health Serv Res 41(4):410–428, 2014 24833486

Bond Edmond M, Aletraris L, Roman PM: Rural substance use treatment centers in the United States: an assessment of treatment quality by location. Am J Drug Alcohol Abuse 41(5):449–457, 2015 26337202

Bradford H: Marijuana law enforcement cost states an estimated $3.6 in 2010: ACLU. Huffpost, June 4, 2013. Available at: www.huffpost.com/entry/marijuana-arrests-cost-racially biased_n_3385756. Accessed August 29, 2019.

Carr DB: Patients with pain need less stigma not more. Pain Med 17(8):1391–1393, 2016 27418318

Centers for Disease Control and Prevention: Alcohol Related Disease Impact (ARDI) application. Atlanta, GA, Centers for Disease Control and Prevention, 2013. Available at: www.cdc.gov/ARDI. Accessed August 29, 2019.

Centers for Disease Control and Prevention: Multiple cause of death, 1999–2017. CDC Wonder database, 2018. Available at: www.drugabuse.gov/related-topics/trends-statistics/overdose-death-rates. Accessed December 29, 2019.

Centers for Medicare and Medicaid Services: The Mental Health Parity and Addiction Equity Act (MHPAEA). Atlanta, GA, Centers for Disease Control and Prevention, 2019. Available at: www.cms.gov/cciio/programs-and-initiatives/other-insurance-protections/mhpaea_factsheet.html. Accessed August 29, 2019.

CO*RE: Data trends: opioid prescribing, overdose deaths, and more. San Francisco, CA, Collaborative for Relevant Education, July 12, 2018. Available at: http://core-rems.org/data-trends-opioid-prescribing-overdose-deaths-and-more. Accessed August 29, 2019.

Dangor G: "Mental health parity" is still an elusive goal in U.S. insurance coverage. Washington, DC, NPR, June 7, 2019. Available at: www.npr.org/sections/health-shots/2019/06/07/730404539/mental-health-parity-is-still-an-elusive-goal-in-u-s-insurance-coverage. Accessed August 29, 2019.

DISA Global Solutions: Map of marijuana legality by state. Houston, TX, DISA Global Solutions, 2019. Available at: https://disa.com/map-of-marijuana-legality-by-state. Accessed August 30, 2019.

James K, Jordan A: The opioid crisis in black communities. J Law Med Ethics 46(2):404–421, 2018 30146996

Kelly JF, Westerhoff CM: Does it matter how we refer to individuals with substance-related conditions? A randomized study of two commonly used terms. Int J Drug Policy 21(3):202–207, 2010 20005692

Kristoff N: How to win the war on drugs. New York Times, September 22, 2017. Available at: www.nytimes.com/2017/09/22/opinion/sunday/portugal-drug-decriminalization.html. Accessed August 30, 2019.

Kunz K: The addiction medicine physician as a change agent for prevention and public health, in The ASAM Principles of Addiction Medicine, 6th Edition. Edited by Miller SC, Fiellin DA, Rosenthal RN, et al. Philadelphia, PA, Lippincott Williams & Wilkins, 2019, pp 83–88

Kunz K, White W: Addiction medicine in America: its birth, early history, and current status, in The ASAM Principles of Addiction Medicine, 6th Edition. Edited by Miller SC, Fiellin DA, Rosenthal RN, et al. Philadelphia, PA, Lippincott Williams & Wilkins, 2019, pp 381–388

Kurtzleban D: Data shows racial disparity in crack sentences. US News and World Report, August 3, 2010. Available at: www.usnews.com/news/articles/2010/08/03/data-show-racial-disparity-in-crack-sentencing. Accessed August 30, 2019.

Lagisetty PA, Ross R, Bohnert A, et al: Buprenorphine treatment divide by race/ethnicity and payment. JAMA Psychiatry May 8, 2019 [Epub ahead of print] 31066881

Lexico: Stigma definition. Lexico.com, 2019. Available at: https://en.oxford dictionaries.com/definition/stigma. Accessed August 30, 2019.

Lyapustina T, Alexander GC: The prescription opioid addiction and abuse epidemic: how it happened and what we can do about it. Pharmaceutical Journal 294:7866, 2015

Mack KA, Jones CM, Ballesteros MF: Illicit drug use, illicit drug use disorders, and drug overdose deaths in metropolitan and nonmetropolitan areas—United States. MMWR Surveill Summ 66(19):1–12, 2017 29049278

Mokdad AH, Marks JS, Stroup DF, et al: Actual causes of death in the United States, 2000. JAMA 291(10):1238–1245, 2004 15010446

National Institute on Drug Abuse: Overdose Death Rates, Figure 3. Bethesda, MD, National Institute on Drug Abuse, January 2019. Available at: www.drugabuse.gov/related-topics/trends-statistics/overdose-death-rates. Accessed August 28, 2019.

Novins DK, Aarons GA, Conti SG, et al; Centers for American Indian and Alaska Native Health's Substance Abuse Treatment Advisory Board: Use of the evidence base in substance abuse treatment programs for American Indians and Alaska Natives: pursuing quality in the crucible of practice and policy. Implement Sci 6:63, 2011 21679438

Providers Clinical Support System: Waiver training for physicians. East Providence, RI, Providers Clinical Support System, 2019. Available at: https://pcssnow.org/medication-assisted-treatment/waiver-training-for-physicians. Accessed August 30, 2019.

Robert Wood Johnson Foundation: Substance abuse: the nation's number one health problem. Princeton, NJ, Robert Wood Johnson Foundation, 2001. Available at: www.ncjrs.gov/pdffiles1/ojjdp/fs200117.pdf. Accessed December 29, 2019.

Saitz R, Miller SC, Fiellin N, et al: Recommended use of terminology in addiction medicine, in The ASAM Principles of Addiction Medicine, 6th Edition. Edited by Miller SC, Fiellin DA, Rosenthal RN, et al. Philadelphia, PA, Lippincott Williams & Wilkins, 2019, pp 24–26

Shatterproof: A public health crisis with an enormous cost. New York, Shatterproof, 2019. Available at: www.shatterproof.org/about-addiction/public-health-crisis-with-an-enormous-cost. Accessed August 30, 2019.

Stancliff S, Phillips BW, Maghsoudi N, et al: Harm reduction: front line public health. J Addict Dis 34(2–3):206–219, 2015 26080038

Substance Abuse and Mental Health Services Administration: The TEDS Report: a comparison of rural and urban substance abuse treatment admissions. July 31, 2012. Available at: www.samhsa.gov/sites/default/files/teds-short-report043-urban-rural-admissions-2012.pdf. Accessed August 30, 2019.

Substance Abuse and Mental Health Services Administration: Key substance use and mental health indicators in the United States: results from the 2017 National Survey on Drug Use and Health (HHS Publ No SMA 18-5068, NSDUH Series H-53). Rockville, MD, Center for Behavioral Health Statistics and Quality, Substance Abuse and Mental Health Services Administration. 2018. Available at: https://www.samhsa.gov/data/sites/default/files/cbhsq-reports/NSDUHFFR2017/NSDUHFFR2017.htm. Accessed August 30, 2019.

Szalavitz M: Insurance is supposed to cover addiction treatment but it's still a nightmare. Vice, December 10, 2018a. Available at: www.vice.com/en_us/article/mbyxgx/insurance-covers-opioid-addiction-treatment-but-its-a-nightmare. Accessed August 30, 2019.

Szalavitz M: There's no rational way to justify America's drug laws. Vice, July 13, 2018b. Available at: https://tonic.vice.com/en_us/article/kzy87z/americas-drug-laws-racism-versus-science. Accessed August 30, 2019.

Szalavitz M: Walmart's dumb new opioid policy could cost lives. Vice, May 8, 2018c. Available at: www.vice.com/en_us/article/nekj7d/walmarts-dumb-new-opioid-policy-could-cost-lives. Accessed August 30, 2019.

Volkow ND, Fowler JS, Wang GJ: The addicted human brain viewed in the light of imaging studies: brain circuits and treatment strategies. Neuropharmacology 47(suppl 1):3–13, 2004 15464121

Wakeman SE, Rich JD: Barriers to medications for addiction treatment: how stigma kills. Subst Use Misuse 53(2):330–333, 2018 28961017

Walley AY, Stancliff S, Perez-Urbano I: Harm reduction, overdose prevention, and addiction medicine, in The ASAM Principles of Addiction Medicine, 6th Edition. Edited by Miller SC, Fiellin DA, Rosenthal RN, et al. Philadelphia, PA, Lippincott Williams & Wilkins, 2019, pp 473–482

Wang TW, Asman K, Gentzke AS, et al: Tobacco product use among adults—United States, 2017. MMWR Morb Mortal Wkly Rep 67(44):1225–1232, 2018 30408019

16

Advocacy for Military Service Members

John Chaves, M.D.
Rohul Amin, M.D., FAPA, FACP

Learning Objectives

By the end of this chapter, readers will be able to:

- Summarize three unique advocacy considerations when caring for military personnel with psychiatric illness
- Identify two opportunities for population-based advocacy for military psychiatric patients
- Describe clinical and nonclinical triggers for referring military personnel to a military psychiatrist
- Identify two military resources available for military personnel with psychiatric needs

This chapter is written with the nonmilitary psychiatrist in mind: your advocacy is desperately needed for active duty service members, considering their tremendous mental health needs and, in some cases, their

The views expressed in this chapter are those of the authors and do not reflect the official policy of the Department of the Army, Department of Defense (DoD), or U.S. government.

specific needs for civilian advocacy. Advocacy on an individual and population level starts with understanding the health system that your patients navigate as well as their culture and environment. Because we realize that many civilian providers are not familiar with military culture and structure, we describe some of these specifics throughout the chapter to build a groundwork for advocacy. We then describe several individual advocacy issues relevant to military patients and suggest points to consider when advocating on these issues. Occasionally through the chapter, we mention the patient in the following case.

Case Example 1

Sergeant (SGT) Smith, a 32-year-old married white man, is referred to your community-based practice by his civilian primary care doctor. SGT Smith is an Army recruiter at a local recruiting station a few blocks from your office. On interview, he seems severely depressed and endorses being overwhelmed by the demands of his new job as a recruiter. He started this job 4 months ago and has seen his family once during that time. He is married but geographically separated from the rest of his family, who remain in Fort Hood, Texas, to avoid school disruptions for their children. He reports significant guilt over his three prior deployments and his continued absence from his children's lives. He denies any past psychiatric treatment, but he endorses wishing that he were dead for the past 2 months, saying, "If I didn't wake up in the morning, it would be better for everyone."

You assess that SGT Smith is not at imminent risk for self-harm and does not meet criteria for inpatient hospitalization. However, he states that his situation is hopeless and he feels completely overwhelmed. During the safety assessment, he says, "If it gets bad enough, I can always just shoot myself." He says that he has three firearms at home. You have a lot of questions for him, but before you can form a safety plan and schedule a follow-up, SGT Smith asks, "Do you need to tell my command?"

Military Personnel as a Special Population

Military cultural competency includes understanding common military customs, courtesies, language, and other human elements. It also requires administrative and medicolegal knowledge, such as recognition of the formal and informal limitations on a military member's potential to engage in advocacy (Department of Defense 2008). In this chapter, we understate the heterogeneity among different branches of the military and instead paint the military as a singular group with administrative uniqueness—a subgroup of the population needing special advocacy. Our intent in the current section is to introduce the processes, procedures, and policies that will impact a patient who is a service member. However, to understand the human elements of each of the subcultures within the military, you will have to make yourself accessible to service members, be curious, and interact as much as possible with this group both within and outside of your clinic. Unless you are a service member or veteran yourself and already have some of this knowledge, we hope that the perspective you gain will enable you to be a more effective advocate for your service member patients.

Service Members as Patients

Service members might present to civilian psychiatrists for several reasons. SGT Smith and other recruiters might be working a considerable distance from any military providers. Other service members might live relatively close to a military treatment facility or clinic but much closer to a civilian provider who accepts military insurance, and thus they might choose the civilian provider out of convenience. Service members might present to civilian providers urgently or emergently. Finally, because of stigma or fear of career repercussions or misperceptions of the military exceptions to the Health Insurance Portability and Accountability Act of 1996 (HIPAA; P.L. 104-191)—topics that are discussed later in this chapter (see sections "Chain of Command and the Limits of Confidentiality" and "Impact of Psychiatric Diagnoses on Military Careers")—some service members might prefer seeing a civilian rather than a uniformed provider.

At the population level, the prevalence of mental illness is greater in the military than among sociodemographically matched civilians (Kessler et al. 2014; Trautmann et al. 2017). In one study, one-fourth of Army soldiers met criteria in the previous month for a DSM-IV mental disorder (Lazar 2014). From a mission perspective, mental illness is the leading cause of evacuation from the battlefield in Iraq and Afghanistan among female service members and the fourth leading cause among male service members (Armed Forces Health Surveillance Center 2011).

At an individual level, mental illness can be disabling and deadly. In one study of military suicide deaths, 79.3% of soldiers who died from suicide had a previously identified mental health disorder (Nock et al. 2014). In another internal study, suicides were found to be second (28.5%) only to accidental deaths (32.3%) as the cause of death among U.S. service members (Armed Forces Health Surveillance Center 2014). Mental illness may also result in service members' inability to perform in their occupational roles, leading to medical retirement or administrative separation from duty.

In 2010, about 34% of U.S. Army soldiers had at least one clinical encounter in the military outpatient behavioral health clinics, and more than 97% of this care was delivered by the military health system (Hoge et al. 2016). Although these figures indicate superb access to care, there are still significant challenges with maintaining this needed access to care. One issue is retention of military psychiatrists due to a civilian-military pay differential (Mundell 2010). Although the Patient Protection and Affordable Care Act of 2010 (P.L. 111-148) has had a positive impact on mental health access for many Americans, it also may have contributed to a significant increase in civilian psychiatrist pay, thus widening the pay gap between uniformed and civilian psychiatrists (Peckham 2018; Thomas et al. 2018). An unintended consequence of this may be increased attrition of military psychiatrists to the civilian sector.

Advocacy for service members also includes considering the needs of military families and retirees, which are beneficiary groups served by TRICARE, the military health insurance. TRICARE reimbursements are tied by law to Medicare's allowable charges. Therefore, changes in reimbursement policy can have a significant impact on access to mental health care for this population. (Of note, TRICARE is not synonymous with the Department of Veterans Affairs [VA] health care system. More information on advocacy for veteran patients within the VA system can be found in Chapter 17, "Advocacy for Veterans and Their Families.")

Service Members as Advocates

Active duty military psychiatrists exercise various levels of influence in the military health and leadership enterprise. Advocating simultaneously for patients and the mission of the military is an expectation of duty. Psychiatrists have an impact on and advocate for service members through participation in research, informing and developing policies, and direct communication to other service members. For instance, military psychiatrists have access to a process for internal advocacy for policy change, by which a service member may follow the designated chain of command to the Assistant Secretary of Defense (Health Affairs), the senior health policy maker in the Department of Defense (DoD; Department of Defense 2006). Military psychiatrists may also practice advocacy outside of the military by participating in local and national organizations, in both official and unofficial capacities.

However, political influence and advocacy on behalf of service members must be the realm of civilian advocates. This is because there are restrictions on military personnel related to political engagement. Generally, a service member may endorse a political candidate, party, or cause as a private citizen but not in an official capacity or while in uniform. For example, service members may write letters to the newspaper voicing support for a particular policy as a private citizen, but whether in or out of uniform, they may not participate in public discussions or allow to be published any content that promotes a partisan or political cause (Department of Defense 2008). Considering these limitations, military psychiatrists must rely on and collaborate with their civilian counterparts for lobbying at the state and federal levels for system change. An additional way for civilian psychiatrists to advocate for their military patients is to involve or refer to military psychiatrists when appropriate (as further described in the section "When to Refer to a Military Psychiatrist").

Military Accessions and Medical Retention Standards

The accessions process is part of the selection process that occurs before someone joins the military. (The word *accessions* is used because an individual is accessing the system.) The guidelines for accession standards outline specific medical conditions that are disqualifying for military service. Physical conditions, given their more objective nature, are screened more reliably. For example, sickle cell anemia is detected with an objective blood test that has a low margin of error. Psychiatric illnesses, on the other hand, are more subjective and rely on self-disclosure.

A citizen requiring evaluation for military service is seen by trained military entrance processing station providers to determine eligibility. Many patients with common psychiatric diagnoses may receive a waiver from a specialist, indicating that they are still eligible to serve despite their condition. Conditions for which individuals may receive waivers

include attention-deficit/hyperactivity disorder and a history of an anxiety disorder, among others (these conditions are noted in Table 16–1).
Potential recruits may choose to conceal their psychiatric histories because military recruiters and physicians rely on self-report; however,
fraudulent enlistment is a legal violation with potentially severe legal
ramifications.

After being accepted into the military and making it past basic training, an individual must meet medical retention standards, which are
less strict than accession standards. In terms of psychiatric conditions,
any service member who is found to have significant dysfunction and
poor prognosis for recovery despite sufficient treatment trials may fall
below the retention standards. This results in medical separation from
the military. Table 16–1 shows diagnoses and conditions that are disqualifying for military service.

Accession standards are a fluid part of military policy, and the issu-
ance of waivers varies with the needs of the military. In 2018, *USA Today* reported on a Freedom of Information Act request showing that
more than 700 recruits received waivers for histories of mood disorders,
and nearly 100 received waivers for a history of self-injurious behavior
(Brook 2018). Bringing attention to this subject and advocating to legislators for more inclusive accessions may mean opening up the opportunity for military service, an occupation that offers financial security
and many other benefits, to people with a psychiatric history. In addition, receiving a waiver for a psychiatric condition is not associated with
suicidal ideation or behavior during service (Ursano et al. 2014). Alternatively, advocating for stricter accessions guidelines means protecting
patients from being exposed to the stressors of military service that
could cause relapse or worsening of symptoms. Throughout the years,
psychiatrists and military leaders have advocated successfully for both
the loosening and the tightening of accession standards (Cardona and
Ritchie 2007). Accession standards must balance the mission of the military with the risks of allowing those at high risk for future psychiatric
issues to enlist.

Chain of Command and the Limits of Confidentiality

Responsibilities of the Commander

Military professionals perform many technical jobs. One of the most
recognizable is that of an infantryman. The word *infantry* originates

TABLE 16–1. **Learning, psychiatric, and behavioral conditions that may affect military service opportunity**

History or current occurrence of the following disorders:

Attention-deficit/hyperactivity disorder

Learning disorders after the 14th birthday

Autism spectrum disorders

Disorder with psychotic features

Bipolar and related disorders and affective psychoses

Depressive disorders

Adjustment disorder if current, recurrent, or chronic

History of disruptive, impulse control, or conduct disorders

Any personality disorder

Encopresis after the 13th birthday

Any feeding or eating disorder

Any communication disorder that interferes with speech or repeating commands

Suicidality or self-injury

Obsessive-compulsive disorder

Posttraumatic stress disorder

Anxiety disorders

Dissociative disorders

Somatic symptom and related disorders

Paraphilic disorders

Substance-related and addictive disorder

Any "mental disorders that may reasonably be expected to interfere with or prevent satisfactory performance of military duty"

Prior psychiatric hospitalization for any cause

Source. Department of Defense 2018.

from the word *infant,* with the natural consequence of this being that there must be a *parent*. Military hierarchy, referred to as chain of command, is a tribal ladder with numerous fatherly and motherly figures.

This ladder goes all the way up to the commander-in-chief, the President of the United States. *Command* is military vernacular for a service member's chain of command.

SGT Smith's commanding officer, or commander, is fully responsible for the well-being and accountability of SGT Smith 24 hours a day. A *commander*, by definition, is an individual with legal authority over a soldier. The commander is responsible for everything a unit does or fails to do, which, unlike in the civilian world, includes all unit members' *personal* as well as professional well-being, including their mental health. Various military leadership doctrines encourage delegation of authority to the lowest level possible, but the commander cannot delegate responsibility. Because of this special nature of the relationship between service members and their commanders, the only way to ensure effective advocacy for a patient is by understanding the unique role of the commander and communicating with cultural competence. Engaging another person while caring for an adult can be an uncomfortable concept for physicians, for whom patient autonomy and confidentiality are sacred. Without the full buy-in and engagement of the commander, however, a psychiatrist is unlikely to secure optimal advocacy for a service member.

What Information You Can Share With the Commander

Commanders' exceptions to HIPAA exist. These exceptions are designed to allow commanders to better support the requirements of military operations. This necessity is counterbalanced by the need to protect service members' privacy, which is done by limiting mandatory disclosed personal health information to the "minimum amount of information" required for a given situation (Office of the Surgeon General 2016). This "minimum amount" includes a description of the prescribed medication(s) and treatment plan, the impact of this plan on the service member's ability to work, recommended duty restrictions or limitations, prognosis, and implications for the safety of the service member and others; notably, a diagnosis is not explicitly included in this information. Table 16–2 presents examples of situations in which there is a HIPAA exception for commanders. (For a full list of commander exceptions to HIPAA, see Department of Defense 2009, 2011.) Discussion of any information outside of the scope of the HIPAA exceptions requires that the service member sign a release of information.

Generally, we recommend disclosing only information that is "need to know" for the safety of service members and their units and for the

TABLE 16–2. **Examples of selected military exceptions to the Health Insurance Portability and Accountability Act of 1996 (HIPAA)**

Exception to confidentiality	Example
Harm to self and/or harm to others such as suicide, homicide, or other violent action	A soldier endorses suicidal ideation with plan
Medication that could impair duty performance	A soldier is newly prescribed a possibly sedating medication
Harm to mission; condition impairs the soldier's performance of duty	A soldier becomes psychotic and is unable to continue service without treatment
Coordination of care, including hospitalization and care from civilian providers	A soldier requires inpatient hospitalization for suicidal ideation or continued outpatient treatment for PTSD
Screening and providing updates for an individual in personnel reliability/special programs, such as biological surety, nuclear surety, chemical surety, and personnel security programs	Several sensitive military occupations require clearance for psychiatric illnesses and substance use disorders—most commonly done by military health system providers
Carrying out activities to safeguard the health of the military community, such as reviewing and reporting HIV infection	A soldier reports risky sexual behavior with colleagues from their unit, and an HIV test is positive
Reporting mental status evaluations	A commander asks for a formal evaluation of a soldier—most commonly done by military health system providers
Providing initial and follow-up reports on substance use	A soldier engages in substance use that puts self, others, or the mission of the Department of Defense at risk

Note. Efforts will be made to provide only *minimum necessary* personal health information of an individual that is required to carry out activities necessary to the proper execution of the mission of the military.
Source. Office of the Surgeon General 2016.

execution of the mission of the military. When making need-to-know decisions, you can ask yourself these questions: Does the commander need to know the information to keep the service member or other service members safe and healthy? Would withholding the information put anyone in harm's way or prevent your patient or anyone else from performing their job responsibilities? In many cases, answering these questions requires a discussion with the service member about the specifics of their work duties. Figure 16–1 provides a template letter for communicating the minimum necessary personal health information to a service member's commander.

Officials who are entitled to minimal personal health information are first-line commanders and higher. These officials must be identified and authenticated prior to disclosure, preferably with the name and contact information provided by the service member. First-line commanders may designate others in the military unit in writing to be responsible for requesting and receiving a soldier's personal health information. All of these personnel may be contacted by phone. Disclosing personal health information to commanders or designated members from the patient's unit requires that you explicitly review with them the sensitive nature of this information because command officials typically are not trained in HIPAA policy.

Safety, Suicide, and Means Restriction

A safety assessment of a patient like SGT Smith is critical. As discussed earlier in this chapter, in the relatively healthy and young population of military personnel, suicide ranks among the top causes of death (Hyman et al. 2012). Suicide has been a well-documented, growing, and persistent problem in the military and veteran populations for the past two decades (Ursano et al. 2015). The predominant method of suicide by military personnel is by firearm, and military personnel own firearms at a higher frequency than civilians (Armed Forces Health Surveillance Center 2014). More than 97% of suicides by active and reserve military members occur in the United States rather than during deployment (Pruitt et al. 2019). Given these statistics, a psychiatric evaluation of any service member is incomplete without asking about firearm access and ownership. Understanding this difference in risk between military personnel and civilians, using the knowledge to approach service members with due cultural competency, and disseminating this knowledge to colleagues and trainees is a vital advocacy tool.

Dear Commander:

Your service member (Rank, Name) was seen today in my psychiatry clinic. I diagnosed him/her with a behavioral health condition. This condition requires treatment with medications and talk therapy. It will need to be continued for ____ months. Your service member will need to be able to see me ____ times per week/month. Your service member does/does not have any indications of self-harm. I conclude that (Rank, Name) is low/intermediate/high risk for self-harm. Based on this assessment, I recommend (the following duty restrictions OR no duty restrictions)...

FIGURE 16–1. **Template for communicating to a service member's commander.**

Recommending firearms restriction is a necessary step in ensuring the safety of a high-risk service member. For low-risk service members, however, any recommendations for firearms restriction must be balanced with the stigma of means restriction in military culture (Ritchie 2014). First of all, recommending restriction of a service member's access to firearms is equivalent to saying that the service member cannot do their job, a statement that will have implications for the patient and personnel concerns for the commander. Additionally, confiscation of firearms may lead to disruption of the therapeutic alliance between you and your patient and may fracture trust between service member and commander. It may also have a negative impact on the identity of the service member and affect recovery.

Suffice it to say that your recommendation of means restriction should not be done lightly, and you should keep in mind that it is an appropriate part of the treatment plan for individuals at imminent risk of harm to self or others, for hospitalized individuals, and those for whom a formal thought disorder has not been excluded. Means restriction is ultimately the commander's decision, as is the duration for which firearms are limited. Military psychiatric wards commonly recommend 30-day restrictions on firearms at the time of discharge.

Commanders can physically restrict individuals' access to service rifles and handguns by removing their ability to access the unit's armory. Commanders are also authorized to remove any firearms stored in an on-post residence. However, commanders cannot remove by force firearms that are stored by service members in community dwellings. That being said, in most cases commanders may convince service members to temporarily store their firearms in their unit's armory, effectively removing access.

When caring for service members, you can depend on the command for attention, support, intervention, and means restriction, but these factors never substitute for inpatient hospitalization. An individual's command reserves the right to house service members in the barracks for increased supervision. However, the idea of a "suicide watch" by other soldiers is typically not meaningful because neither the commander nor other soldiers are likely to have expertise in behavioral health treatment and diagnosis.

When to Refer to a Military Psychiatrist

When you treat a patient like SGT Smith, advocating may involve ensuring that the individual follows up with a military psychiatrist. A service member's commander may be informed of such a referral to ensure that the service member follows up with appointments or presents to a walk-in clinic. Additionally, if a patient presents with government-issued paperwork for a recruiter's evaluation, reliability evaluation, or administrative separation evaluation, these situations are best handled by military behavioral health providers, who undergo specialized training to conduct these evaluations. A service member's responsibilities may include handling firearms, costly machinery, and classified information, and military psychiatrists are more familiar with these responsibilities. Furthermore, the information found on official government documents may have ramifications for a service member's career, and therefore they should be completed by evaluators with a thorough understanding of these ramifications. Military psychiatrists may also help civilian psychiatrists by guiding them as to what information may be shared with command officials and by confirming that the content and manner in which personal health information is shared is compliant with laws and regulations. See also the next section, which covers diagnostic considerations for when to refer to a military psychiatrist.

Impact of Psychiatric Diagnoses on Military Careers

In military psychiatry, every assessment is a fitness-for-duty assessment. Providers must be aware that every psychiatric patient may require temporary duty limitations, and a fraction of presenting patients will require permanent duty limitations. Fear of duty limitations secondary to seeking treatment for psychiatric illness is a key contributor to the stigma that service members must overcome when they seek care (Cozza et al. 2014).

Those service members who require permanent duty limitations are evaluated for fitness for duty and potential compensation through the Integrated Disability Evaluation System (IDES; Department of Defense 2014). The role of a psychiatrist in this process is to determine when a service member must be referred to a medical board to determine whether the individual continues to meet medical retention standards. Severe diagnoses, including bipolar disorder, schizophrenia, and other psychotic spectrum disorders, result in automatic entrance into the disability process. For this reason, a military psychiatrist should be consulted immediately when military patients are treated for psychosis or bipolar disorder. An even wider array of psychiatric diagnoses may lead to a medical board if the service member's symptoms do not respond to treatment (see Table 16–1 earlier in this chapter). These diagnoses include chronic adjustment disorder, posttraumatic stress disorder, major depressive disorder, generalized anxiety disorder, and many more.

Some conditions that are disqualifying for continued military service will not result in medical separation. Instead, service members with these conditions are considered for administrative separation from the military, which does not result in medical compensation. Such conditions include acute adjustment disorder, personality disorders, and substance use disorders when they do not respond to sufficient treatment. Administrative separation should not be pursued for patients with disabling psychiatric illnesses, nor should it be a punitive measure by command. If, as a civilian provider, you feel that a service member has not received standard-of-care treatment prior to administrative separation or that psychiatric treatment was withheld punitively, this would be another reason to consult a military psychiatrist or to state your concerns to the patient's commander. Uniformed psychiatrists have multiple options for advocating for their patients in this situation, including speaking directly to the service member's chain of command or placing a new referral through IDES.

Some experts assert that the military disability system is predisposed to exploitation and might reward and thus incentivize sustained or exaggerated symptoms of psychiatric illness (O'Donnell et al. 2015). Opportunities for improvement of IDES include advocating for legislation that incentivizes treatment rather than emphasizing illness severity for treatable conditions and documenting any evidence of malingering or of administrative or political pressure for inaccurate diagnosis (Hart et al. 2018).

Additional Treatment Resources

Despite some improvements in recent years, seeking treatment remains stigmatized by members of the military (Quartana et al. 2014). One way to counter stigma has been to implement confidential resources that, when used, will not be part of a service member's medical or military record. Because providers of these resources do not report information to the patient's command and do not write notes that are readily accessible to DoD providers or military authorities, the use of these programs is a way for service members to receive care through the DoD that is relatively anonymous but still within the military infrastructure and conveniently located on military posts or via telecommunication. Table 16–3 describes some of these confidential resources. Also, seeing civilian providers will generally be more confidential than seeing uniformed providers because the only documentation from civilian encounters that is accessible by DoD providers is prescribed medications paid for by military insurance—medications paid for out of pocket at outside pharmacies would be unknown to the system.

Additional Advocacy Considerations

Besides the opportunities for advocacy described in previous sections, there are many other topics important to advocacy in military psychiatry that are grounds for active debate.

Scope of Practice

At the time of this writing, both the Army and the Navy allow for the training and practice of prescribing psychologists in an effort to increase the number of total uniformed prescribers and to bolster military readiness (Department of the Army 2009; Department of the Navy 2015). Although this is an effort to preserve fighting force, it is important to note that the American Psychiatric Association has opposed legislation in several states granting prescribing power to psychologists (Levin 2017). The argument against psychologist prescribing is, at its core, patient safety. In the military context, this argument must be weighed carefully because military prescribers may be responsible for prescribing without supervision or backup in austere environments.

TABLE 16–3. Anonymous, confidential resources for service members with psychiatric needs

Resource	Eligibility	Phone	Website	Notes
Military OneSource/ Military and Family Life Counseling	AD, family members (all branches)	1-800-342-9647	www.militaryonesource.mil	One-stop source for various confidential services, including behavioral health
Safe Helpline	AD (all branches)	1-877-995-5247	www.safehelpline.org	Sexual assault support for the Department of Defense community
Veterans Crisis Line	Veterans, AD	1-800-273-8255, press 1	www.veteranscrisisline.net	Resource for veterans in crisis and their family and friends; also available for AD service members
Unit Ministry Team	AD, family members (all branches)	Obtain from commander	Obtain from commander	Spiritual advice frequently less stigmatized than treatment for behavioral health

Note. AD = active duty.

Military Sexual Trauma

Case Example 2

Specialist (SPC) Johnson, a 25-year-old single woman with no significant past medical or psychiatric history, presents for an outpatient evaluation a week after being seen in the emergency department for a sexual assault. SPC Johnson, after asking multiple times about limits of confidentiality, confides to you that her assailant is an acquaintance and she chose to make a "restricted report" of the assault in order to get medical care without pressing charges against him. She explains that she was seen with her assailant at a party on the night of the assault and that he is well known and well trusted in their field. Although he is not in her direct chain of command, they are in the same field, and he outranks her. She worries that allegations against him would not be believed, would be "toxic" to her command, would limit her potential for promotion and success in her field, and would require her to relive the details of the assault.

Six months after her initial visit, SPC Johnson reports sustained issues with hypervigilance, avoidance, nightmares, and interpersonal conflict at work. SPC Johnson's commander, aware only that she is having personal problems, works with her to coordinate a permanent change of station. Although her new command is aware that personal issues led to this move, they are unaware of the details.

High rates of sexual trauma in service members, also known as military sexual trauma (MST), are an unfortunate reality in the U.S. military (Department of Defense 2017a). Treating sexual trauma in the military setting is a special challenge because the victim and perpetrator may have power relationships, work and live together, and expect to deploy together. Also, although the above vignette depicts a female survivor, it is important to remember that male and transgender service members are also at risk of experiencing MST (Matthews et al. 2018), and one should not make assumptions about who may or may not be an MST survivor.

MST survivors may choose to avoid reporting harassment or assault because of stigma and barriers to care. Policies enable a service member to file what is known as a *restricted report*, which allows for the victim to receive medical care, counseling, and legal aid, although no official investigation is conducted and chain of command is not made aware of the incident. In contrast, when an *unrestricted report* is made by a service member, the incident is reported formally by a sexual assault prevention and response representative to the service member's commander, who mandatorily reports to his superior officers. This report includes the service member's identity, allowing the commander to advocate for the service member with additional medical, emotional, and administrative support.

When caring for a victim of MST, you should first clarify whether the service member filed the incident. If so, it is important to know if the incident report was restricted or unrestricted. This fact should be clearly documented so that subsequent medical caregivers do not accidentally disclose any reference to a sexual trauma event. Any accidental disclosure can lead to loss of the patient's trust as well as potential social and career ramifications for the patient.

Regardless of whether a service member's report is restricted or unrestricted, support from command can include facilitating the transfer of the service member to another unit or even to another geographic location. The role of a military psychiatrist may include clinical care for the victim or consultation to the commander.

The 2012 Kirby Dick documentary *The Invisible War* brought renewed attention to MST (Jenkins 2012). The film can be considered as a form of media advocacy because the publicity it received played a role in galvanizing several changes that have since been made in DoD policy and programming to combat MST and to encourage service members to report MST (Department of Defense 2017b). Unfortunately, MST rates continue to rise, and the results of these programs and policies have not been rigorously studied (Orchowski et al. 2018). One possible explanation for this continued trend is that the DoD efforts are paying off with improved reporting. A better understanding of MST and of the effects of these policy changes is needed to fully evaluate the problem and develop a way forward.

The current state of reporting sexual trauma in the military is imperfect. Presently, there are political efforts under way to improve adjudication of MST by *professionalization* of the process. Currently, commanders, who are not professional judges and have no formal legal training, adjudicate MST. Some political leaders are arguing that these cases should be handled by specialized MST judges. Others argue that this will result in an inability of commanders to instill order and discipline in their units. The verdict on this issue is still out at the time of this writing. Advocating for MST-surviving service members means understanding these nuances and additional challenges the victim will face because of the unique legal and administrative hurdles of the military. Even considering the weaknesses of the current system, the clearly defined difference between restricted and unrestricted reporting of sexual assault and the emphasis of allowing the survivor to choose whether or not there is an investigation while prioritizing medical and psychological care could be adopted as a template by other organizations that do not have a system in place.

Transgender Service Members

Until 2015, "transgender conditions" were disqualifying conditions for accession and cause for administrative separation from the military (Virupaksha et al. 2016). Two common arguments among advocates against allowing openly transgender individuals to serve are that transgender service members negatively affect morale and that the medical and psychiatric treatment of transgender service members would dramatically impact the DoD budget. However, the recorded and estimated numbers of transgender active duty personnel are low, and allowing transgender individuals to serve openly would have "marginal impact on health care costs and the readiness of the force" (Schaefer et al. 2016, p. 69). For those transgender service members who are actively receiving care, there is also a lack of expertise in the military health care system regarding their care, and clinical decisions that benefit transgender patients may compete with military readiness considerations (Ford and Schnitzlein 2017).

Although allowing transgender individuals to serve may be considered a mostly administrative issue, shifting sociopolitical views can increase stigma or worsen barriers to care for these service members. At the time of this writing, the final verdict on this issue remains undecided in U.S. courts. Through the study of existing policies and data in the United States and the 18 other countries that permit transgender individuals to serve openly, an individual or organization may come to an informed opinion about the issue and then raise public awareness and contact policy makers to comment on this ongoing debate (Schaefer et al. 2016). Further research to dispel some of the fears related to transgender service would also help policy makers with improving the work climate for transgender Americans who want to serve.

Conclusion

Approximately a quarter of a million active duty service members come into contact with mental health providers each year. Advocating for service members in your care requires appropriate liaison with a service member's commander or mindful deferment of this contact, an understanding of the implications of certain diagnoses and medication recommendations, and a cursory knowledge of available resources. Military psychiatry is at the center of several undecided policy issues, and an individual could affect these issues by raising public awareness or contacting legislators.

References

Armed Forces Health Surveillance Center: Causes of medical evacuations from Operations Iraqi Freedom (OIF), New Dawn (OND) and Enduring Freedom (OEF), active and reserve components, U.S. Armed Forces, October 2001–September 2010. MSMR 18(2):2–7, 2011 21793603

Armed Forces Health Surveillance Center: Surveillance snapshot: manner and cause of death, active component, U.S. Armed Forces, 1998–2013. MSMR 21(10):21, 2014 25357142

Brook TV: Army issues waivers to more than 1,000 recruits for bipolar, depression, self-mutilation. USA Today, April 26, 2018. Available at: www.usatoday.com/story/news/politics/2018/04/26/army-issues-waivers-1-000-recruits-history-bipolar-depression-self-mutilation/554917002. Accessed August 31, 2019.

Cardona RA, Ritchie EC: U.S. military enlisted accession mental health screening: history and current practice. Mil Med 172(1):31–35, 2007 17274262

Cozza SJ, Goldenberg M, Ursano RJ (eds): Care of Military Service Members, Veterans, and Their Families. Arlington, VA, American Psychiatric Publishing, 2014

Department of the Army: Policy and Procedures for Credentialing and Privileging Clinical Psychologists to Prescribe Medications. Houston, TX, Department of the Army, 2009

Department of Defense: Policy on Military Health System (MHS) Decision-Making Process. Health Affairs Policy 06-009. Washington, DC, Department of Defense, 2006

Department of Defense: Political Activities by Members of the Armed Forces. DoD Directive 1344.10. Washington, DC, Department of Defense, 2008

Department of Defense: Privacy of Individually Identifiable Health Information in DoD Health Care Programs. DoD Instruction 6025.18. Washington, DC, Department of Defense, 2009

Department of Defense: Command Notification Requirements to Dispel Stigma in Providing Mental Health Care to Service Members. DoD Instruction 6490. Washington, DC, Department of Defense, 2011

Department of Defense. Disability Evaluation System (DES). DoD Instruction 1332.18. Washington, DC, Department of Defense, 2014

Department of Defense: Annual report on sexual assault in the military. 2017a. Available at: www.sapr.mil/public/docs/reports/FY17_Annual/DoD_FY17_Annual_Report_on_Sexual_Assault_in_the_Military.pdf. Accessed December 30, 2019.

Department of Defense: Sexual Assault Prevention and Response (SAPR) Program. DoD Directive 6495.01. Washington, DC, Department of Defense, 2017b

Department of Defense: Medical Standards for Appointment, Enlistment, or Induction in the Military Services. DoD Instruction 6130.03. Washington, DC, Department of Defense, 2018

Department of the Navy: Credentialing and Privileging Program. BUMEDINST 6010.30. Falls Church, VA, Department of the Navy, 2015

Ford S, Schnitzlein C: Gender dysphoria in the military. Curr Psychiatry Rep 19(12):102, 2017 29110095

Hart D, Zavyalov E, Ritchie E, et al: De-incentivizing disability: providing long-term care without promoting long-term illness. Workshop presented at the 171st American Psychiatric Association Annual Meeting, New York, May 5–9 2018

Hoge CW, Ivany CG, Brusher EA, et al: Transformation of mental health care for U.S. soldiers and families during the Iraq and Afghanistan wars: where science and politics intersect. Am J Psychiatry 173(4):334–343, 2016 26552941

Hyman J, Ireland R, Frost L, et al: Suicide incidence and risk factors in an active duty U.S. military population. Am J Public Health 102(suppl 1):S138–S146, 2012 22390588

Jenkins M: "Invisible War" documentary examines rape in the military. Washington Post, June 21, 2012. Available at: www.washingtonpost.com/entertainment/movies/invisible-war-documentary-examines-rape-in-the-military/2012/06/21/gJQAcGqhtV_story.html?noredirect=onandutm_term=.ac93cd1fcaef. Accessed September 1, 2019.

Kessler RC, Heeringa SG, Stein MB, et al; Army STARRS Collaborators: Thirty-day prevalence of DSM-IV mental disorders among nondeployed soldiers in the U.S. Army: results from the Army Study to Assess Risk and Resilience in Servicemembers (Army STARRS). JAMA Psychiatry 71(5):504–513, 2014 24590120

Lazar SG: The mental health needs of military service members and veterans. Psychodyn Psychiatry 42(3):459–478, 2014 25211433

Levin A: Psychologist prescribing bills defeated in many states. Psychiatric News, July 27, 2017. Available at: https://psychnews.psychiatryonline.org/doi/10.1176/appi.pn.2017.8a2. Accessed September 1, 2019.

Matthews M, Coreen F, Margaret T, et al: Needs of male sexual assault victims in the U.S. Armed Forces. Santa Monica, CA, RAND Corporation, 2018. Available at: www.rand.org/pubs/research_reports/RR2167.html. Accessed September 1, 2019.

Mundell BF: Retention of military physicians: the differential effects of practice opportunities across the three services. Santa Monica, CA, RAND Corporation, 2010. Available at: www.rand.org/pubs/rgs_dissertations/RGSD275.html. Accessed September 1, 2019.

Nock MK, Stein MB, Heeringa SG, et al; Army STARRS Collaborators: Prevalence and correlates of suicidal behavior among soldiers: results from the Army Study to Assess Risk and Resilience in Servicemembers (Army STARRS). JAMA Psychiatry 71(5):514–522, 2014 24590178

O'Donnell ML, Grant G, Alkemade N, et al: Compensation seeking and disability after injury: the role of compensation-related stress and mental health. J Clin Psychiatry 76(8):e1000–e1005, 2015 26335085

Office of the Surgeon General: Release of protected health information to unit command officials. Medical Command Policy Memo 16-087. Washington, DC, Office of the Surgeon General, 2016

Orchowski LM, Berry-Caban C, Prisock K, et al: Evaluations of sexual assault prevention programs in military settings: a synthesis of the research literature. Mil Med 183(suppl 1):421–428, 2018 29635603

Peckham C: Medscape psychiatrist compensation report 2018. Medscape, April 18, 2018. Available at: https://medscape.com/slideshow/2018-compensation-psychiatrist-6009671. Accessed September 3, 2019.

Pruitt LD, Smolenski DJ, Bush NE, et al: Suicide in the military: understanding rates and risk factors across the United States' Armed Forces. Mil Med 184(suppl 1):432–437, 2019 30423136

Quartana PJ, Wilk JE, Thomas JL, et al: Trends in mental health services utilization and stigma in U.S. soldiers from 2002 to 2011. Am J Public Health 104(9):1671–1679, 2014 25033143

Ritchie EC (ed): Forensic and Ethical Issues in Military Behavioral Health. Fort Sam Houston, TX, Borden Institute, U.S. Army Medical Department Center and School; Office of the Surgeon General, United States Army, 2014. Available at: www.cs.amedd.army.mil/borden/FileDownloadpublic.aspx?docid=ce8d4a48-96c1-4292-8282-93ce9dd8b9bb. Accessed December 30, 2019.

Schaefer AG, Iyengar R, Kadiyala S, et al: Assessing the implications of allowing transgender personnel to serve openly. Santa Monica, CA, RAND Corporation, 2016. Available at: www.rand.org/pubs/research_reports/RR1530.html. Accessed September 3, 2019.

Thomas KC, Shartzer A, Kurth NK, et al: Impact of ACA health reforms for people with mental health conditions. Psychiatr Serv 69(2):231–234, 2018 29137555

Trautmann S, Goodwin L, Höfler M, et al: Prevalence and severity of mental disorders in military personnel: a standardised comparison with civilians. Epidemiol Psychiatr Sci 26(2):199–208, 2017 27086743

Ursano RJ, Colpe LJ, Heeringa SG, et al; Army STARRS collaborators: The Army Study to Assess Risk and Resilience in Servicemembers (Army STARRS). Psychiatry 77(2):107–119, 2014 24865195

Ursano RJ, Heeringa SG, Stein MB, et al: Prevalence and correlates of suicidal behavior among new soldiers in the U.S. Army: results from the Army Study to Assess Risk and Resilience in Servicemembers (Army STARRS). Depress Anxiety 32(1):3–12, 2015 25338964

Virupaksha HG, Muralidhar D, Ramakrishna J: Suicide and suicidal behavior among transgender persons. Indian J Psychol Med 38(6):505–509, 2016 28031583

17

Advocacy for Veterans and Their Families

Harold Kudler, M.D.

Learning Objectives

By the end of this chapter, readers will be able to:

- Trace the history of advocacy for veterans and their families

- Appraise obstacles facing veterans and their families as they pursue optimal mental wellness, including those obstacles inherent in military culture

- Identify areas for improvement in professional training and clinical practice regarding veterans and their families

- Consider new opportunities for advocacy on behalf of veterans and their families within their own practices and communities

In order to advance advocacy for veterans of the United States military and their families in the twenty-first century, it is necessary to appreciate a rich history reaching back to the nation's colonial period. In every generation, veterans have faced significant challenges in their pursuit of mental, physical, and family well-being. With each generation and each new war, the nation has deepened its understanding of the sacrifices made by those who serve and broadened the range of benefits for veterans and their families. These advances have required coordinated efforts on behalf of the government, health care professionals, community organizations, and private citizens. The national challenge of war unfailingly spurs new concepts, discoveries, and clinical practices that, in turn, advance understanding and treatment not only for veterans but for all citizens. This chapter builds on almost three centuries of American military experience to point toward new opportunities in advocacy on behalf of veterans and their families.

Case Example

Ms. A, an otherwise healthy 25-year-old nursing school student, presents for evaluation and reports that although her marriage is going well and she had always looked forward to motherhood, she is now "afraid of becoming pregnant." She describes significant anxiety associated with thoughts about "taking responsibility for a child" and reports fears that "haunt her" during the day and become still more intense at bedtime. She denies nightmares but endorses significant trouble falling and staying asleep coupled with daytime somnolence. Ms. A describes frequent tearfulness and pervasive doubts about her self-worth. Her most painful fear is that her child will be "born damaged." You ask about other history of anxiety or depression and carefully inquire about possible precipitants, including past pregnancies or history of childhood sexual abuse, but she denies any such problems.

After ensuring that Ms. A is not currently pregnant, you prescribe a selective serotonin reuptake inhibitor and initiate cognitive-behavioral therapy for depression. It is not until your fifth meeting that a chance remark by Ms. A prompts you to ask whether she has ever served in the military. She responds that she was an Army medical technician who served two tours in Afghanistan. Among those she cared for was a group of critically injured children who had survived a terrorist attack. Despite her best efforts, one of those children, a 6-year-old boy, died of his wounds. Ms. A was devastated by his death and felt tortured by thoughts that perhaps she could have prevented it. She hid these feelings from the other members of her team because they didn't seem to be as affected by the child's death as she and she didn't want to be "that girl" who "let others down." When asked why she had not mentioned this incident or her military service earlier, she responded, "Well, you never asked and, quite frankly, I wasn't sure how you felt about the military or the war in Afghanistan. I didn't want anything to get in the way of our work."

A Brief History of Advocacy for Veterans and Their Families

Advocacy for U.S. veterans and their families is an ever-evolving, reciprocal process between them, the government, and the public at large that proceeds at a pace determined by the frequency and intensity of new military challenges. Its beginnings predate the American Revolution: in 1636, several colonies passed legislation establishing their first formal militias and providing pensions for those who became disabled in the colony's defense (U.S. Department of Veterans Affairs 2019a).

The Continental Congress defined benefits for disabled veterans in 1776, but whereas Congress promised pensions to officers before the American Revolution ended, it did not grant them to enlisted service members (many of whom had gone unpaid during the war itself) until 1832. Teipe (2002) suggested that although there had been many enlisted Revolutionary service members, they were too small a component of the electorate to advocate effectively for themselves.

The Civil War

Although the concept of posttraumatic stress disorder is often traced to Da Costa's (1871) study of Civil War veterans, "On Irritable Heart," a close reading makes it clear that Da Costa, a cardiologist, understood this as a heart problem. Similarly, neurologist Silas Weir Mitchell understood the exhaustion reported by veterans as a physiological depletion of the nervous system. His book *Fat and Blood: and How to Make Them* (Mitchell 1877) and "the rest cure" he developed for Civil War veterans focused on how to reconstitute that vital energy. Psychiatry was not yet ready to articulate the impact of war theoretically or clinically. It fell to government, veterans' organizations, and the public to advocate for veterans in terms of gratitude and social justice. In 1865, President Abraham Lincoln eloquently summed up this obligation in his second inaugural address: "[L]et us strive on to finish the work we are in; to bind up the nation's wounds; to care for him who shall have borne the battle, and for his widow, and his orphan." His words now comprise the mission statement of the United States Department of Veterans Affairs (VA). Their deep humanity continues to inform advocacy for veterans.

Public awareness of the challenges faced by Civil War veterans was amplified by new modes of communication, including the telegraph and photography, and the high casualty rate of a prolonged, industrialized war fought across much of the homeland. Contemporary authors including Walt Whitman, Samuel Clemens (Mark Twain), and Ambrose Bierce (each of whom served in some capacity during the war) provided new psychological context for the problems facing veterans and their families, and later generations of writers, including Stephen Crane and William Faulkner, deepened the imprint of the Civil War on the American psyche. Even today, the nation continues to struggle with the legacy of that war. As Faulkner observed in his 1951 novel *Requiem for a Nun*, "The past is never dead. It's not even past" (Faulkner 1951).

Because of public advocacy for Civil War veterans, Congress established the first federal cemeteries in 1862 and, in 1865, the first federal facility for Union Army volunteers, the National Asylum for Disabled Volunteer Soldiers in Togus, Maine (still in operation today as part of the Department of Veterans Affairs [VA] medical system). There were no corresponding federal benefits for Confederate veterans. Ironically, the origin of the national holiday of Memorial Day (originally Decoration Day) can be traced, at least in part, to April 25, 1866, when a group of local women visited a cemetery in Columbus, Mississippi, to decorate the graves of Confederate soldiers with spring flowers. According to the history maintained by the VA, "Nearby were the graves of Union soldiers, neglected because they were the enemy. Disturbed at the sight of the bare graves, the women placed some of their flowers on those graves, as well" (U.S. Department of Veterans Affairs 2019b). Often, it is the moral act of a few individuals that inspires national awareness and action.

The Mental Hygiene Movement

The most important mental health advocacy program in U.S. history, the Mental Hygiene Movement, sprang from a personal event: On June 23, 1900, Clifford Beers (1876–1943), then 24 years old and gripped by psychosis, attempted suicide by hurling himself out of an upper-story window. After 2 years in private and public mental hospitals where treatment was rarely helpful and frequently brutal, Beers wrote a book for the general public titled *A Mind That Found Itself: An Autobiography* (Beers 1908), with the aim of galvanizing action on behalf of individuals with mental illness. His basic message was that if this could happen to him, it could happen to the reader or a loved one.

Beers, a consumer advocate, engaged help from William James and Adolf Meyer. James was the nation's greatest authority on mental health at the time, and Meyer, as chief psychiatrist at Johns Hopkins Hospital, was to become one of the most influential psychiatrists in U.S. history. In 1909, this triumvirate founded the National Committee for

Mental Hygiene (later the National Mental Health Association and now Mental Health America). The National Committee coordinated a network of state and local mental hygiene associations (members of which had been inspired by Beers's book). Together, they successfully advocated for reforms in psychiatric facilities, model legislation governing involuntary commitment, and the establishment of child guidance clinics across the United States.

Perhaps the most unique feature of the Mental Hygiene Movement was its focus on the mental health of populations rather than of individuals. Beers (quoted by Bertolote 2008) put it this way:

> [The Mental Hygiene Movement] visualized, not a single patient, but a whole community; and it considered each member of that community as an individual whose mental and emotional status was determined by definite causative factors and whose compelling need was for prevention rather than cure. The Mental Hygiene Movement, then, bears the same relation to psychiatry that the public-health movement, of which it forms a part, bears to medicine in general. It is an organized community response to a recognized community need.... At the present time both psychiatrists and mental hygienists are more than ever conscious that their objectives are in fact identical and that each group needs the other for the fulfilment [sic] of their common task. (p. 114)

The mental hygiene movement insisted that the nation had a fundamental responsibility to identify specific stressors facing defined populations and, whenever possible, act to prevent mental illness. This principle positioned the National Committee to define psychiatric advocacy on behalf of American veterans.

Thomas Salmon, World War I, and the Founding of the VA

Although the concept of mental hygiene was framed by Beers, James, and Meyer, much of the credit for its successful implementation belongs to the man they hired as their first executive director, psychiatrist Thomas Salmon (1876–1927). Salmon was a "horse and buggy" general practitioner in rural New York until he developed tuberculosis in 1901. While recuperating, he worked for the New York State Health Department tracking infectious diseases in state mental hospitals. This led him to undertake psychiatric training.

By 1903, Salmon was working on Ellis Island conducting psychiatric examinations of newly arrived immigrants for the U.S. Public Health Service, where his persistent advocacy for reform of that process led to a brief suspension for insubordination. In 1911, he was lent to the New

York State Commission in Lunacy as its chief medical examiner and statistician. This brought him to the attention of the National Committee for Mental Hygiene, which hired him in 1912.

Soon after World War I broke out in Europe in 1914, a new diagnosis, *shell shock*, emerged as a leading cause of casualties other than physical wounds. Although psychiatrists around the world argued whether shell shock was a neurological disorder or a psychiatric one, all agreed that it was an urgent health crisis. Salmon turned his attention to shell shock long before the United States entered the war in 1917, perhaps because he understood that this international phenomenon provided a unique opportunity to demonstrate the power of mental hygiene.

Two months before the United States declared war, Salmon met with Army Surgeon General William Gorgas to offer plans for the prevention of shell shock among members of the American Expeditionary Forces (AEF). Gorgas, a public health pioneer whose work on preventing yellow fever and malaria helped enable completion of the Panama Canal, sent Salmon to meet with General John J. "Blackjack" Pershing. Pershing, who would soon lead the AEF, knew that 10% of all disability discharges among his troops in the Mexican Border War were for mental health problems. He must have been impressed with Salmon's vision because he appointed Salmon director of psychiatry for the AEF; this was the first psychiatric posting in the history of the U.S. Army.

Salmon retained Pershing's confidence throughout the course of his military service, as documented in a letter from Pershing to Salmon after the end of WWI:

> My Dear Colonel:
>   The activities of the A.E.F. are now drawing to a close and you will soon return to the U.S.... You have achieved remarkable success in a comparatively new field of the medical science, one which modern warfare has shown merits a most important consideration, and one which should be carefully developed. By your excellent service you have done much to conserve manpower for the fighting units.
>   Believe me,
>   Very sincerely,
>   John J. Pershing (Bond 1950, p. 118)

Pershing was referencing Salmon's invention of military combat stress control based on proactive engagement of service members 1) in close proximity to the front, 2) with immediacy at first sign of onset, and 3) with high expectancy of recovery. This so-called PIE model remains core to combat stress control doctrine for the United States and for militaries around the world.

The War Ends, But Its Mental Health Burden Lingers On

When WWI ended in 1918, Salmon transitioned to the Army Surgeon General's office, where he assumed responsibility for 2,000 psychiatrically hospitalized American troops still in France. Concerned about the lack of preparations for the soldiers' return home, Salmon conducted a public debate with Navy leadership over their "obsolete and inhumane" attitudes and practices, which included restricting mental health casualties to below decks during their voyage home.

Having consistently called for enhancement of the nation's capacity to receive returning psychiatric casualties, Salmon blasted the findings of a September 11, 1918 joint report of Army, Navy, and Public Health Service officers, which held that "the number of soldiers that will require hospital accommodations…will probably be small and can be taken care of in existing hospitals." Ironically, the Public Health Service reported just 6 days later that their stateside psychiatric units were already filled beyond capacity.

Salmon vented his frustration in a letter to a colleague:

> If any soldier who fought in France and received an invisible wound that has darkened his mind now lies in a county jail or almshouse or is for any reason deprived of the best treatment that the resources of modern psychiatry can provide, our national honor is compromised. (Bond 1950, p. 114)

In 1918, the Bureau of War Risk Insurance and the U.S. Public Health Service were responsible for the care of new veterans but lacked the capacity to meet their mental health needs. The branches of the National Home for Disabled Volunteer Soldiers, originally called the National Home Asylum for Disabled Volunteer Soldiers when it was developed for Union Civil War veterans, were domiciliaries rather than mental health hospitals.

In desperation, Salmon planned to retain WWI Army psychiatrists in the military and distribute them and their patients to mental hospitals across the nation. This idea was predicated on his realization that successful treatment demanded a level of military cultural and clinical competence unavailable in civilian hospitals. This plan, however, was rejected by veterans and their families who insisted that the government that sent these troops to war must now provide federal psychiatric facilities for their treatment.

In 1919, the Surgeon General of the Public Health Service asked five leading psychiatrists (including Salmon) to draft a mental health plan for WWI veterans. Their report called for a new veterans hospital system. Government action was not forthcoming, so Salmon partnered with the American Legion (a veterans service organization chartered by Congress that same year) to advocate for the veterans hospitals.

In his January 1921 testimony, Salmon urged Congress to create

> a real unified agency that can reach into these men's houses, take them out, and put them into Government hospitals established, built and maintained solely for their benefit; not constructed to care for dying, demented old people, but to care for young men in full vigor, who, nevertheless are suffering from this disease.... Unless something is done within the present year to improve conditions under which insane ex-service men are receiving treatment, hundreds who now stand a fair chance of being cured, will be doomed to permanent insanity. In spite of the fact that on December 16, 1920, 5,500 ex-service men were in neuropsychiatric hospitals, the Government has not spent a dollar for the construction of a single hospital for the insane up to date. Only one-third of these men are in hospitals owned by the Government. (Bond 1950, p. 175)

Salmon and the American Legion held a rally at Carnegie Hall at which General Pershing, by then a national icon, joined them in lambasting the government for broken promises and political posturing.

Finally, in August 1921, Congress consolidated three disparate WWI programs into a single agency: the Veterans Bureau. It would oversee the largest federal hospital construction program in U.S. history. By 1930, forty-nine hospitals had been built, with more in progress, despite the corruption of the Bureau's first director, who went to prison for misappropriating $200 million (in 1921 dollars) in a scandal that almost brought down President Warren Harding's administration (Stevens 2016).

Salmon stepped away from the National Committee in 1922 to promote the establishment of departments of psychiatry within medical schools across the nation. Until then, psychiatry did not have a defined role in most medical schools. Salmon played a prominent role at Columbia University, where he helped found the New York State Psychiatric Institute. In 1923, he became president of the American Psychiatric Association (APA)—the first since its founding who had not been superintendent of a mental hospital. He died at age 51 in a 1927 boating accident.

One lesson from this history is that even as the nation embraces a new generation of veterans, it often fails to generalize newly conceived benefits to *all* veterans. The Veterans Bureau served only WWI veterans, whereas older programs continued to serve only Civil War veterans. It was not until 1930 that these programs were merged to serve all veterans as the new Veterans Administration. In 1988, President Ronald Reagan elevated the VA to a cabinet agency, the Department of Veterans Affairs, comprising the Veterans Health Administration, the Veterans Benefits Administration, and the National Cemetery Administration. The VA is now the second-largest U.S. government agency in budget and personnel and, at the time of this writing, operates 172 medical centers, 1,069 outpatient clinics, and 300 readjustment counseling centers (Vet Centers) (U.S. Department of Veterans Affairs 2019c). It offers the nation's largest integrated mental health system and one of the world's most productive research and education programs dedicated to the specific mental health needs of service members, veterans, and their families.

World War II: The Cycle Repeats

Those who study the history of military mental health know that advances of the previous war tend to be forgotten until they are rediscovered in the next. Had Salmon lived another 14 years, he almost certainly would have jump-started the mental health response to World War II. Instead, it was left to William Menninger, still in medical school at the end of WWI, to reinstitute the advances made by Salmon. After WWII ended, Menninger followed Salmon's path to become APA president in 1948 and championed its first *Diagnostic and Statistical Manual of Mental Disorders* (DSM-I; American Psychiatric Association 1952). DSM-I was based on Menninger's 1945 revision of the *Army Mental Health Diagnostic Manual* (War Department Technical Bulletin, Medical 203), which was necessitated by the military's responsibility to consistently and accurately diagnose and track mental disorders on a worldwide front. This significant advance did not come easily. It required the creation of the Group for the Advancement of Psychiatry (GAP), with members drawn from psychiatrists who had served under Menninger during the war. Menninger wrote,

> [T]he founding group was seeking a way in which American psychiatry could give more forceful leadership, both medically and socially. Although the name may sound presumptuous, it was chosen because of the sense of great urgency that psychiatry should advance, and the belief that by hard work, and teamwork, we could help it do so. Those early years of GAP were marked by the feeling on the part of its membership that much needed to be done, and quickly. (Group for the Advancement of Psychiatry 2018)

Despite Salmon's efforts in the 1920s, until the end of WWII, most American medical schools did not have departments of psychiatry. It was the efficacy of psychiatric treatment as documented in case reports and theoretical constructs such as those reported by then military psychiatrists Roy Grinker and John Spiegel in their landmark 1945 work, *Men Under Stress*, that helped inspire this significant change in American medicine. Grinker and Spiegel's (1945) core message was that given enough pressure, *anyone* can break. That, in addition to the fact that one in five casualties of WWII was psychiatric, created a new national appreciation of the importance of psychiatry. Furthermore, because effective treatments were based on psychoanalytic principles, American psychiatry took a dramatic turn toward psychoanalysis.

Many postwar leaders of American psychiatry (including Theodore Lidz, Stephen Fleck, Jerome Frank, and Lawrence Kolb) were shaped by their experiences as military psychiatrists in WWII. In addition, many had been trained either by Adolf Meyer or by his former residents who carried forward core principles of the Mental Hygiene Movement.

Advocacy for Veterans in the Vietnam Generation and Its Ongoing Impact

The Vietnam War inspired a new wave of psychiatric advocacy on behalf of veterans that continues to have significant impact on psychiatry and the nation. Much of this sprang from the decision of psychiatrists/psychoanalysts Robert Lifton and Chaim Shatan to accept an invitation from the organization Vietnam Veterans Against the War to sit in on veteran "rap groups" during the early 1970s. That experience led them to formulate what DSM-III introduced in 1980 as posttraumatic stress disorder (PTSD; American Psychiatric Association 1980). Establishing PTSD as a mental disorder in turn initiated a rich cascade of innovation and advocacy on behalf of veterans and their families.

Arthur S. Blank, a psychiatrist who served with the Army in Vietnam and an early proponent of the PTSD diagnosis, went on to become the first national director of the VA's Readjustment Counseling Service. The Vet Centers coupled professional and peer support with community-level service to veterans and their families. Blank also cofounded what is now the International Society for Traumatic Stress Studies, the world's largest interdisciplinary professional organization promoting knowledge about traumatic stress.

In 1989, psychiatrist Matthew Friedman became the first executive director of the VA's National Center for PTSD, which had been mandated by Congress and is now the world leader in promoting PTSD treatment, research, and training. As part of its advocacy for veterans and their family members receiving treatment outside of the VA (only about one-third of veterans currently receive VA health care, and many of these also receive at least some health services in the community), the

National Center for PTSD offers a Community Provider Toolkit (www.mentalhealth.va.gov/communityproviders) and a PTSD Consultation Service for community providers (www.ptsd.va.gov/professional/consult/index.asp).

VA mental health leaders successfully advocated for creation of the VA's Mental Illness Research, Education and Clinical Centers (MIRECCs) as a means of significantly accelerating mental health research on behalf of veterans. These translational research programs generate new knowledge about the nature of mental disorders, apply findings to develop new treatments, and educate providers across VA and other health systems. Because the VA is the largest provider of clinical training in the United States, such advances disseminate rapidly across the country and around the world.

Special mention should be made of psychiatrist Aphrodite Matsakis's (1988) book *Vietnam Wives*. Written in lay terms, it opened a new window on the lives of veterans and their families and provided both validation and practical advice. The rapid acceptance of Matsakis's grassroots approach demonstrates the power of effective advocacy.

Because of the many efforts by individuals and organizations, PTSD, originally referred to as Vietnam stress syndrome (Figley 1978) and largely limited to veterans of that war, is now a major focus of mental health care, research, and education around the world and has been expanded to all generations of veterans and to new populations including (but not limited to) survivors of childhood and adult sexual trauma, man-made and natural disasters, genocide, human trafficking, and historical trauma. New models of mind and brain and new clinical delivery systems have grown out of this advocacy, as have new public awareness and policy.

Following the Thread to the Nation's Most Recent Wars

Psychiatrists continue to lead in support of service members, veterans, and their families. The Uniformed Services University (USU) School of Medicine, founded by Congress during the Vietnam War, focuses on military and public health medicine to educate uniformed physicians in support of all military branches and the general public. Among other foci, USU's Center for the Study of Traumatic Stress, founded by psychiatrist Robert Ursano, advances research and care for military service members and families. The Walter Reed Army Institute of Research, has followed in Salmon's footsteps by combining expertise in psychiatry and epidemiology to define and address psychiatric consequences of the wars in Iraq and Afghanistan (Hoge et al. 2016).

The Defense Centers of Excellence for Psychological Health and Traumatic Brain Injury (DCoE) were created by Congress in 2007 to provide guidance across Department of Defense (DoD) programs in advancing prevention and care of psychological health and traumatic brain injury (TBI). Since 2016, the DCoE's founding director, psychiatrist and retired Brigadier General Loree Sutton, has served as Commissioner for New York City's Department of Veterans' Services, the nation's first municipal-level agency devoted solely to advocacy for veterans and their families.

Although space will not allow a full account of psychiatric advocacy on behalf of veterans and their families in recent years, the following are some highlights that provide an overview of the scope. (Websites for the organizations listed are provided in "Recommended Additional Resources" later in the chapter.)

- Army Colonel (retired) Norman Camp, who served as a psychiatrist in Vietnam, authored *U.S. Army Psychiatry in the Vietnam War* (Camp 2014), a comprehensive review published by the U.S. Army Medical Department that lays out mental health lessons learned (and not learned) from that war.
- Army Colonel (retired) Elspeth Cameron Ritchie, a psychiatrist who served as chief behavioral health consultant to the Army Surgeon General, is a prolific writer and editor who has addressed a wide range of issues in military behavioral health, including forensic and ethical issues and gender and sexual issues (see Recommended Additional Resources). She has also collaborated with former U.S. Army Preventive Medicine Officer Dr. Remington Nevin to call attention to possible long-term psychiatric and neurological effects of the antimalarial mefloquine (a drug developed by the DoD and used in recent military operations) among service members and veterans (Nevin and Ritchie 2016).
- Captain William Nash, Navy Medical Corps (retired), pioneered combat and operational stress control in the U.S. Marine Corps and, as a VA psychiatrist, continues to champion the recognition of moral injury (Nash and Litz 2013).
- As director of the Deployment Health Clinical Center at Walter Reed and associate chair for research in the department of psychiatry at USU, Army Colonel (retired) Charles Engel developed a collaborative care approach to the recognition and management of depression and PTSD in primary care settings. His research demonstrating the

power of such programs has led to their adoption in military, VA, and community health systems around the world (Curry et al. 2014).

- Navy Captain (retired), psychiatrist, and preventive medicine physician Robert Koffman advanced TBI assessment and treatment as the first medical director of the National Intrepid Center of Excellence at the Walter Reed National Military Medical Center. As medical director of the Semper Fi Fund, a nonprofit organization that supports combat wounded, critically ill, and catastrophically injured members of the U.S. Armed Forces and their families, he continues to advocate for complementary and integrative health approaches, including acupuncture and animal assisted therapies, for injured and critically ill service members.

- Psychiatrist Jonathan Shay, author of *Achilles in Vietnam: Combat Trauma and the Undoing of Character* (Shay 1994) and *Odysseus in America: Combat Trauma and the Trials of Homecoming* (Shay 2002) and self-described "missionary" on behalf of veterans, champions prevention of psychological and moral injury by maximizing unit cohesion and promoting ethical leadership in the military.

- Veterans service organizations such as the American Legion, Veterans of Foreign Wars, Disabled American Veterans, and Vietnam Veterans of America maintain their vigilant advocacy. More recently founded organizations, including the Code of Support Foundation and the Iraq and Afghanistan Veterans of America (IAVA), have sprung up in support of our newest generation of veterans. IAVA achieved a major legislative victory with the passage of the Clay Hunt Suicide Prevention for American Veterans Act (P.L. 114-2) in 2015. The act links civilian mental health programs and communities with VA suicide prevention efforts to create a broad web of support for veterans in danger of suicide.

- Following the suicide of their son Sergeant Daniel Somers, who returned from Iraq with invisible wounds including PTSD and TBI, Howard and Jean Somers have become highly effective advocates for suicide prevention by collaborating with leaders at all levels of government while engaging individuals and families at the grassroots level. The Somers' 2014 statement to the House Committee on Veterans Affairs about their son's struggles and their subsequent mission can be found at https://docs.house.gov/meetings/VR/VR00/20140710/102444/HHRG-113-VR00-Wstate-SomersMDH-20140710-SD004.pdf.

- The Military Child Education Coalition, a unique coalition of public and private schools, colleges and universities, small businesses and corporations, military commands, families and individuals, advocates for U.S. military children and their families around the world.

- Give an Hour, originally designed to coordinate donated mental health services for veterans and their families, has spun off another initiative, the Campaign to Change Direction, which takes on the challenge once addressed by the National Committee for Mental Hygiene by helping veterans and all citizens gain the mental health literacy needed to have words for intense and painful feelings, better understand and accept mental health problems, know that effective help is available, and know where to get it.
- PsychArmor Institute bridges the military/veteran-civilian divide through free online education about military culture and mental health challenges. Self-paced courses are geared to health care providers, employers, educators, caregivers, and transitioning service members.
- Spurred by the federal Substance Abuse and Mental Health Services Administration (SAMHSA), a number of states have developed DoD/VA/state and community partnerships. Among the most productive and sustained of these is the North Carolina Governor's Working Group, established in 2006 to advance health and wellness, job creation, legal and financial services, and benefits for service members, veterans, and their families. This coalition has evolved into an advocacy and referral network that connects veterans and their families with services and supports while cutting red tape across systems.
- Finally, several professional organizations, including the Group for the Advancement of Psychiatry and the American Psychoanalytic Association, maintain standing committees to advance military cultural competence among members and trainees and to assist providers and stakeholders in improving the mental health, resilience, and well-being of service members, veterans, and their families. The APA—through its Society of Uniformed Services Psychiatrists (a district branch), professional publications, annual conferences (which have featured a special military and veterans track), and federal advocacy programs—dramatically amplifies the voice of military and VA psychiatrists, informs policy, and expands the knowledge base of mental health professionals and the general public to ensure that medical and mental health support services are responsive to the needs of veterans and their families.

Thinking About the Future

The principles of mental hygiene are now echoed in the term *population health*, which is defined by the Centers for Disease Control and Prevention (2019) as an interdisciplinary, customizable approach that...utilizes non-traditional partnerships among different sectors of the community—public health, industry, academia, health care, local government entities, etc.—to achieve positive health outcomes.

A population health approach demands that these outcomes be measured not simply in terms of symptom reduction but also by wellness, quality of life, and coping ability across an entire life trajectory. The concepts and definitions of PTSD and TBI have spurred critically important research and new clinical approaches, but a population health approach demands that outcomes be measured not simply in terms of symptom reduction but also by wellness, quality of life, and coping ability across an entire life trajectory.

With the achievements of the mental hygiene movement as an exemplar, might it be possible to create new national partnerships of veterans, their families, professionals, nonprofit organizations, and government? Ideally, veterans and those close to them would play a central role in such partnerships, such that military cultural competence would be infused across it. This is critically important because, as portrayed in the opening vignette of this chapter, military culture itself mitigates against veterans talking with civilians about problems related to their military service (even when it is in their own interest to do so). In part, this stems from a sense that talking about military experience violates the warrior ethos by causing the individual to appear needy or even weak. Veterans are uncomfortable with the idea that others might think that they are trading on their military experience to obtain special treatment. Furthermore, a significant proportion of the veteran population is concerned about sharing any aspect of classified information with civilians, even within the context of treatment. On the other hand, many veterans who might not share their military experience and related problems on their own behalf would readily speak up on behalf of other veterans and their families. This is an aspect of military culture that could empower new population health enterprises. In this way, military culture could become a driver of population health rather than an obstacle to it.

It is essential that health care providers and other community resources, including employers, educators, members of law enforcement and judicial systems, and the public at large, have a better understanding of military culture and the potential effects of deployment stress on service members, veterans, and their families. As documented in the RAND Corporation's report *Ready to Serve* (Tanielian et al. 2014), the vast majority of community mental health providers are severely lacking in the capabilities, attitudes, and behaviors necessary to deliver high-quality, culturally appropriate care to veterans and their families.

One example of advocacy to address this problem would be a national program by which veterans and their families and friends launch a grassroots campaign, planned around kitchen tables across the United States, to approach neighborhood health providers at routine appointments with a deceptively simple observation: "You've never asked me if I served in the military." In follow up, that advocate would say, "Because you're my health care provider, you need to know that I'm one of millions of Americans who face potential health risks and that I'm probably not the only service member, veteran, or family member that you see in your practice. I also need you to know that I may be eligible for enhanced health resources and benefits because either I or someone close to me served in the military. You will only know this about me if you ask."

This brief intervention would end with a call for action on the part of the provider and/or health system: "As your patient, I want you to start asking *all* of your patients if they or someone close to them has served in the military. I'm not asking this for myself but for my buddies and their families."

Other forms of advocacy within a population health model could include the following:

- Disseminating suicide prevention training (which has already been developed for the lay public, professionals, and policy makers and is readily accessible through the VA, PsychArmor Institute, and other venues)
- Alerting veterans that they and their family members may be eligible for federal VA benefits as well as additional state and local government benefits including but not limited to housing and vocational assistance, educational benefits for children, special tax exemptions, and access to adaptive sports equipment
- Identifying and supporting veterans and their dependents in schools, on college campuses, and in small and large businesses by creating veterans' forums and social organizations within these settings and linking them to national organizations such as the Student Veterans of America, the Military Child Education Coalition, and the Employee Assistance Professionals Association

At a time when fewer than 1% of all Americans currently serve in the military, it is important to clarify that the United States has a huge military subculture, including almost 2.5 million current service members and 20 million veterans. Together, they comprise one of the largest components of American society, yet they remain largely invisible within it. When their dependents are included (using a conservative estimate of 1.5 dependents per service member or veteran), more than 56 million Americans (roughly 1 out of every 6 American men, women, and children) would answer "Yes" to the question "Have you or someone close to you served in the military?"

It is worth considering whether the exponential growth of the VA and of veterans service organizations since WWI may have unintentionally lulled veterans, policy makers, and the public into reliance on government and large organizations to solve the challenges facing today's veterans. If so, this is truly a paradoxical consequence of Salmon's success in pushing the federal government to accept responsibility for the mental health of veterans in the aftermath of WWI. Furthermore, the very size, scope, and expertise of the VA may have inadvertently predisposed other sectors of American health care to become complacent in the belief that the health and well-being of veterans and their families are solely the VA's responsibility. This may help explain why community clinicians and health systems do not act on the realization that most veterans (including many who receive at least some of their treatment through the VA) receive care in non-VA settings and are, in fact, their patients, too. Clearly, a new birth of advocacy is needed to ensure proactive identification of veterans and their family members in non-VA practices and health systems, development of greater military cultural and clinical competence across all sectors of society, enhanced awareness of services and resources, and significantly greater integration of care and services.

Another inadvertent but likely inevitable consequence of building the VA to the necessary scale is a complex bureaucracy that can make navigating the system a challenge for veterans and health care professionals alike. Veterans are often confused about what benefits they are eligible for and may feel daunted in attempts to access care. Because the VA has more than a thousand sites that provide care, even the most advanced policies and practices may not penetrate the VA system uniformly, resulting in concern about the quality of VA care.

Such concerns are often complicated by politics. Journalist Suzanne Gordon (2017) documented one such instance: In an effort to gain support for the Affordable Care Act, the Obama administration trumpeted the VA as a federal agency that delivers outstanding care at significantly lower cost than the private sector. This placed the VA squarely in the sights of political groups who oppose government-run health care, and Gordon described a coordinated national effort launched in 2014 to undermine faith in VA care. Studies such as that of the National Academies of Sciences, Engineering, and Medicine (2018), which found that VA care is generally equal to or better than the care in the community, did little to change public perceptions or stem the political push for urgent "improvement" of VA care. One result is the VA Mission Act of 2018 (U.S. Congress 2018), which is framed as enhancing timely access to care but will send veterans to community providers who, as RAND research has shown (Tanielian et al. 2014), usually lack the military cultural or clinical competence required to effectively care for veterans. Given that the VA is a U.S. Cabinet agency, political considerations often vie with clinical and research concerns in establishing policies, implementing practices, and evaluating outcomes.

New generations of veterans often face unique challenges requiring new programs and resources, but the ongoing needs of older generations should not be overshadowed when new veterans come home. Veterans of past eras have raised concern about losing priority as the VA receives new generations of veterans. Furthermore, as knowledge advances with each new war (e.g., the recognition of PTSD among Vietnam veterans and of TBI among soldiers returning from Afghanistan and Iraq), it is a matter of clinical sense (and of justice) to consider whether such discoveries are relevant to earlier generations. Advocates and VA leaders must work together to ensure that clinical advances and program innovations are harnessed for the good of *all* veterans.

Conclusion

Turning back to the vignette at the opening of this chapter, if Ms. A's doctor had asked her if she or someone close to her had served in the military as a routine part of the clinical intake examination, it might have quelled the patient's concerns about the doctor's interest and empathy toward service members and veterans and facilitated more focused and effective treatment. Alternatively, if Ms. A. had been an empowered advocate who, when her doctor failed to ask about military service, spoke up, not just on her own behalf, but on behalf of other service members, veterans, and their family members, she might have inspired a significant improvement in her doctor's practice. The fact that neither of them addressed the issue at the outset of care was perhaps the single greatest obstacle to their work together. Thus far, lectures, editorials, and research publications have failed to get clinicians across the country to reliably ask, "Have you or someone close to you served in the military?" It may be that advocacy by patients and family members in one-to-one interactions with their doctors will be the swiftest, surest path to this next important step in advocacy for veterans and their families.

Recommended Additional Resources

Books

Ritchie EC (ed): Forensic and Ethical Issues in Military Behavioral Health. Fort Sam Houston, TX, Borden Institute, U.S. Army Medical Department Center and School; Office of the Surgeon General, United States Army, 2014. Available at: www.cs.amedd.army.mil/borden/FileDownloadpublic.aspx?docid=ce8d4a48-96c1-4292-8282-93ce9dd8b9bb. Accessed September 3, 2019.

Ritchie EC: Intimacy After Injury: Restoring Sexual Health on Return From Combat. New York, Oxford University Press, 2017

Ritchie EC, Llorente MD (eds): Veteran Psychiatry in the US: Optimizing Clinical Outcomes. New York, Springer, 2019

Ritchie EC, Naclerio AL (eds): Women at War. New York, Oxford University Press, 2015

Ritchie EC, Wise J, Pyle B (eds): Gay Mental Healthcare Providers and Patients in the Military: Personal Experiences and Clinical Care. New York, Springer, 2018

Websites and Other Resources

American Legion: www.members.legion.org

Campaign to Change Direction (a coalition of concerned citizens, non-profit leaders, and leaders from the private sector seeking to change the culture in America about mental health, mental illness, and wellness): www.changedirection.org

Coaching Into Care (a national telephone service of the VA for family members and friends concerned about a veteran): www.mirecc.va.gov/coaching

Code of Support Foundation (dedicated to leveraging the full spectrum of national resources to ensure that all military members, veterans, and their families receive the support they need and have earned): www.codeofsupport.org

Disabled American Veterans: www.dav.org

Employee Assistance Professionals Association: www.eapassn.org

Give an Hour (a nonprofit organization that develops national networks of volunteer professionals who help meet the mental health needs of service members, veterans, and their families): https://giveanhour.org

International Society for Traumatic Stress Studies: www.istss.org

Iraq and Afghanistan Veterans of America: https://iava.org

Make the Connection (a VA engagement website in support of veterans of all eras, and their friends and family): https://maketheconnection.net

Military Child Education Coalition: www.militarychild.org

Military OneSource (provider of DoD-funded 24/7 live and Web-based assistance on a wide range of issues from identifying a mental health problem to changing a flat tire. Now available to new veterans and their family members for the first year after separation): 1-800-342-9647 or www.militaryonesource.mil

PsychArmor Institute (a nonprofit organization that bridges the civilian-military gap by offering free online training courses and resources): https://psycharmor.org

Semper Fi Fund: https://semperfifund.org

Student Veterans of America: https://studentveterans.org

VA National Center for PTSD: www.ptsd.va.gov

VA Suicide Prevention website (offers programs and resources for veterans and their loved ones, friends, and health care providers): www.mentalhealth.va.gov/suicide_prevention

Veterans Crisis Line (connects veterans in crisis and their families and friends with qualified, caring VA responders through a confidential toll-free hotline, text, or chat services): 1-800-273-8255 or www.veteranscrisisline.net

Veterans of Foreign Wars: www.vfw.org

Vietnam Veterans of America: https://vva.org

References

American Psychiatric Association: Diagnostic and Statistical Manual: Mental Disorders. Washington, DC, American Psychiatric Association, 1952

American Psychiatric Association: Diagnostic and Statistical Manual of Mental Disorders, 3rd Edition. Arlington, VA, American Psychiatric Association, 1980

Beers CW: A Mind That Found Itself: An Autobiography. New York, Longmans, Green, & Company, 1908

Bertolote J: The roots of the concept of mental health. World Psychiatry 7(2):113–116, 2008 18560478

Bond ED: Thomas W. Salmon, Psychiatrist. New York, WW Norton, 1950

Camp NM: US Army Psychiatry in the Vietnam War: New Challenges in Extended Counterinsurgency Warfare (Textbooks of Military Medicine). Fort Sam Houston, TX, Borden Institute, U.S. Army Medical Department Center and School, 2014

Centers for Disease Control and Prevention: What is population health? Atlanta, GA, Centers for Disease Control and Prevention, 2019. Available at: www.cdc.gov/pophealthtraining/whatis.html. Accessed December 16, 2019.

Curry J, Engel CC, Zatzick DF: Mitigating stigma and other barriers to care through mental health service delivery in primary care settings, in Care of Military Service Members, Veterans, and Their Families. Edited by Cozza S, Goldenberg M, Ursano R. Washington, DC, American Psychiatric Publishing, 2014, pp 203–221

Da Costa JM: On irritable heart: a clinical study of a form of functional cardiac disorder and its consequences. Am J Med 11(5):559–567, 1871

Faulkner W: Requiem for a Nun. New York, Random House, 1951

Figley CR (ed): Stress Disorders Among Vietnam Veterans: Theory, Research, and Treatment. New York, Brunner/Mazel, 1978

Gordon S: The Battle for Veterans' Healthcare: Dispatches From the Front Lines of Policy Making and Patient Care. Ithaca, NY, Cornell University Press, 2017

Grinker RR, Spiegel JP: Men Under Stress. Philadelphia, PA, Blakiston, 1945

Group for the Advancement of Psychiatry: History. Dallas, TX, Group for the Advancement of Psychiatry, 2018. Available at: https://ourgap.org/History. Accessed September 3, 2019.

Hoge CW, Ivany CG, Brusher EA, et al: Transformation of mental health care for U.S. soldiers and families during the Iraq and Afghanistan Wars: where science and politics intersect. Am J Psychiatry 173(4):334–343, 2016 26552941

Matsakis A: Vietnam Wives: Women and Children Facing the Challenge of Living With Veterans With Post-Traumatic Stress Disorder. Kensington, MD, Woodbine House, 1988

Mitchell SW: Fat and Blood: and How to Make Them. Philadelphia, PA, JB Lippincott, 1877

Nash WP, Litz BT: Moral injury: a mechanism for war-related psychological trauma in military family members. Clin Child Fam Psychol Rev 16(4):365–375, 2013

National Academies of Sciences, Engineering, and Medicine: Evaluation of the Department of Veterans Affairs Mental Health Services. Washington, DC, The National Academies Press, 2018

Nevin RL, Ritchie EC: FDA black box, VA red ink? A successful service-connected disability claim for chronic neuropsychiatric adverse effects from mefloquine. Fed Pract 33(10):20–24, 2016 30766139

Shay J: Achilles in Vietnam: Combat Trauma and the Undoing of Character. New York, Scribner, 1994

Shay J: Odysseus in America: Combat Trauma and the Trials of Homecoming. New York, Scribner, 2002

Stevens R: A Time of Scandal: Charles R. Forbes, Warren G. Harding and the Making of the Veterans Bureau. Baltimore, MD, Johns Hopkins University Press, 2016

Tanielian T, Farris C, Batka C, et al: Ready to serve: community-based provider capacity to deliver culturally competent, quality mental health care to veterans and their families. Santa Monica, CA, RAND Corporation, 2014. Available at: www.rand.org/pubs/research_reports/RR806.html. Accessed September 3, 2019.

Teipe EJ: America's First Veterans and the Revolutionary War Pensions. Lewiston, NY, Edwin Mellen Press, 2002

U.S. Congress: VA Mission Act of 2018, Pub. L. No. 115-182, 2018.

U.S. Department of Veterans Affairs: History—VA history. Washington, DC, U.S. Department of Veterans Affairs, 2019a. Available at: www.va.gov/about_va/vahistory.asp. Accessed December 16, 2019.

U.S. Department of Veterans Affairs: Memorial Day history. Washington, DC, U.S. Department of Veterans Affairs, 2019b. Available at: www.va.gov/opa/speceven/memday/history.asp. Accessed September 3, 2019.

U.S. Department of Veterans Affairs: Veterans Health Administration. Washington, DC, U.S. Department of Veterans Affairs, 2019c. Available at: www.va.gov/health. Accessed September 3, 2019.

18

Advocacy for Patients in Medical Settings

Kaila Rudolph, M.D., M.P.H., M.B.E.
Rebecca Weintraub Brendel, M.D., J.D.

Learning Objectives

By the end of this chapter, readers will be able to:

- Identify advocacy opportunities for psychiatric patients receiving care within the medical setting across the spectrum of physician advocacy domains and clinical care provision levels

- Develop strategies to engage medical teams in the medical and mental health care of psychiatric patients

- Employ strategies to engage stakeholders and legislators to support institutional and population-level advocacy initiatives targeting psychiatric patients receiving care within medical settings

- Identify barriers to the engagement of advocacy efforts for psychiatric patients within the medical setting

- Form partnerships with medical colleagues to develop and implement collaborative advocacy education initiatives for psychiatric and medical trainees

Need for Advocacy in the Consultation-Liaison Psychiatry Context

Advocacy has become increasingly recognized as a central role of medical practitioners and is identified both as a core competency by the Academy of Consultation-Liaison Psychiatry (formerly the Academy of Psychosomatic Medicine) and an ethical imperative by the American Medical Association (Earnest et al. 2010; Leentjens et al. 2011). *Advocacy* has been defined as "action by a physician to promote social, economic, educational, and political changes that ameliorate suffering and threats to human health and well-being" (Earnest et al. 2010, p.63). Prominence of the biopsychosocial model within psychiatry, and in particular within the consultation-liaison subspecialty, necessitates that physicians possess skills to address both biological health interventions and social determinants of health at the patient, institution, and population levels (Engel 1977).

Advocacy is required in consultation-liaison psychiatry practice to address the health inequities observed in patients with comorbid medical and psychiatric illnesses. Compared with the general population, psychiatric patients with comorbid medical illness have reduced access to medical care, higher rates of undiagnosed and untreated physical illness, and poorer health outcomes (De Hert et al. 2011a, 2011b). Patients with severe and persistent mental illness have been found to have reduced life expectancy by 13–30 years, with 60% of this excess mortality attributable to physical health conditions (De Hert et al. 2011b).

For example, persons with schizophrenia have been shown to receive inadequate medical management of vascular risk factors, with 30%, 62%, and 88% of patients with schizophrenia not receiving medical treatment for diabetes, hypertension, and dyslipidemia, respectively (Nasrallah et al. 2006). Such treatments are critical because psychotropic medications are linked to cardiovascular disease, a leading cause of premature death for patients with schizophrenia (Bushe et al. 2010). The health inequities observed in access to medical care and treatment outcomes for patients with severe and persistent mental illness are multifactorial and present opportunities for psychiatrists to serve as advocates for their patients within the medical setting (De Hert et al. 2011a).

Conversely, patients with chronic medical conditions have increased rates of mental health concerns, such as depressive disorders (Katon

2003). The presence of depression in medically ill patients is associated with poorer health outcomes, increased mortality, and greater health care costs (Katon 2003). These outcome disparities have been linked to patient health behaviors, such as treatment nonadherence (DiMatteo et al. 2000). In the medical setting, treatment nonadherence has been found to be three times more likely in medically ill patients with depression than in those who are not depressed (DiMatteo et al. 2000). Psychiatrists are needed to advocate for enhanced clinical care of patients with medical illnesses complicated by psychiatric challenges, to educate medical teams to recognize psychiatric conditions, and to improve health system functioning for psychiatric patients in the medical setting.

All psychiatrists working within the medical setting can become health advocates. Advocacy at the patient level is most emphasized in clinical practice, whereas in order to enhance population health, clinical initiatives must be combined with advocacy involvement in community, state, and federal settings.

Case Example: Ms. F's Need for Advocacy

Ms. F is a 48-year-old female with a past psychiatric history significant for schizophrenia and a medical history notable for chronic obstructive pulmonary disease (COPD) and a smoking history of 25 pack-years. Ms. F immigrated as a refugee from Ethiopia in 1995; she speaks Amharic and has limited English proficiency. She receives Supplemental Security Income assistance and Medicaid health coverage. She was brought to the hospital by emergency medical services after a concerned bystander found her wandering in the street appearing confused and short of breath. At the time of her last outpatient mental health assessment 9 months ago, Ms. F's schizophrenia was well controlled with olanzapine (10 mg nightly). Since that time, she has missed two mental health appointments and had six emergency room presentations, each of which resulted in discharge to a shelter. She was last assessed in the emergency department 2 weeks earlier, when she presented with a cough and seeking food and assistance with housing resources.

Case Example: Ms. F's Need for Advocacy *(continued)*

You receive a page from Dr. W, the internal medicine attending physician, who was consulted by the emergency room physician for management of Ms. F's shortness of breath. Dr. W reports that Ms. F has improved after receiving nebulizer treatment in the emergency department and describes her dyspnea as chronic in the setting of COPD with continued cigarette smoking, despite repeated recommendations by care providers to quit. Dr. W indicates uncertainty about whether psychiatry needs to become involved but notes that Ms. F seems "somewhat odd" and was mildly agitated during the evaluation, and Dr. W concludes that it would be reassuring for psychiatry to assess Ms. F prior to hospital discharge. When asked about medical interpreter involvement in the evaluation, Dr. W noted that the medicine service has been very busy and therefore was unable to assess Ms. F with an interpreter because of time constraints. Her test results are not yet available, but Dr. W anticipates they will be within normal limits given her unremarkable medical evaluation. You agree to assess Ms. F and obtain Dr. W's pager number to continue to discuss Ms. F's care.

How to Use This Chapter

This chapter is intended to serve as a general guide for physicians advocating for psychiatric patients within the medical setting. We hope that the content of this chapter can help psychiatrists tailor advocacy initiatives to complement their clinical practices and academic interests. We consider potential opportunities and strategies to complete advocacy initiatives, as well as existing barriers preventing advocacy initiative engagement and optimal patient health. We structure this chapter using a socioecological framework to consider advocacy interventions at various levels of implementation, from direct patient care to federal initiatives (McLeroy et al. 1988). Although this chapter is organized by health care intervention levels, it is critical to appreciate that core advocacy actions in psychosomatic medicine may occur across all health care levels. For example, increasing care access, combating mental health stigma, addressing social determinants of health, and promoting positive health behaviors may occur at multiple implementation levels.

Advocacy in the Clinical Setting

Patient-Level Interventions

Advocacy interventions are required on a daily basis to promote the health of psychiatric patients in medical settings. Patient advocacy may be achieved by providing psychoeducation to enable patient autonomy and informed decision making, screening for the presence of drug interactions between medical and psychiatric medications, and completion of capacity evaluations to ensure that decisionally impaired adults have appropriate support. Patient advocacy interventions are grounded in the use of person-centered communication to provide care in accordance with patient goals and to motivate engagement in medical and mental health care (for additional information about patient-level advocacy, see Chapter 5, "Patient-Level Advocacy").

Person-centered communication refers to obtaining clinical information that facilitates understanding of patient preferences within their social and cultural context and then applying this knowledge to arrive at shared treatment goals (King and Hoppe 2013). Effective communication should be simple, communicate specific key messages with use of repetition to enforce central themes, and avoid medical jargon (King and Hoppe 2013). To ensure patient understanding, a teach-back approach may be implemented, in which patients are instructed to repeat key medical information to allow prompt detection and correction of any misconceptions (King and Hoppe 2013).

In addition to having direct patient contact, psychiatrists in the medical setting can advocate for their patients by educating medical teams about the use of person-centered communication. As the case of Ms. F highlights, interpreters are underutilized in medical settings even though Title VI of the Civil Rights Act of 1964 requires that recipients of federal financial assistance take reasonable steps to make their programs, services, and activities accessible by eligible persons with limited English proficiency (Juckett and Unger 2014). Ms. F's clinicians can prompt medical teams to engage with interpreter services and provide education to promote their effective use.

Clinicians can encourage person-centered communication to effectively meet six key goals in patient encounters: 1) build therapeutic alliance, 2) gather information, 3) educate patients about their health and appropriate health resources, 4) empower informed decision making, 5) respond to emotional reactions, and 6) facilitate engagement in treatment and health-promoting behaviors (King and Hoppe 2013). Advocating for enhanced patient-clinician communication can promote patient trust, care engagement, and increased care quality to reduce suffering and improve health (Street et al. 2009).

Current barriers to the completion of patient-level advocacy interventions include a lack of access to psychiatric services within the medical setting, clinician time constraints and lack of training in patient advocacy, prohibitive medical and mental health care costs, reduced government investment in mental health services as compared with physical health care, and absence of social programming resources to address social determinants of health (World Health Organization 2003). Many of these barriers are impossible to resolve at the patient level alone and require systemic solutions.

Case Example:
Patient-Level Advocacy for Ms. F

You schedule an in-person Amharic medical interpreter. You inform the medical team of the need to assess Ms. F with an interpreter and invite them to the assessment so they may complete their evaluation and provide medical information in the presence of the interpreter. During the patient assessment with the interpreter, you encourage the medical resident to speak directly to Ms. F, request sentence-by-sentence interpretation, and have the interpreter write down short, simple key medical messages to help Ms. F understand her medical information (Juckett and Unger 2014). You also encourage the medical team to engage in a postinterview discussion with the interpreter to assist in detection of any mental status concerns or behavior outside of cultural norms (Juckett and Unger 2014). The medical resident acknowledges the helpful information gained from in-person interpreter evaluation but notes time constraints as a primary barrier to consistently using this approach. You discuss the use of phone interpreter services paired with serial short evaluations in the hospital. You highlight the need for hospital-wide advocacy to address widespread challenges balancing hospital and systemic pressures to maximize efficiency with high clinician workload and the time it takes to communicate well with patients.

> ## Case Example:
> ## Patient-Level Advocacy for Ms. F *(continued)*
>
> During your psychiatry consultation, Ms. F is unable to provide a coherent narrative, even with the Amharic medical interpreter present. Across serial brief evaluations, Ms. F demonstrates fluctuations in her mental status ranging from somnolence to mild agitation. On cognitive testing, she is inattentive and disoriented.
>
> During your chart review, you locate a telephone number for Ms. F's sister and contact her to obtain collateral history. She reports uncertainty regarding the nature of her sister's medical problems, outside of her having "mental issues." She indicates becoming overwhelmed by attempting to care for her sister and not being able to provide care or housing for her over the past year. Limited understanding of Ms. F's care needs, competing responsibilities to her two children, becoming a guardian to Ms. F's 9-year-old son, and having limited financial means are identified as barriers to aiding Ms. F. The sister denies any ongoing child protective services involvement or any concern for the child's safety. She discusses experiencing anxiety, insomnia, and feelings of guilt due to her concerns for Ms. F's health. She denies access to any care provider supports or her own primary care physician. She is agreeable to meeting with the team social worker to discuss these challenges and appropriate community resources, including family physician referral sources. You provide education regarding signs and symptoms of care provider burden and community support resources.

Family-Level Interventions

Care provider burden is common and may be heightened in settings of comorbid medical and psychiatric illness because of the requirement for family members to attend to both medical and psychiatric care needs of the patient (Awad and Voruganti 2008). Psychiatrists in the medical setting can advocate for family members through direct assessment and through liaison with medical teams.

Advocating for families is critical because it can reduce family distress, enhance patient well-being, and enable and empower patients and families to become health advocates (Awad and Voruganti 2008). Patients and families can serve important roles in advocacy, including raising awareness about the importance of mental health care engagement, developing health consumer and family support advocacy groups, linking psychiatrists to these community initiatives, and supporting mental health public policy initiatives (World Health Organization 2003). To advocate for family member well-being, psychiatrists in the medical setting can consider the completion of four CARE tasks: **c**ollaborate, **a**sk, **r**efer, and **e**ducate.

Collaboration with medical teams, particularly social work colleagues, is essential for evaluating and addressing family-level advocacy. Partnerships rely on mutual respect and effective communication to establish care goals and equitable task delegation (Haig et al. 2006). Such partnerships can facilitate routine screening for family challenges in consultation settings. For children or other dependents, the primary advocacy goal is to ensure their safety and well-being while their guardian is receiving medical and psychiatric care. When dependents are present, assessing challenges to providing care to dependents, establishing the current guardian, and ascertaining any history of abuse or protective services involvement is required. Screening resources such as the Zarit Caregiver Burden Scale can be administered to assess the presence of care provider burden (Awad and Voruganti 2008).

Asking family members about their experience provides an opportunity to discuss their goals as care providers and for their loved ones. This information can facilitate appropriate *referral* to family resources, such as community care provider support programs, family care provider reimbursement programs, and child and elder protective services. Appropriate referrals for the patient may also emerge from care provider discussions. Eligible patients may be transitioned from hospital to short-term facilities, such as rehabilitation centers, skilled nursing facilities, or outpatient day programs, for ongoing care and care provider respite. Promoting the safety and well-being of family members in the medical setting also involves *educating* family members by supporting them in care-related problem solving, stress management, affect regulation, and provision of psychoeducation about their loved one's illness course and treatment (Awad and Voruganti 2008).

Barriers to achieving family advocacy include the perception that family member well-being is a secondary priority to direct patient care, lack of access to community programming to support family members, poor communication with family member health care teams about the need for child care or care provider supports, and lack of standardized burden screening of care providers in medical settings. Routine care provider burden screening, hospital-wide care provider education initiatives, and development of care provider specialty medical teams would help to address the care needs of both patients and their care providers.

Medical Team–Level Interventions

Psychiatric patient well-being in the medical setting is founded on the establishment and maintenance of effective collaborations with medical teams. Effective psychiatry consultation, ongoing clinical involvement, and provision of psychoeducation are dependent on high-quality psychiatry-medicine liaisons.

The psychiatric care provider may promote medical team engagement through clinical practice enhancement, teaching, and mentorship advocacy activities. Successful medical team liaisons are supported by collaborative engagement with patient, family, and health care teams to elicit their knowledge and preferences, followed by assessment of care needs and available resources. The SBARE communication framework—situation, background, assessment, and recommendation, with an e added for education within the medical setting—can be implemented to support provider consultation discussions and ongoing communication between health care professionals (Table 18–1) (Haig et al. 2006). Integrating knowledge of stakeholder preferences and available medical resources is then used to develop an evidence-based mental health care strategy. Reflection on the quality and success of medical team liaisons is critical for addressing potential conflicts and improving collaboration expertise.

Psychiatrists may advocate for effective patient care by providing short, relevant clinical pearls pertinent to the clinical encounter during medical team interactions. Effective communication and psychoeducation can address medical provider barriers to engagement in the care of psychiatric patients in the medical setting. Such barriers include lack of confidence in engaging psychiatric patients, presence of mental health stigma, limited support to manage distress or frustration in clinical encounters with psychiatric patients in the medical setting, and uncertainty of the role of psychiatry consultants in medical settings. Supporting medical teams and educating them about mental health stigma and the use of psychiatry services, countertransference management, and difficult family interactions as well as providing a rationale for medication recommendations may reduce distress and promote engagement with psychiatric patients. These interventions can foster a sense of efficacy and capability for medical teams, leading to improved care of the patient and increased medical provider capacity going forward through individual and team learning and skill development.

TABLE 18–1. A collaborative model for clinician-to-clinician communication

Communication strategy	Definition	Psychiatry consultation
Situation	Describe the present clinical circumstance leading to communication encounter	Reframe the consultation question (e.g., "Is Ms. F's mental status change due to an underlying psychiatric etiology or an acute medical concern?")
Background	Describe circumstances prior to the present situation	Describe pertinent findings from preadmission, past psychiatric history, and mental status evaluation
Assessment	Describe your understanding of the current clinical concern	Provide the diagnostic formulation and provisional psychiatric diagnosis
Recommendation	Describe what might be done to address the clinical concern	Provide verbal and written instructions outlining a plan for mental health care in the medical treatment setting (e.g., pharmacology treatment, development of an individualized behavioral plan)
Education	Describe any relevant learning points or clinical pearls	Concisely describe key psychiatry learning points for the medical consultant (e.g., rationale for recommendations, referral to journal article, tips for medical interpreter use, impact of mental health stigma)

Source. Adapted from Haig et al. 2006.

Case Example: Medical Team Interventions to Help Ms. F and Others

You page Dr. W to discuss Ms. F's clinical case. You inform Dr. W that your evaluation aimed to assess psychiatric contributions to Ms. F's altered mental status. You state your impression that Ms. F is experiencing a mixed delirium, suspected in the setting of community-acquired pneumonia given evidence of consolidation on chest radiograph, and that her acute presentation is not consistent with an exacerbation of her underlying psychiatric disorder.

You highlight that consistent with many patients with severe and persistent mental illness, Ms. F has had limited engagement with medical and mental health care and nonadherence to both schizophrenia and COPD treatment regimens. Given Ms. F's altered mental status, dyspnea with COPD and pneumonia, unstable housing, and limited social supports, you and Dr. W agree on admission for acute medical treatment with psychiatry involvement and reengagement with her outpatient care teams. You thank Dr. W for this referral and normalize Dr. W's uncertainty about placing psychiatry consultations. You provide Dr. W with an article outlining the role of psychiatry in the general medicine setting (Lokko and Stern 2015).

You take this opportunity to discuss mental health stigma and diagnostic overshadowing with Dr. W (Knaak et al. 2017). You explain that all persons have implicit biases of which they are unaware and that negative perceptions of persons with mental illness are common in both society and medical care settings. It is common to focus on mental health symptoms, such as schizophrenia, and to overemphasize these symptoms above acute medical illnesses, such as delirium; this can contribute to medical misdiagnosis and therefore to reduced access and quality of care for patients with mental illness (Knaak et al. 2017). Mental health stigma is common in your hospital's workplace culture, and you invite Dr. W to consider collaboration with you on a psychiatry-medical education initiative. Dr. W is supportive of this idea and agrees to consider it further.

Advocacy Beyond the Clinical Setting: Organization- and Population-Level Considerations

Advocacy at organization and population levels generally requires more time and intensive preparation than advocacy initiatives at the clinical level. However, such initiatives can have a wider-reaching degree of influence, impacting public policies and the health of entire communities and populations. Advocacy at this level may involve direct appeal to and education of policy makers, as well as the implementation of improved health care programs and policies.

Advocacy at the Organization (Health System) Level

The World Health Organization (2019) defines a *health system* as "the people, institutions and resources, arranged together in accordance with established policies, to improve the health of the population they serve." Organizational advocacy for institution-wide initiatives that enhance health care access, coverage, quality, or efficiency can strengthen the health system to improve the health of the targeted population (World Health Organization 2019). Examples of psychiatric health system advocacy initiatives include hospital-wide educational campaigns to reduce mental health stigma; the development and implementation of hospital policies in safe use of restraints; mental health screening initiatives in primary care and medical units; hospital-wide delirium prevention initiatives; and standardized patient discharge protocols.

One example of organization-level advocacy for psychiatric patients in the medical setting is advocacy for safe, comprehensive discharge planning to facilitate efficient care transitions and reduce risks of lengthy hospital stays, medical errors, and readmissions (Jack et al. 2008). Standardized discharge initiatives are emerging to produce hospital-wide discharge protocols; discharge training manuals for health care providers; and templates for individualized discharge plans documenting patient medication schedules, upcoming follow-up appointments, and discharge diagnosis information (Jack et al. 2008). Such discharge initiatives may begin with acknowledgment by key stakeholders that inefficient discharge planning can contribute to discharge delays and readmissions. These stakeholders may include the department heads of hospital admitting services, the heads of the nursing and social work departments, hospital administrators, the hospital's chief executive officer, information technology personnel, and the head of outpatient primary care (Jack et al. 2008). Small interdisciplinary working groups may be used to outline draft discharge frameworks, with integration of team proposals into one comprehensive discharge protocol (Jack et al. 2008). The discharge protocols may be piloted on selected units as a quality improvement initiative, with further modifications based on clinical feedback and investigation results prior to hospital-wide rollout.

Case Example: Organization-Level Advocacy for Ms. F

Following Ms. F's admission to the general medical unit, the psychiatry team remains closely involved for management of her delirium and intermittent agitation. Because patients with psychiatric and medical comorbidities can have complex discharge plans, you attend interdisciplinary team medicine rounds to facilitate discharge planning on the second day of Ms. F's admission. At the interdisciplinary meeting, a social work colleague asks about peer support initiatives that might promote Ms. F's engagement with mental health and medical services. The medicine team is unfamiliar with this care model and asks for further information.

You explain that peer support workers are persons recovering from mental health experiences who may also have concurrent substance use and medical challenges and who have training in peer support competencies (Gagne et al. 2018). Mental health recovery models and peer support initiatives have grown from the grassroots mental health consumer survivor movement, which has gained widespread public and political support (Gagne et al. 2018). Peer support workers have been implemented in integrated care settings, such as primary care clinics providing mental health services, to reduce stigma surrounding mental health care engagement, provide health education, and link to community care resources (Gagne et al. 2018). Peer support programs also foster the reintegration of persons recovering from mental health challenges into the workforce. Presently, 40 states have peer support worker training certification, and 36 states have Medicaid billing processes for peer support workers (Gagne et al. 2018).

> ### Case Example: Organization-Level Advocacy for Ms. F *(continued)*
>
> You inform the team that your hospital has developed a partnership with a community affiliate of a large nonprofit organization and that organizations such as the National Alliance on Mental Illness (www.nami.org/find-support/nami-programs/nami-peer-to-peer) and Mental Health America (www.mentalhealthamerica.net/center-peer-support) are helpful resources for developing community partnerships. Monthly information sessions are held in the outpatient primary care clinic to link patients to community mental health resources and community reintegration opportunities, such as peer support employment. These sessions are facilitated by the community organization and peer support workers employed by the hospital. You provide the team social worker with contact information for the community program affiliate and encourage dissemination of this information to social workers from medical and surgical departments.

Advocacy at the Community Level

Community-based initiatives, such as nonprofit patient advocacy organizations, provide important opportunities for political and health policy reform (World Health Organization 2003). Such collective efforts may occur through faith-based organizations, racial and ethnic cultural groups, and social justice initiatives. Community organizations can empower patients and families to become mental health leaders and encourage creation of and participation in health consumer–led initiatives (World Health Organization 2003).

Psychiatrists in the medical setting can advocate for community organizations through encouragement of patient and family involvement in community initiatives, support of existing community and academic partnerships (e.g., existing peer support worker initiatives), and promotion of the formation of new community liaisons. Initiating new community partnerships is a time-consuming, long-term process that requires community engagement planning (Israel et al. 1998).

Community engagement begins with clearly defining the purpose and expectations of the community-academic partnership (Israel et al. 1998). Clinician-community collaborations may be pursued to reduce mental health stigma, encourage treatment engagement in targeted patient populations, integrate mental health care into community organizations such as homeless shelters and hospices, and seek community stakeholder guidance on proposed mental health care reforms.

Case Example: Community-Level Advocacy for Ms. F

As Ms. F stabilizes clinically, you and her team continue her discharge planning. You decide that referral to an outpatient integrated care clinic, a primary care clinic with specialty mental health services, is most appropriate given her history of follow-up nonadherence and limited access to transportation. Although your hospital is equipped with an integrated care clinic, Ms. F hopes to find housing close to her sister, in an area that is a significant distance from the hospital and has no local integrated care clinic. As you continue your search, you learn that integrated care clinic access is limited throughout your state.

You recall that Minnesota has successfully implemented a statewide evidence-based treatment protocol for depression in the primary care setting across 75 clinics (Solberg et al. 2013). The Institute for Clinical Systems Improvement, a Minnesota nonprofit quality improvement organization, sponsored this initiative. Stakeholders, including physician-advocates, patients, health payers, and employers, were identified and recruited. The consolidated primary care practice organization and health plan coverage in the state facilitated the health care payer's agreement to provide a per-participant monthly bundled payment for standardized depression care. A working group was formed to review pertinent literature and develop a protocol for depression care in the primary care setting. Primary care clinics were recruited and trained in the depression treatment protocol. Monthly meetings were held postimplementation to support participating clinics and address emergent challenges. Researchers performed primary care site visits to collect patient health data and provider surveys to evaluate patient outcomes and provider experience (Solberg et al. 2013).

You decide to contact your state legislator to discuss the potential for increasing integrated care access for patients with mental illness in the primary care setting in your state. With Ms. F's case present in your mind, you decide to prepare talking points for a meeting with your state legislator.

Advocacy at Local, State, and Federal Legislative Levels

Physicians can serve as bipartisan advocates using their medical expertise and direct patient knowledge to enhance population health through efforts at local, state, and federal legislative levels. As collaborators, educators, and patient advocates, psychiatrists have highly developed skills that can be harnessed to execute successful advocacy initiatives at the population level. Advocacy opportunities applicable to all legislative levels may include direct contact with legislators to advocate for mental health policy reform; participation as a committee member or stakeholder in a local, state, or national medical association task force; composing health commission reports; and participation in publicized media coverage to promote health awareness.

At the local community or city level, psychiatrists have opportunities to build relationships with legislators through public and academic events, which offer valuable opportunities to discuss community advocacy (Hofford 2001). Local-level psychiatry initiatives may include enhanced transportation support for mental health patients to attend their medical appointments, recruitment of mental health care providers to provide services in local hospitals, and expanding access to community hospital telepsychiatry services.

State-level advocacy opportunities include testifying before the committee debating a new bill, obtaining legislative support to fund a state-level initiative, and drafting a bill to have new state legislation introduced (Hofford 2001). Psychiatrists may advocate for initiatives to increase mental health care provider training and access, such as statewide dissemination of integrated care models. Patient safety may be promoted through development of state laws to guide use of restraints in medical settings. Autonomy may also be enhanced through state adoption of laws recognizing psychiatric advance directives and supporting funding to enhance availability of public guardians for incapable adults with no health care proxy.

At the federal level, psychiatry advocacy initiatives may involve appeal for increased mental health care coverage for Medicaid recipients, augmentation of federal parity laws to increase employer mental health service coverage, and increasing the amount of federal budget spending dedicated to social programming. Social determinants of health, "the conditions in which people are born, grow, live, work and age," highlight the impact that social factors such as poverty, homelessness, limited health literacy, and inadequate care access have on mental and physical health (Commission on Social Determinants of Health 2008, p. 1). Psychiatrists can educate legislators on the need to enhance social supports, such as subsidized housing, to reduce the impact of social factors, such as homelessness, on physical and mental health (World Health Organization 2003).

Case Example

Government-Level Advocacy for Ms. F and Others

Your telephone call to your state legislator's office facilitates an in-person meeting with your state legislator, who greets you and asks to hear more about your integrated care initiative proposal.

You: Patients with mental health conditions complicated by medical illness have poor health outcomes, and the scientific literature supports that providing medical and mental health care in the same environment can improve those outcomes. Other states, such as Minnesota, have successfully implemented statewide integrated care clinics that include comprehensive outpatient care. Unfortunately, there are few integrated care clinics in our state, so most of my patients are unable to access these services. One of my patients, a woman with schizophrenia, has limited support and is having difficulty getting to appointments, which contributed to her being hospitalized with confusion and pneumonia. This is a very common story in my practice, and I would like to work with you to consider funding an integrated care initiative in our state to help provide comprehensive care in a single location.

Legislator: Investing in integrated care seems like a promising idea. Can you tell me more about the Minnesota model and potential implementation costs in our state?

You: I have brought educational materials that outline how the Minnesota model could be modified for our state. I haven't completed a cost-effectiveness analysis, so I cannot accurately comment on implementation costs. I will contact the Minnesota authors for information about potential costs and will contact you to arrange a follow-up meeting to discuss this further.

Your state legislator indicates that this is a promising beginning and suggests that after your completion of further research, the two of you schedule serial follow-up meetings to outline a specific implementation plan.

Case Example *(continued)*

Ms. F's Discharge

As Ms. F is being discharged from the hospital, she and her sister thank you for your help. Dr. W subsequently approaches you and indicates that seeing Ms. F's improved mental status with antipsychotic treatment has changed his perception of patients with schizophrenia. Dr. W indicates interest in collaborating on an advocacy education initiative addressing mental health stigma at your hospital. The goals of this curriculum are to promote positive attitudes toward psychiatric patients in the medical setting and instill provider hope for patient care engagement and recovery.

You conduct background research and discover a free online antistigma resource, Understanding Stigma, recently developed by the Mental Health Commission of Canada (Center for Addiction and Mental Health 2019). You and Dr. W arrange a meeting with the psychiatry and medicine residency program directors, who agree to support psychiatry and medicine residents independently completing this training, with a 1-hour lunchtime session for both specialties to collaboratively discuss the course content. You plan to administer a pre- and postintervention stigma scale, the Opening Minds Scale for Health Care Providers, to all psychiatry and medicine residents, via e-mail, to assess program efficacy (Knaak et al. 2017). If this pilot stigma intervention is successful, you hope to initiate mandatory training for all new hospital employees and apply for continuing medical education certification.

Advocacy in Medical Education

The World Health Organization has proposed that medical education must fulfill an obligation to social accountability, dedicating resources to address health concerns identified as a priority by key stakeholders, such as the government and local communities served by the health system (Boelen and Heck 1995). Addressing not only the health needs of individuals but also the needs of communities and populations at large requires the inclusion of advocacy within the medical curriculum (Boelen and Heck 1995).

The recognition of the need to integrate psychiatry and medicine parallels the important interplay between biological and social factors in the etiology and maintenance of illness in this population. Advocacy curricula are needed to provide clinicians with the knowledge and skills required to address the presence of health inequities within the health care delivery system and society due to the impacts of race, socioeconomic status, education, and housing (Basu et al. 2017). Components of an advocacy curriculum may include training on social determinants and social service provision models, health care system development, public health research methods, and the processes of policy development and political advocacy (Basu et al. 2017; Bhate and Loh 2015). Although advocacy curricula remain in their infancy, they are being devised and disseminated in emerging scientific literature (Basu et al. 2017). (For more information on advocacy education, see Chapter 8, "Education as Advocacy.")

The Accreditation Council for Graduate Medical Education and American Board of Psychiatry and Neurology (2014) recognize advocacy achievements as important consultation-liaison trainee milestones. Although there is limited literature on a formal consultation-liaison advocacy curriculum, this specialty is well positioned to provide advocacy training to both psychiatry and medical trainees through liaisons with diverse hospital teams. Formation of advocacy educational partnerships may propel the development of psychosomatic medicine advocacy curricula and increase the quality and impact of advocacy education initiatives.

Conclusion

In this chapter, we have explored advocacy for psychiatric patients in the medical setting from clinical, institutional, and population perspectives. Through close collaboration with medical colleagues, psychiatric care providers can aid patients and families in receiving high-quality care and navigating complex health care systems. Promoting the development and implementation of improved health care programs and hospital-level educational campaigns can enhance patients' health at the institution level. Local, state, and federal health reforms can be achieved by collaborating with key stakeholders to augment existing health laws, policies, funding, and social programming models to enhance population health.

Psychiatry providers in the medical setting, through their hospital-wide partnerships and liaison skills, are well situated to develop relationships with stakeholders and medical advocates to serve as leaders across the continuum of advocacy levels and domains. Psychiatry providers serve a complex patient population, requiring innovative approaches and increased emphasis on advocacy initiatives to promote the health of current and future generations.

References

Accreditation Council for Graduate Medical Education, American Board of Psychiatry and Neurology: The Psychosomatic Medicine Milestone Project. Chicago, IL, Accreditation Council for Graduate Medical Education, October 2014. Available at: www.acgme.org/Portals/0/PDFs/Milestones/ PsychosomaticMedicineMilestones.pdf. Accessed September 4, 2019.

Awad AG, Voruganti LN: The burden of schizophrenia on caregivers: a review. Pharmacoeconomics 26(2):149–162, 2008 18198934

Basu G, Pels RJ, Stark RL, et al: Training internal medicine residents in social medicine and research-based health advocacy: a novel, in-depth curriculum. Acad Med 92(4):515–520, 2017 28145945

Bhate TD, Loh LC: Building a generation of physician advocates: the case for including mandatory training in advocacy in Canadian medical school curricula. Acad Med 90(12):1602–1606, 2015 26200573

Boelen C, Heck J: Defining and measuring the social accountability of medical schools. Geneva, Switzerland, World Health Organization, 1995. Available at: http://apps.who.int/iris/bitstream/handle/10665/59441/?sequence=1. Accessed September 5, 2019.

Bushe CJ, Taylor M, Haukka J: Mortality in schizophrenia: a measurable clinical endpoint. J Psychopharmacol 24(4)(suppl):17–25, 2010 20923917

Center for Addiction and Mental Health: Understanding stigma. Toronto, ON, Canada, Center for Addiction and Mental Health, 2019. Available at: www.camh.ca/en/education/continuing-education-programs-and-courses/ continuing-education-directory/understanding-stigma. Accessed September 5, 2019.

Commission on Social Determinants of Health: Closing the gap in a generation: health equity through action on the social determinants of health. Final report of the Commission on Social Determinants of Health. Geneva, World Health Organization, 2008

De Hert M, Cohen D, Bobes J, et al: Physical illness in patients with severe mental disorders, II: barriers to care, monitoring and treatment guidelines, plus recommendations at the system and individual level. World Psychiatry 10(2):138–151, 2011a 21633691

De Hert M, Correll CU, Bobes J, et al: Physical illness in patients with severe mental disorders, I: prevalence, impact of medications and disparities in health care. World Psychiatry 10(1):52–77, 2011b 21379357

DiMatteo MR, et al: Depression is a risk factor for noncompliance with medical treatment: meta-analysis of the effects of anxiety and depression on patient adherence. Arch Intern Med 160(14):2101–2107, 2000 10904452

Earnest MA, Wong SL, Federico SG: Physician advocacy: what is it and how do we do it? Acad Med 85(1):63–67, 2010 20042825

Engel GL: The need for a new medical model: a challenge for biomedicine. Science 196(4286):129–136, 1977 847460

Gagne CA, Finch WL, Myrick KJ, et al: Peer workers in the behavioral and integrated health workforce: opportunities and future directions. Am J Prev Med 54(6S3):S258–S266, 2018 29779550

Haig KM, Sutton S, Whittington J: SBAR: a shared mental model for improving communication between clinicians. Jt Comm J Qual Patient Saf 32(3):167–175, 2006 16617948

Hofford RA: Seven tips for effecting legislative change. Fam Pract Manag 8(4):35–38, 2001 11331980

Israel BA, Schulz AJ, Parker EA, et al: Review of community-based research: assessing partnership approaches to improve public health. Annu Rev Public Health 19:173–202, 1998 9611617

Jack B, Greenwald J, Forsythe S, et al: Developing the tools to administer a comprehensive hospital discharge program: the ReEngineered Discharge (RED) Program, in Advances in Patient Safety: New Directions and Alternative Approaches, Vol. 3. Edited by Henriksen K, Battles JB, Keyes MA, et al. Rockville, MD, Agency for Healthcare Research and Quality, 2008

Juckett G, Unger K: Appropriate use of medical interpreters. Am Fam Physician 90(7):476–480, 2014 25369625

Katon WJ: Clinical and health services relationships between major depression, depressive symptoms, and general medical illness. Biol Psychiatry 54(3):216–226, 2003 12893098

King A, Hoppe RB: "Best practice" for patient-centered communication: a narrative review. J Grad Med Educ 5(3):385–393, 2013 24404300

Knaak S, Mantler E, Szeto A: Mental illness-related stigma in healthcare: barriers to access and care and evidence-based solutions. Healthc Manage Forum 30(2):111–116, 2017 28929889

Leentjens AF, Rundell JR, Wolcott DL, et al: Reprint of: Psychosomatic medicine and consultation-liaison psychiatry: scope of practice, processes, and competencies for psychiatrists working in the field of CL psychiatry or psychosomatics: a consensus statement of the European Association of Consultation-Liaison Psychiatry and Psychosomatics (EACLPP) and the Academy of Psychosomatic Medicine (APM). J Psychosom Res 70(5):486–491, 2011 21511080

Lokko HN, Stern T: Collaboration and referral between internal medicine and psychiatry. Prim Care Companion CNS Disord 17(1):1–23, 2015 26137348

McLeroy KR, Bibeau D, Steckler A, et al: An ecological perspective on health promotion programs. Health Educ Q 15(4):351–377, 1988 3068205

Nasrallah HA, Meyer JM, Goff DC, et al: Low rates of treatment for hypertension, dyslipidemia and diabetes in schizophrenia: data from the CATIE schizophrenia trial sample at baseline. Schizophr Res 86(1–3):15–22, 2006 16884895

Solberg LI, Crain AL, Jaeckels N, et al: The DIAMOND initiative: implementing collaborative care for depression in 75 primary care clinics. Implement Sci 8:135–146, 2013 24238225

Street RL Jr, Makoul G, Arora NK, et al: How does communication heal? Pathways linking clinician-patient communication to health outcomes. Patient Educ Couns 74(3):295–301, 2009 19150199

World Health Organization: Advocacy for mental health: mental health policy and service guidance package. Geneva, Switzerland, World Health Organization, 2003. Available at: www.who.int/mental_health/policy/services/1_advocacy_WEB_07.pdf. Accessed September 4, 2019.

World Health Organization: Health systems: health systems strengthening glossary. Geneva, Switzerland, World Health Organization, 2019. Available at: www.who.int/healthsystems/hss_glossary/en/index5.html. Accessed September 4, 2019.

19

Community and Public Sector Advocacy

Jeanne Steiner, D.O.
Allison Ponce, Ph.D.
Michael Rowe, Ph.D.
Kenneth Thompson, M.D.

Learning Objectives

By the end of this chapter, readers will be able to:

- Identify social determinants of health and structural factors that inequitably shape the distribution of health and illness

- Discuss the importance of a population health perspective within community and public sector systems of care

- Describe examples of innovative programs and initiatives that promote social justice and inclusion

- Promote the central importance of advocacy roles for public sector mental health professionals

In this chapter, we focus on the critical importance of advocacy at the level of communities and across the public sector. Our definition of *community* includes neighborhoods, towns, cities, and regions, encompassing the multiple domains of individuals who live and work there, as well as transportation and education systems, cultural activities, economic status, and employment opportunities. We also consider the *public sector*, referring to the wide array of clinical and other services that are funded through state and federal mechanisms for individuals who experience serious mental health disorders. Our basic assertion is that in order to improve the lives of the individuals we serve, we must consider our roles as advocates within a population health context, that is, the "upstream" conditions in which members of our community live and the public policies that exert enormous influence on these conditions. We discuss the centrality of social determinants of health and their connections to health equity and assert that the framework of social justice is the basis of several overarching goals of community and public advocacy (Shim and Compton 2018).

The actions we can take support the following goals:

- Ensure access to health care for all—including individuals who are uninsured, poorly insured, and/or undocumented
- Promote access to treatment for substance use and other mental health disorders that is recovery oriented, person centered, and culturally competent
- Address the inequities in care that affect underrepresented minorities, regardless of race, gender, sexual orientation, gender identity or expression, and immigration status
- Address critical issues of social justice, including poverty and access to affordable housing
- Promote policies, funding mechanisms, and education and training opportunities that will address the workforce shortage that is particularly relevant for persons with serious illness who are served by the public sector

In this chapter, we provide background on and evidence for the centrality of a focus on social justice and present two examples of successful initiatives that involve advocacy and the pursuit of creative partnerships across agencies and funding sources. The first example, the Citizens Project, illustrates the importance of social inclusion for individuals who are typically marginalized and the use of specific mechanisms to promote engagement and empowerment in their community. The second example is a model program for homelessness services that harnessed the power of public-private partnerships to develop and bolster person-centered services. These comprehensive programs demonstrate effective approaches to promoting social inclusion and support for housing, education, and vocational services for individuals who are traditionally underserved. Each of these examples was built on a foundation of social justice that values advocacy by mental health professionals in partnership with community members and institutions.

The following are key concerns for individuals receiving services in public and community settings, several of which are highlighted in more detail in this chapter:

- Affordable and supportive housing opportunities
- Food insecurity
- Supported education and employment
- Financial health/literacy
- Legal services
- Integrated care for physical health
- Social inclusion and community integration
- Self-advocacy

Social Justice and Health/ Mental Health Inequities

Beginning with the epidemiological work of Rudolph Virchow (Brown and Fee 2006) and Friedrich Engels (Engels 1958) working in the middle of the nineteenth century up to the recent extraordinary work of Sir Michael Marmot (Marmot 2017), it has long been understood and repeatedly observed that health and illness, well-being and suffering, are not randomly distributed through the population. Instead, with the exception of the rare diseases of affluence, health and illness follow the changing stratification of society according to evolution of social status and power through history. This means that at any given moment, the social/cultural process of exercising power results in the distribution of health and illness based on wealth and income and sets the terms of how people live according to socially constructed categories such as gender, sexual orientation, race/ethnicity, occupation, unemployment, and geographic location. These are all determinants of health, along with more concrete factors such as housing, food, air quality, and transportation, because in toto they create the social/environmental niche that particular groups of people inhabit. This nonrandom distribution of health and illness has also been found repeatedly in the subfield of psychiatric epidemiology, beginning with the work of Robert Faris and Warren Dunham (Faris and Dunham 1939); progressing through Alexander Leighton (Leighton 1959), the Midtown Manhattan study (Srole et al. 1962), August Hollingshead and Frederick Redlich (Hollingshead and Redlich 1958), and the Epidemiologic Catchment Area study (Klerman 1986);

and continuing on to the work of Bruce Link, Ronald Kessler, David Williams, and many others (Dohrenwend et al. 1992; Kessler and Cleary 1980; Williams 2017).

The distribution of health and illness—and mental health and mental illness—is neither random nor just. It specifically burdens the people and the communities with the fewest resources and least power and is created by policies and actions that inflict trauma or deny needed resources. The exercise of power, unless carefully attended to, is easily abused to empower some and disempower others. Throughout history, it has created neglect, exclusion, oppression, and exploitation. The dynamic process of social power and its impact on general health and mental health is continually evolving in interaction with the society it creates. The fact that the exercise of social power and the structure it creates are fluid, no matter how solid they appear to be at the moment, creates the room for advocacy for social justice and health and mental health equity.

As might be expected, there have been attempts by those in power to defuse the observations described above. The most prevalent approach, still common today, is to blame the victim. Usually, this is done by tying the distribution of ill health, including mental ill health, to "lifestyle choices," thereby implicitly endorsing the idea that a well-resourced life (exercise, healthy diet, no stress, good sleep) is the way to live. There is little attention to how certain lifestyle choices may be determined by the social structure (e.g., individuals choosing unhealthy fast food because it is affordable), and there is a lack of full exploration to see if these lifestyle choices are in fact the primary determining factor in the occurrence of illness. Another way the victim is blamed is by ascribing the nonrandom distribution of health and illness to the idea that people with illness and disability "drift" into poverty. In this case, the inequity in the distribution of illness is blamed on the illness itself rather than on social policies that ensure that many people with disabilities must live in poverty.

Another historical tendency has been to blame the unfair distribution of ill health on the unfair distribution of health care resources. For generations, Americans have been led to believe that the cure for the country's health inequalities lies in obtaining equal access to health care. Although this explanation does not blame the victim, it does subsume a tremendous amount of energy and keeps the focus on the distribution of and access to health care rather than on the circumstances in which people live and the exercise of power that excludes or oppresses them. Hard as it has been to achieve change, the power structure has proven to be much more willing to concede resources for health care access than to address, for example, childhood poverty. It is interesting to note that since the passage of the Patient Protection and Affordable Care Act of 2010 (ACA; P.L. 111-148) and the expansion of access to most people in some states, people in the United States have begun to more fully appreciate the concept of the *social determinants of health*, but in a manner that can serve to avoid its larger implications. Clinicians are being taught to survey their individual patients to determine what their social determinants of health are—whether they have money for food, a place to live, and so forth—with the goal of solving a person's particular problems rather than to think of the life circumstances of their patients as a social problem requiring broad social action. Despite the passage of the ACA, the struggle for universal access to health care continues to face a great deal of resistance. Efforts to dismantle the ACA persist, and 14 states, mostly in the South, have refused to extend Medicaid. Efforts to move to Medicare for All generated controversy in the months leading up to the 2020 presidential elections.

Overcoming these arguments and pushing for significant changes to the social order and to how power is exercised to create greater social justice and achieve health equity in the ongoing construction of our society has been a time-consuming effort. Attempts at change have required many decades of struggle on personal, civil, and political levels and many movements, including labor, racial justice, gender and sexual orientation equity, social welfare provision (including health and mental health care), and environmental protection, to name the most obvious.

It is worthwhile noting that advocacy for social justice in mental health (including substance use) has faced an additional hurdle. Power structures, including some in the profession of psychiatry, have made it easy to discount the voices of people with mental health challenges—people in charge have simply pointed to individuals' mental illness as a way to disqualify their observations and demands. Some in the profession have reacted by taking the opportunity to speak "for the voiceless," whereas others have worked to partner with the people who are speaking up. Most of the struggle in mental health advocacy has focused, as might be expected, on the issues of how services are delivered. There have been two distinct branches to this advocacy: how to make services accessible and how to deal with coercion in care. The former has not been controversial in the profession or the field or even among consumers of services. The latter, however, has been extremely controversial. Somewhere in the middle of these two large streams of advocacy is a third stream focused on improving the care provided, which may or may not make the care more or less paternalistic and coercive. In the meantime, larger campaigns to address the social inequities in society that foster and abet psychiatric challenges have, until recently, gone largely unaddressed.

Two things have changed to open up and broaden advocacy for social justice in mental health. The first is growing evidence that the United States is experiencing a wave of psychiatrically caused premature death unlike anything observed previously. The explosive increases in deaths due to opioid use along with lesser but still noticeable increases in alcohol-related deaths and suicide that are occurring among people with less education have given rise to the notion of "the deaths of despair" in communities where industry has collapsed (Case and Deaton 2015). Although efforts to stem the tide of deaths have focused on increasing access to substance use treatment services and the availability of naloxone, there also has been an increasing awareness that broad social and economic issues need to be addressed.

A second development is a growing appreciation by local governments that attending to the mental health of their populations requires more from them than providing psychiatric services, important as that is. Communities need to be developed in such a way that needed resources and opportunities are available to everyone, and although government cannot provide all that is needed, it can serve as a convener and point of accountability. In such communities, advocacy for health equity and social justice in mental health is firmly expanded beyond provider, family, consumer, and government payer to include the community and all its stakeholders. ThriveNYC is the prime example of this approach (https://thrivenyc.cityofnewyork.us).

The struggle for social justice and mental health, like the struggle for social justice and health overall, is clearly not won, but successes occur, despite persisting resistance. Even so, it is easier now than it has been in the past to advocate *against* racism, classism, homophobia, and so on and *for* democracy, good government, housing, food, education, family supports, and jobs as key elements of what produces health, mental health, and wellness.

Advocates for social justice and mental health need to be in the struggle for the long haul, with a sense of radical perseverance, and be ready for the next opportunity to move forward, whether at the local, national, or international level. Advocates must be creative. The struggle goes through ever-changing cycles, and each cycle requires something different. People who aspire to be advocates and who care deeply about these issues need to find ways to mutually support each other and help each other hone their efforts. They need to keep their eye on the prize—to constantly imagine how things could be different. They also need to know that the path will be challenging, and they may need to step aside briefly to recuperate from time to time. They need to know that they cannot and will not stop. They must organize! Power concedes nothing without a fight. Also, as Sigmund Freud would have advised, they must allow joy and love in their work and lives.

Example 1: Citizens Project

Citizenship, as we define it, is a person's strong connection to the 5 Rs that society offers its members—**r**ights, **r**esponsibilities, **r**oles, **r**esources, and **r**elationships—and a sense of belonging that is validated by others. Access to the 5 Rs supports a sense of belonging, and a sense of belonging supports a person's connection to the 5 Rs (Rowe 2015). To become this type of citizen requires both practical assets—legal citizenship, yes, but also knowledge and skills to gain access to tangible resources and opportunities—and symbolic (or emotional) assets, such as the experience of having a valued role in society. Citizenship refers to all people, although its approach is applied, as discussed here, to support the 5 Rs and the sense of belonging of people with psychiatric disorders. Citizenship is citizenship; a special form of citizenship for people with psychiatric disorders is a contradiction in terms. (There is no "psychiatric citizenship.")

The inspiration for this conceptual framework of citizenship as social inclusion of people with mental illnesses originated in the 1990s from the activity of mental health outreach to people who were homeless (Rowe 1999). In this type of service, clinicians, case managers, and others leave their offices to look for people who are not receiving mental health treatment. In many cases, these individuals have endured previous negative experiences with mental health care, such as involuntary hospitalization, and are not looking to be found by mental health staff. Outreach workers attempt to gain trust slowly with prospective clients, building on the person's strengths and honoring the person's first choices for help (e.g., dental vs. mental health care) whenever possible, and gradually persuading the person to accept mental health and primary care, as well as housing. Outreach is often successful in that it connects most clients with care and vital resources, although where it reaches the limits of its effectiveness relates to the long-term challenge inherent, for example, in the community mental health movement's dual goals of effective treatment and creating a life in the community (Kennedy 1963). Some formerly homeless individuals feel isolated and out of place and sometimes contemplate returning to a life on the street. Outreach work can do much, but it cannot confer on recipients the status of neighbor, community member, and citizen.

The Citizens Project, initiated in 2001, is the longest-standing citizenship intervention (Rowe 2015). The project takes the 5 Rs plus belonging and translates them into a 6-month intervention with four moving and integrated parts:

1. Classes on one's rights and responsibilities in relation to mental health and other systems (e.g., criminal justice, entitlement programs), resources such as employment and housing, intimate and casual relationships, roles including advocacy, and many other topics
2. Valued role projects in which students take what they have learned from the classes and put it into practice through individual projects such as hosting a Thanksgiving dinner for family members, thus "doing for" others instead of being the one who has to be "done for" (i.e., by attending the dinner but not being expected to bring a dish or to contribute in other ways), or group projects such as teaching police cadets what it is like to be homeless and on the streets with active symptoms of mental illness and to be approached by a police officer
3. "Wraparound" peer mentor support
4. Student-led, nontherapy discussions about "what's up?" in students' lives, in which everyone speaks and everyone gives feedback

The Merriam-Webster definition of *advocacy* is "the act or process of supporting a cause or proposal" (www.merriam-webster.com/dictionary/advocacy). Advocacy can be performed by an individual, a group, or an organization; in any case, the definition assumes the capacity or skill to perform the actions of advocacy, whether or not the actions lead to the desired objectives. The Citizens Project is an advocacy building and doing project in at least five ways.

1. Advocates need to know what they are advocating for and why. Included among the 20 or so class topics (which change somewhat with each cohort on the basis of students' knowledge, interests, and pressing needs) are the Americans With Disabilities Act, patients' rights as recipients of services and ways to assert those rights, and more general knowledge and skills that undergird the actions of the advocate, such as training and practice in the fine skills of assertiveness versus aggressiveness with others.
2. The Citizens Project changes the framework of services that participants are accustomed to receiving from "care" and "supports" to the building of citizenship and social participation. The Citizens Project starts from the idea that the person with mental illness is a person first and then a recipient of mental health services and posits that the

person's role is first as a member of society rather than as a client or patient.

3. The Citizens Project offers students opportunities for both preparation for and acts of advocacy, including training in public speaking; visits to state legislators to practice and demonstrate their capacities and capabilities as citizens in presenting recommendations as concerned citizens; and valued role projects in which, as in the police cadet example mentioned earlier, they advocate for others and themselves.

4. By building broader citizenship skills, the Citizens Project contextualizes advocacy for students. People who run their own group support component ("What's up?") develop and act out the rules and guidelines of group support (e.g., no "cross talking," no "war stories") and thereby become better prepared for, comfortable with, and likely to gravitate toward advocacy roles and topics.

5. Advocacy and other citizenship skills have components that are both instrumental (skills and *factual* knowledge) and affective (the empowerment and *affective* knowledge that come with instrumental capacities). Voters, for example, are people who cast their votes with others. Voters are also people who know that they can vote, even when no election is upcoming and even when they do not vote. The Citizens Project provides opportunities for both instrumental and affective empowerment that support people's advocacy orientation and acts.

Example 2: Collaboration to Fund and Implement a Model Program for Homelessness Services

The literature has long addressed a clear relationship between mental illness and homelessness (Caton et al. 2005; Creech et al. 2015; Struening and Padgett 1990). In addition to the psychosocial factors that may lead to and maintain homelessness for individuals with mental illness, there are structural factors that create barriers to housing. For example, a report from the U.S. Department of Housing and Urban Development (2017) carefully detailed the forms and prevalence of housing discrimination against individuals with disabilities, including mental illness. It appears that the mere fact that a person has mental illness is sufficient to hamper access to housing at appalling rates.

In addition to having challenges with entering housing, individuals who experience homelessness have difficulty accessing a variety of services despite having serious health care needs. Those who are homeless also experience barriers to employment and access to disability income (Lowder et al. 2017). All of these obstacles converge to limit opportunity for these individuals to obtain the necessary tools to exit homelessness, obtain income to support themselves, and receive the services needed to improve health on multiple dimensions. It is incumbent on psychiatrists and other mental health professionals to lead advocacy efforts to address homelessness and to participate in the creation of solutions to address the associated issues.

The Pathways to Independence (PTI) project is an example of one such program that was designed by mental health professionals in conjunction with community service providers to provide integrated services to individuals experiencing chronic homelessness. Creating such partnerships is a crucial form of advocacy work for psychiatrists and other mental health professionals. In this case, faculty from the Yale School of Medicine's department of psychiatry, through the publicly funded Connecticut Mental Health Center, brought crucial skills to bear to collaborate with Columbus House, a private nonprofit homelessness services organization, to provide support to some of the most vulnerable individuals in the community. Through the use of grant-writing, evaluation, and clinical and education skills to cocreate a public-private partnership, the group developed a program based on recovery and citizenship principles that has had very promising results (Brown et al. 2018). This is a case study in attending in very intentional ways to increasing access to a life in the community for individuals living with mental illness.

Starting in 2011, PTI was funded by a $1.5 million Cooperative Agreements to Benefit Homeless Individuals (CABHI) grant from the Substance Abuse and Mental Health Services Administration (SAMHSA) to provide a package of recovery-oriented services to support chronically homeless individuals in meeting their self-articulated goals related to living a meaningful life in the community. The program was designed to provide comprehensive, specialized, person-centered services based on the wishes of each individual participant. These services included supported employment; help applying for federal benefits through SAMHSA's SOAR (SSI/SSDI Outreach, Access, and Recovery) Technical Assistance Center (Kauff et al. 2016); support in accessing and maintaining housing; financial literacy classes; and colocated mental health and medical services. PTI services were offered in a framework that allowed individual participants to determine what supports they desired and when.

PTI differed in notable ways from standard case management and assertive community treatment (Lehman et al. 1997), which are common interventions for individuals who experience chronic homelessness, with regard to how the staff functioned and the priorities of the program. Each PTI team member specialized in a single service area, allowing them to achieve considerable depth of expertise in their area. The small staff worked within a tight-knit structure with a focus on offering highly individualized services. The team included specialists in SOAR, employment, and housing; a patient navigator for health care services; and a psychology postdoctoral fellow to address mental health concerns.

Quantitative and qualitative findings indicate that PTI was a promising model leading to success in housing, employment, and attainment of benefits (Brown et al. 2018) and largely resulting in a positive impression of the program among a variety of stakeholders (Ponce et al. 2018). Advocacy was a grounding principle of the program from the outset. A social justice framework undergirded the structure of the intervention, with a focus on collaboration to draw on the strengths of organizations and ensure a culture in which participants' goals and priorities were prioritized. The voices of mental health professionals, in collaboration with those of community partners and individuals with lived experience of mental illness and homelessness, can support the creation of powerful opportunities to enhance the recovery and citizenship of those members of communities who have systematically and historically been silenced.

Conclusion

In this chapter, we assert the fundamental value and critical importance of advocacy in communities and in the public sphere. We know that poverty, racism, exposure to violence, and lack of affordable housing—to name just a few of the societal issues that our nation is experiencing— have a significant impact on the mental and physical health and opportunities to lead meaningful lives of all members of our communities. We offer arguments to support the efforts of mental health professionals to become advocates for the people they serve in an expansive array of contexts—not just by treating individuals but also by forming community partnerships to develop innovative approaches and opportunities for the people they serve and by raising their collective voices to influence state and national policies.

References

Brown TM, Fee E: Rudolf Carl Virchow: medical scientist, social reformer, role model. Am J Public Health 96:2104–2105, 2006

Brown M, Rowe M, Cunningham A, Ponce AN: Evaluation of a comprehensive SAMHSA service program for individuals experiencing chronic homelessness. J Behav Health Serv Res 45(4):504–613, 2018 29435863

Case A, Deaton A: Rising midlife morbidity and mortality in midlife among white non-Hispanic Americans in the 21st century. Proc Natl Acad Sci 112(49):15,078–15,083, 2015 26575631

Caton CL, Dominguez B, Schanzer B, et al: Risk factors for long-term homelessness: findings from a longitudinal study of first-time homeless single adults. Am J Public Health 95(10):1753–1759, 2005 16131638

Creech SK, Johnson E, Borgia M, et al: Identifying mental and physical health correlates of homelessness among first-time and chronically homeless veterans. J Community Psychol 43(5):619–627, 2015

Dohrenwend B, Levav I, Shrout PE, et al: Socioeconomic status and psychiatric disorders: the causation-selection issue. Science 255(5047):946–952, 1992 1546291

Engels F: The Condition of the Working Class in England. Redwood City, CA, Stanford University Press, 1958

Faris REL, Dunham HW: Mental Disorders in Urban Areas: An Ecological Study of Schizophrenia and Other Psychoses. Chicago, University of Chicago Press, 1939

Hollingshead AB, Redlich FC: Social Class and Mental Illness: Community Study. New York, Wiley, 1958

Kauff JF, Clary E, Lupfer KS, Fischer PJ: An evaluation of SOAR: implementation and outcomes of an effort to improve access to SSI and SSDI. Psychiatr Serv 67(10):1098–1102, 2016 27133724

Kennedy JF: Special message to the Congress on mental illness and mental retardation. Santa Barbara, CA, American Presidency Project, February 5, 1963. Available at: www.jfklibrary.org/asset-viewer/archives/JFKPOF/052/JFKPOF-052-012. Accessed January 10, 2020.

Kessler RC, Cleary PD: Social class and psychological distress. Am Sociol Rev 45(3): 463–478, 1980 7406359

Klerman G: Epidemiologic Catchment Area (NIMH-ECA) program: background, preliminary findings and implications. Soc Psychiatry 21(4):159–166, 1986 3024327

Lehman AF, Dixon LB, Kernan E, et al: A randomized trial of assertive community treatment for homeless persons with severe mental illness. Arch Gen Psychiatry 54(11):1038–1043, 1997 9366661

Leighton AH: My Name is Legion. New York, Basic Books, 1959

Lowder EM, Desmarais SL, Neupert SD, Truelove MA: SSI/SSDI Outreach, Access, and Recovery (SOAR): disability application outcomes among homeless adults. Psychiatr Serv 68(11):1189–1192, 2017 28760095

Marmot M: The health gap: the challenge of an unequal world: the argument. Int J Epidemiol 46(4):1312–1318, 2017 28938756

Ponce AN, Brown M, Cunningham A, Rowe M: Stakeholder perspectives on integrated services for people who experience chronic homelessness. J Soc Distress Homeless 27(2):126–134, 2018

Rowe M: Crossing the Border: Encounters Between Homeless People and Outreach Workers. Berkeley, University of California Press, 1999

Rowe M: Citizenship and Mental Health. New York, Oxford University Press, 2015

Shim RS, Compton MT: Addressing the social determinants of mental health: if not now, when? If not us, who? Psychiatr Serv 69(8):844–846, 2018 29852822

Srole T, Langner S, Michael ST, et al: Mental Health in the Metropolis: The Midtown Manhattan Study, Vol 1. New York, McGraw-Hill, 1962

Struening EL, Padgett DK: Physical health status, substance use and abuse, and mental disorders among homeless adults. J Soc Issues 46:65–81, 1990

U.S. Department of Housing and Urban Development: Rental housing discrimination on the basis of mental disabilities: Results of pilot testing, 2017. Washington, DC, U.S. Department of Housing and Urban Development. Available at: www.huduser.gov/portal/sites/default/files/pdf/Mental Disabilities-FinalPaper.pdf. Accessed January 10, 2020.

Williams DR: From disparity to equity, in Knowledge to Actions: Accelerating Progress in Health, Well-Being, and Equity. Edited by Plough AL. New York, Oxford University Press, 2017, pp 21–30

20

Advocacy for People With Mental Illness at Risk for Criminal Justice Involvement

Debra A. Pinals, M.D.
Danna E. Mauch, Ph.D.

Learning Objectives

By the end of this chapter, readers will be able to:

- Describe current trends in the prevalence rates of people with mental illness and co-occurring substance use disorders who are involved with the criminal justice system

- Describe major policy frameworks related to reducing justice system involvement for people with substance use disorders or other mental illness

- Delineate the roles of advocacy from the patient level and the system level in effecting change for patients involved with the justice system

- Describe how to advocate on behalf of patients to reduce the likelihood of their involvement in the criminal justice system

Setting the Stage: Advocacy at Different Levels for Patients in Criminal Justice Settings
Patient-Level Advocacy

Case Example

Mr. O, a patient with schizophrenia complicated by a co-occurring substance use disorder, is admitted to a community hospital. He has had 10 previous hospitalizations, including one in the state hospital after he was found incompetent to stand trial, in addition to four criminal charges of assault with jail time within the last 4 years. He has gone on and off psychotropic medications. This hospitalization, like many of his others, was precipitated by a worsening of psychiatric symptoms, including hearing voices and believing that neighbors are monitoring his actions, which has resulted in intermittent aggressive episodes.

On the inpatient unit, Mr. O is disorganized and exhibits behavioral dysregulation. He breaks lighting on the unit and then has an assaultive episode. After the assaultive episode, Mr. O's team wants to move quickly toward discharging him. Some of the staff are asking the psychiatrist to facilitate Mr. O's arrest because they believe this course of action would make the most sense as a way to "manage" him.

The psychiatrist reviews Mr. O's history and sees that he has done remarkably well in the past when taking clozapine. However, Mr. O then lost his housing, moved to a new community, ran out of his medication, and destabilized. Since then, his hospitalizations have been too short to try clozapine again. After considering this information, the psychiatrist advocates for Mr. O's clinical needs and for the hospital to refrain from pressing charges, despite damage to the unit. The psychiatrist determines that Mr. O would be best served by another proper medication trial and more time to stabilize. The psychiatrist makes this case to the medical director and hospital administrators, who agree with the plan.

In this example of patient-level advocacy for an individual who often engages with both the mental health and criminal justice systems, the psychiatrist combined his clinical judgment, his knowledge of the mental health–criminal justice interface, and the tenets of patient-level advocacy (see Chapter 5, "Patient-Level Advocacy") to act in the patient's best interests, while still being sensitive to staff concerns. He saw in the patient's record a history of successful community-based treatment. He was well aware of the evidence that "managing" mental illness with arrests does not work. Also, he understood that the proper channel for advocacy was to speak with hospital administration because it was clear that there was disagreement among the treatment team members.

Patient-level advocacy in and of itself requires psychiatrists to gather facts about each case as well as evidence from the literature, in addition to understanding which advocacy approaches might be helpful. In work with patients who have criminal justice system involvement, patient-level advocacy further requires a working knowledge of the complexities of the mental health–criminal justice interface.

Systems-Level Advocacy

Case Example

In Massachusetts prior to 2016, women with substance use disorders could be civilly committed for their substance use to the women's prison, the Massachusetts Correctional Institution at Framingham. There had been earlier litigation addressing this practice (the settlement agreement mandate in *Hinckley v. Fair* 1990) but no lasting traction on change. When a new governor came into office in 2015 and new leadership was appointed at the Massachusetts Executive Office of Health and Human Services, new opportunities arose to advocate for moving women from a setting of incarceration to a more treatment-focused setting.

Case Example *(continued)*

Seeing these opportunities, advocates advanced on several fronts at the same time. Legal advocates pursued new litigation, a team of female legislators took up a cause of action, and outside advocates (including chapter author D.M.) initiated dialogue across stakeholder groups and with government leaders. Internal to the state's health and human services agencies, a team of professionals, led by a psychiatrist (chapter author D.P.), was tasked with identifying a plan of treatment that could provide the needed care for these individuals. Through this multifaceted system-level advocacy work, further dialogue ensued between judges, correctional officials, and consumers. With changes in legislation, allocation of funding, and the development of a program model, Massachusetts was ultimately able to end the practice of incarcerating civilly committed women. The Women's Recovery From Addictions Program was fully operational by February 2016, and the governor subsequently signed a bill changing the prior statute to disallow these civil commitments to the prison (Anderson 2016).

This program is an example of systems-level advocacy that spans boundaries and engages multiple stakeholder groups, which is a common and often necessary way to effect change at the mental health–criminal justice interface. The activity represents a combination of external and internal systems-level advocacy and illustrates the positive potential of psychiatric involvement in systems reform.

The psychiatrist and colleagues in this case worked with the advocacy community as well as systems-level administration to develop a treatment model that could meet the needs of the patient population. Knowledge of the criminal justice system and civil commitment processes for stakeholders was instrumental in driving the systems change. In addition, the psychiatrist and others involved in planning engaged professional networks to connect with colleagues who would be interested in this work and to recruit staff who could provide the women with appropriate care. To ultimately effectuate the systems change, the psychiatrist also partnered with administrative staff, who were able to weigh in and work together to create a balanced system of care, as well as legislators, who were aware of the need for funding of such a service.

Other psychiatrists interested in this type of work would do well to develop an area of focus and to work closely within relevant organizations, such as the local psychiatric society, to develop the necessary subject matter expertise as well as professional connections to do boundary-spanning advocacy work. In these ways, they will be able to stay abreast of opportunities for systems change and to be a part of making these changes happen.

Background and Overview of the Issues

It is by now well established that there is an overrepresentation of individuals with substance use disorders or other mental illness in our nation's courts, jails, and prisons. Studies have found, for example, that slightly over 25% of recipients of public mental health services have experienced at least one arrest (Fisher et al. 2006) or have been recently involved in the justice system (Swanson et al. 2013). In another often-cited study, Steadman et al. (2009) reported that nearly 17% of people in jails have serious mental illness, a rate that is at least three to six times higher than the rate of serious mental illness in the general population, and this still might be an underestimate.

The morbidity and mortality of individuals with behavioral health needs in the justice system are serious public health concerns. Among incarcerated individuals, the rates of serious, disabling, or chronic diseases, including co-occurring behavioral health conditions, are higher than those found among the general population. Incarcerated individuals have a 40% greater incidence of chronic health conditions, four times the rate of infectious diseases, and more than four times the rate of serious mental illness, with 72% of individuals with a serious mental illness having a co-occurring substance use disorder (Maruschak et al. 2016). Even after release, individuals with a history of criminal justice system involvement are at greater risk of mortality. In one recent study comparing the opioid overdose death risk of individuals released from North Carolina prisons with that of the general North Carolina population (Ranapurwala et al. 2018), the risk was 40 times higher for the former inmates at 2 weeks after release and 11 times higher at 1 year after release. Those former inmates with an increased risk of opioid overdose death included individuals who had been identified as receiving mental health or substance use treatment while in prison.

Individuals with substance use disorders or other mental illness are also at an elevated risk for criminal recidivism. In fact, the highest rate of recidivism for any group of released jail or prison inmates is 68%, found among individuals with co-occurring behavioral health conditions (Wilson et al. 2011). In a New York City study of more than 10,000 releases, conducted between 2008 and 2013, there were 473 individuals who recidivated more than 18 times. Of those individuals, 85% were incarcerated for misdemeanors or violations of probation or parole, often related to their behavioral health conditions. Twenty-one percent of those individuals had a serious mental illness, and 99.4% had a substance use disorder (NYC Mayor's Office of Criminal Justice 2014; Subramanian et al. 2015).

Numerous systems failures and challenges and complex policy decisions have contributed to how these statistics have unfolded (Lamb and Weinberger 2017; Pinals 2014). Taken together, they support the argument that advocacy is needed for individuals with behavioral health needs and current or past criminal justice system involvement to ensure their appropriate care and treatment across all settings and diversion from the justice system when possible and safe.

Individuals who cross between the mental health and criminal justice systems require careful attention and multiple interventions if the goal is to reduce the penetration of individuals with mental health conditions into the justice system (Pinals 2014). They represent perhaps the most vulnerable among the vulnerable, beset with disparities upon disparities, because of the disproportionate risk of criminal justice involvement for individuals with mental illness and the challenges posed by the settings in which they are incarcerated. Even the U.S. Supreme Court has commented on the "double stigma" for individuals in both the criminal justice and mental health systems (Baxstrom v. Herold 1966).

Implementing solutions is challenging for a host of reasons, not the least of which is the very disenfranchised nature of the population, which often lacks sufficient advocacy. Sound solutions would require a collaborative, multiply dimensioned approach to redirect the numerous individuals with mental illness out of the justice system and into treatment settings. A large part of the challenge in fixing these problems is finding the right voices to advocate for the needs of these individuals. Informed advocates are needed to examine these individuals' conditions of confinement and their journeys from the handcuffs of arrest to the recesses of prisons and then back out into community settings—only all too often to face homelessness, substance use, and victimization before a return to the justice system. Furthermore, to improve outcomes for this population and for individual persons with mental illness involved with the justice system, advocacy at both the patient level and systems level is needed, as illustrated by the preceding case examples. (More information on the fundamental principles of patient-level advocacy can be found in Chapter 5, "Patient-Level Advocacy," and principles of systems-level advocacy can be found in Chapter 6, "Organizational Advocacy," and Chapter 7, "Legislative Advocacy.")

To tease apart the areas of needed advocacy and provide an overview, we first describe some systems frameworks that have been conceptualized to more closely examine the complex interplay of mental illness and the justice system, from police to courts to jails and prisons. We then discuss, with case examples, several ways in which advocacy has been used to address this population's needs. By examining the multiple approaches to advocacy for this population, we provide models that can be used at both the patient level and the systems level to help inspire change for those individuals at this justice intersection. Of note, in this chapter we focus on the interface between the adult criminal legal system and individuals with mental illness. Much could be said about similar issues for youth in the juvenile justice system, but that is beyond the scope of this chapter.

Advocacy Across the Criminal Justice Continuum

The interface between the criminal justice and mental health systems can present unique challenges for advocates because not all stakeholders view improving access to care as a reform priority, and public safety mandates sometimes overshadow other agendas. Yet, even though courts, judges, and correctional systems are oriented toward their own objectives, there is increasing interest in partnering across branches of government and across agencies to turn the tide of criminalization of substance use disorders and other mental illness. These efforts require careful balancing of stakeholder interests because the varied stakeholders have differing opinions about maximizing autonomy and self-reliance, differing conceptualizations of budget and policy priorities, and different vantage points from which they assess which outcomes can be mutually desired and shared.

That said, opportunities to advocate on behalf of individuals with behavioral health conditions abound at this time, in some ways more so than during prior eras. Disparities in access to treatment and in social determinants of health, as drivers of both incarceration and difficulties once incarcerated, can be a source of grave disability, institutional disorder, and human suffering—conditions that are being increasingly recognized as ripe for change through advocacy. However, to effectively advocate across so many systems at the mental health–criminal justice interface, it is important to first have a clear conceptual understanding of how to approach advocacy in this complex continuum.

Model Advocacy Frameworks

At the intersection of the mental health and criminal justice systems, there have been two major frameworks that have helped push advocacy agendas forward in an organized manner. Knowledge of these frameworks is useful when considering approaches to advocacy at either the individual or systems levels.

Model Advocacy Framework 1: The Sequential Intercept Model

The Sequential Intercept Model, illustrated in Figure 20–1, is a framework that was originally developed in 2006 by Munetz and Griffin (2006) and then further developed by researchers at the Substance Abuse and Mental Health Services Administration's (SAMHSA's) GAINS Center (Abreu et al. 2017). (GAINS is an acronym for **g**ather, **as**sess, **i**ntegrate, **n**etwork, and **s**timulate.) The framework posits that there are a series of opportunities, or *intercepts*, during which people with behavioral health conditions can be identified and diverted out of the justice system and into treatment and that working across these intercepts can decrease the penetration of these individuals into the criminal justice system. The model has evolved to include the following intercept components, which apply to individuals in the community with mental health, substance use, or co-occurring behavioral health conditions who are at high risk for criminal justice involvement.

- *Intercept 0 (community services):* individuals exhibit exacerbations of the symptoms of their illness(es), behavioral dysregulation, and/ or role dysfunction
- *Intercept 1 (law enforcement):* individuals engage with 911 first-responder services and/or local law enforcement authorities during a period of crisis, putting them at risk for arrest and incarceration
- *Intercept 2 (initial detention and court hearings):* as a result of contact with the police during a crisis, individuals find themselves detained in jail, awaiting a first court appearance, and then appearing before a judge for either a misdemeanor or a felony charge
- *Intercept 3 (jails or courts):* individuals either 1) have appeared already in court and are in jail awaiting trial or are in jail or prison under sentence for adjudicated misdemeanors or felonies or 2) may be under the direction of a specialty court (mental health court, drug court, homeless court, veterans court) or dispositional court as a result of diversion plans
- *Intercept 4 (reentry stage):* individuals are planning for release from jail or prison
- *Intercept 5 (community corrections:* individuals have been released and are under the direction of probation or parole, the community supervising authorities for the justice system

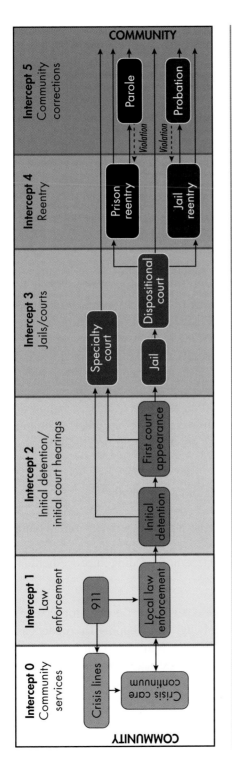

FIGURE 20–1. **Sequential intercept model.**

Source. Reprinted from Abreu D, Parker TW, Noether CD, et al.: Revising the paradigm for jail diversion for people with mental and substance use disorders: intercept 0. *Behavioral Sciences and the Law*, 35:5–6, 380–395, 2017. Available at: https://doi.org/10.1002/bsl.2300. © 2019 Policy Research Associates, Inc. Used with permission.

At each intercept point, there are multiple opportunities to advocate and intervene for people with behavioral health conditions to increase the rates of treatment, reduce the risk of incarceration, mitigate the time and effects of incarceration, maximize appropriate access to quality treatment during confinement, reduce the rates of recidivism, support successful completion of probation or parole, and improve rates of recovery.

Model Advocacy Framework 2: The Stepping Up Initiative

The Stepping Up Initiative (https://stepuptogether.org), supported by the American Psychiatric Association Foundation, the Council of State Governments Justice Center, and the National Association of Counties and promoted by numerous other stakeholders, has inspired 503 counties at the time of this writing (https://stepuptogether.org/what-you-can-do) to sign resolutions indicating their county-level commitments to reducing the numbers of people with mental illness in their county jails. As the number of counties signing these resolutions continues to grow across the United States, this initiative holds significant promise to create further system reform. Using the Stepping Up framework, counties agree to examine several core questions to identify the baseline numbers of individuals with mental illness in their jails, as well as data systems and methods that can help reduce those numbers. The questions include the following (https://stepuptogether.org/toolkit):

1. Is our leadership committed?
2. Do we conduct timely screening and assessments?
3. Do we have baseline data?
4. Have we conducted a comprehensive process analysis and inventory of services?
5. Have we prioritized policy, practice, and funding improvements?
6. Do we track progress?

This type of organizing framework helps to set the stage for further interagency dialogue and problem solving. The Stepping Up model easily ties into other frameworks, including the Sequential Intercept Model. Newer offshoots of Stepping Up include the designation of county innovators who are attempting to do the data work that the model calls for, as well as consideration of the Stepping Up model at the state and national levels.

Approaches to Advocacy

Together, these frameworks can give advocates a road map for strategizing, problem solving, and finding solutions. The approaches to advocacy will vary depending on a number of factors associated with the basic intercept points (that also tie into Stepping Up data), including the following:

- the number of individuals at each intercept point
- the length of time those individuals remain at a particular intercept, available to advocacy and intervention
- the degree of access that the potential advocate has at any particular intercept point
- the authority available to advocate or intervene
- the availability of services to offer the individual
- the degree to which the various systems coordinate and communicate to provide actual alternatives to the criminal justice system

The interaction of these factors, combined with the methods of advocacy used, will determine the impact made at either or both the individual or systems levels.

Effecting Change Through Boundary-Spanning Advocacy

Even with the frameworks discussed in the previous section, advocacy for psychiatric patients in criminal justice settings is far from straightforward, especially when it is focused at the systems level and requires the engagement of multiple stakeholders. Psychiatrists advocating at the systems level must define a need on which their advocacy efforts are focused; design a solution; set an advocacy agenda; and gather the support of executive, judicial, and legislative decision makers who also are interested in the criminal justice and mental health interface. Additionally, because many solutions require funding, attracting philanthropic support to finance the demonstration, evaluation, and proof-of-concept phases of system changes can be critical. Advocacy for individuals with substance use or other mental health conditions who have criminal justice system involvement often requires boundary spanning, meaning working across traditional service lines between the behavioral health system and the justice system. The following subsection provides an example of boundary-spanning advocacy (see also the systems-level advocacy vignette at the beginning of this chapter).

Worcester Initiative for Supported Reentry Program

The Worcester Initiative for Supported Reentry program in Worcester, Massachusetts, is an "in-reach" (vs. outreach) effort at intercept 4 in which clinicians from Advocates, a Massachusetts-based comprehensive community behavioral health organization, are embedded at the Worcester County Jail to work with inmates (Advocates 2019). They work with the inmates for a year or more prior to release, not only on benefits advocacy but also on clinical assessment, treatment plan development, and treatment intervention in the jail. Their efforts include integrated reentry planning to ensure continuity of treatment, case management, and housing and community support services on release.

A Brandeis University evaluation of the program, covering 166 men on superior court probation, found positive outcomes, including that these individuals have approximately one-third the recidivism rate of similar probationers not in the program; the average cost per person is $5,800 per year, compared with $53,040 for incarceration; all participants were housed and not homeless; three out of five have had continuous employment for at least 6 months; 90% have health insurance; and 96% of those who were referred to substance use disorder treatment accessed recommended services (Brolin 2016).

This model reflects a program of advocacy spanning across traditionally siloed operations. A psychiatrist working as a systems-level advocate to address the mental health needs of incarcerated individuals and reduce their recidivism on release would potentially benefit from knowledge about this type of evaluation data and the methods used to assist the patients. Such knowledge could be used as proof-of-concept information to drive further change and, in combination with boundary-spanning advocacy techniques, would prepare psychiatrist-advocates to be a part of the solution in their own jurisdictions.

Other Types of Advocacy at the Mental Health–Criminal Justice Interface

In addition to patient-level advocacy and boundary-spanning, systems-level advocacy, discussed previously, we describe two additional types of advocacy—legislative advocacy and media advocacy—that have a history of success in promoting change for patients traversing the mental health and criminal justice continuum. (For more information on these types of advocacy, see Chapter 7, "Legislative Advocacy," and Chapter 10, "Engaging the Popular Media.")

Legislative Advocacy

Federal Level

Legislative advocacy at the federal level can influence the national policy agenda to prioritize the population of individuals at the intersection of the behavioral health and criminal justice systems. For example, the American Psychiatric Association and a coalition of entities interested in behavioral health were very active in advocating for the 21st Century Cures Act (P.L. 114-255; U.S. Food and Drug Administration 2018), which President Obama signed in 2016 at the end of his administration. The act called for several elements related to the mental health–justice system interface, including codifying into law the Sequential Intercept Model (see subsection "Model Advocacy Framework 1" earlier in the chapter) and focusing efforts and funding on jail diversion. The American Psychiatric Association was also actively involved in crafting and passing the Excellence in Mental Health Act of 2014 (S.264/H.R. 1263; U.S. Congress 2013), which called for the establishment of Certified Community Behavioral Health Clinics (CCBHCs) to provide integrated mental health and addiction treatment in communities across the country. CCBHCs serve as a treatment resource for diversion (intercept 0) and reentry (intercept 4) services to individuals at risk for or having criminal justice involvement. In 2018, the first year, $100 million was appropriated for CCBHCs, followed by $150 million in 2019 and $200 million in 2020.

An earlier example of the effective roles played by psychiatrist-advocates in shaping federal legislation to address the unmet treatment needs of prisoners with behavioral health conditions concerns a single passage in the Second Chance Act of 2007 (P.L. 110-199). Pursuant to research conducted on the treatment of addiction by a psychiatrist and principal investigator at the University of Pennsylvania, the Second Chance Act funded, among other items, the study of depot naltrexone for treatment of heroin-dependent offenders. The legislative language was crafted by a young psychiatrist, trained at the university, who was serving as a psychiatric fellow in a senator's office.

Local Level

Legislative advocacy at the local level can also be powerful. In Washtenaw County, Michigan, for example, a host of community challenges involving the justice-involved population led to growing awareness of the population of individuals with mental illness in the local jail. As a result, the local community mental health director partnered with the sheriff to hold a Sequential Intercept Mapping workshop. With the participation of psychiatric leadership in the area's major departments of psychiatry and their designees, the workshop revealed several areas that could benefit from further improvement. Solutions over the years (some of which predated and inspired the workshop) included training patrol officers with a specialized mental health curriculum, expanding mental health services in the jail, and pursuing a local millage to help fund other services downstream. The millage was successfully passed on a ballot initiative, with the development of an oversight mechanism to ensure that the moneys are appropriately distributed for mental health and public safety needs.

Role of Media as a Catalyst to Advocacy

Media attention to issues at the mental health–criminal justice interface can help to move the advocacy agenda forward in a powerful way. Two examples are presented below.

Rikers Island

A *New York Times* exposé of inmate violence and high rates of inmate mental illness at Rikers Island, a New York City jail complex, created a storm of controversy (Schwirtz 2014), contributing to the formation of a commission and a restructuring of the clinical and correctional services at the facility. Even with these reforms, however, media attention continued to swirl, and political forces ultimately called for the closure of the facility. Further reform was fueled after an independent commission was formed to evaluate the entire justice system in New York City (see A More Just NYC, www.morejustnyc.org).

Bridgewater State Hospital

Bridgewater State Hospital, a Massachusetts psychiatric facility, was known for many years for the fact that it provided secure treatment to individuals with forensic status within the state's Department of Correction. This practice was contrary to that of every other state, in which forensic patients, even those with secure treatment needs, were served in mental health systems. The impact of the media can clearly be seen in the advocacy efforts for this practice to end.

Atrocities at Bridgewater were revealed publicly in *Titicut Follies*, a 1968 documentary by Fredrick Wiseman. After this media attention, the facility came under fire repeatedly over the years for the poor care and treatment delivered to "inmates." Litigation in the 1980s resulted in the establishment of a commission that ultimately recommended system improvements, while keeping Bridgewater State Hospital under the operational authority of the Department of Correction.

When *Boston Globe* journalists (some of whom were from the newspaper's Spotlight investigative team) learned of alleged patient abuse in more recent years, controversy over the facility again swirled, and the media attention stoked further attempts at reform (Rezendes 2015). As legal advocates and patient advocates (including chapter author D.M.) began to take action, several strategies came together, including class action litigation, interagency review of practices using psychiatric (chapter author D.P.) and psychological expertise, and political pressure with important input from high-level stakeholders including the governor and the state secretary of Health and Human Services. Through multifaceted action, correctional officers were eventually removed from roles involving direct "security" management of patient interactions, and a comprehensive, clinically competent staff was installed to operate the treatment program (Governor's Press Office 2017). The *Boston Globe* reported on the success of these reforms (Rezendes 2017).

In sum, there were several exposés of conditions at Bridgewater State Hospital, dating back 50 years to the release of *Titicut Follies*. These were often followed by some action to improve care. A lesson learned from this history is that system reform is generally not a "one-and-done" type of activity. There is always more work to do and further improvements to be made, noted even at the time of this writing. This does not mean, however, that efforts to improve the conditions of confinement for individuals with mental illness in the justice system or efforts to divert them out of the justice system are for naught. Incremental change for the better is still critical change and can lead to further enhancements that ultimately move to solve some of our society's most difficult challenges. The role of the media as a catalyst at Bridgewater State Hospital highlights how the media helped push forward system reform, as well as the important role that psychiatrist-advocates and allied advocates play in trying to achieve that incremental change.

Potential Barriers to Effective Advocacy

Advocacy is not easy and requires concentrated attention to key issues, awareness of shifting priorities and needs, and a commitment to a focused agenda. Potential barriers to successful advocacy at the mental health–criminal justice interface can be daunting.

One such barrier is the *commitment of leadership* to advocacy around any particular topic. A challenge in advocating for individuals with mental illness in the justice system is that leaders in policy development may not consider this area their top priority for advocacy. For example, a leader aiming to help address critical gaps and shortages in the mental health system may not feel that a justice-focused agenda will impact sufficiently on the system to make this a top-priority area. In large administrations with complex functions and competing priorities, not all leaders are aligned with helping underserved and justice-involved individuals. Not all public safety leaders, for example, go into their roles with an idea that mental health issues will be a priority. Elected officials running on a public safety platform might find mental health issues too politically charged to take up. Thus, without sustained commitment from leadership, advocacy for the criminal justice–involved mental health consumer may take a back burner.

A second significant barrier in advocacy is the *need to balance interests with available resources across systems*, in a world where there are never enough resources to meet all needs. For example, in correctional settings, mental health conditions—especially those that require psychotropic medications—can be expensive and chronic, and the associated costs pull from other programs such as education or even basic security needs. Similarly, individuals in the mental health system who have significant justice histories might require approaches and additional staff that have expertise in criminal justice involvement, as was seen with the establishment of a model referred to as forensic assertive community treatment teams (Cuddeback et al. 2013). Although each of these systems may have a will to produce better results, resources are necessary across systems to do so, and decision makers may or may not prioritize the mental health–criminal justice interface as they make those resource allocation decisions.

Workforce shortages are a third major barrier to overcome in this context. Only a subset of psychiatric or mental health trainees will choose to work with the criminal justice population, and by far most general practitioners would rather avoid this population altogether. When staffing is limited and at a critical mass, advocating for more services becomes even more difficult.

Fourth, advocates who are willing to take up social justice issues might need specific *interpersonal and organizational skills* as well as *specialized knowledge* to effectively advocate for the particular needs of individuals with mental illness in the justice system. Although advocates can gain some of the necessary skills and knowledge by going to trainings on topics related to the mental health and justice systems, a significant investment of time and energy is necessary to become an expert at this interface. Furthermore, because these systems cross over into housing, child welfare, and other services, advocates also need to have a wealth of information about other systems to take informed positions and make cogent policy recommendations that will yield the positive outcomes desired. Well-trained and well-suited individuals who have familiarity with these complex systems are necessary to be the agents of change.

Fifth, there are *legislative and regulatory barriers* to effecting change. As described in the case involving civil commitment of women to the Massachusetts Correctional Institution at Framingham (see subsection "Systems-Level Advocacy" earlier in chapter), statutory boundaries needed to shift to ensure that women civilly committed for substance use treatment would not be sent to the women's prison. In another example, there has been increasing discussion about bail reform through legislative change as a targeted strategy to help remove some of the silting in the justice system of individuals who are confined merely because of financial inability to post bail or bond (e.g., Kentucky bail reform; Ragsdale 2019). Without reform of existing practices, such change could not occur, and individuals with mental illness would succumb to these legislative barriers.

Regulatory barriers, though somewhat easier to change than laws, still have their own rigidity and complexity. For example, a great deal has been written about the challenges posed by the Health Insurance Portability and Accountability Act of 1996 (HIPAA; P.L. 104-191) and 42 CFR Part 2, Confidentiality of Substance Use Disorder Patient Records (www.ecfr.gov/cgi-bin/text-idx?rgn=div5;node=42%3A1.0.1.1.2), to clear communication between treatment providers and justice system officials, despite the fact that such communication could actually assist with moving people into the proper treatment system when appropriate (Quantum Units Education 2019). Additional regulatory and statutory barriers can inadvertently silt people more toward the justice system by setting bars too high to access care or by developing protocols that limit options available for systems to manage individuals who are frequently dropping out of care and community supports.

Finally, advocacy at the mental health–criminal justice interface encounters the *core political barriers seen with disenfranchised populations.* Unless a legislator or policy maker has a personal stake in the outcome, there may not be the political will to help a stigmatized population that does not have a powerful constituency. For politicians, public perception on stances can make or break careers. Fear and stigma associated with individuals with mental illness who are involved in the justice system can provide enough negative incentive for politicians to eschew even the most basic of causes for this group of people. Unions that represent the vast numbers of staff working in jails, prisons, and state hospitals can be another challenge for politicians, who are trying to leverage popular support and may not wish to tackle issues that result in pushback from labor and trade associations.

Educating Trainees on Advocacy for Justice-Involved Persons With Mental Illness

Trainees within psychiatry may not have exposure to advocacy. At the patient level, they will hopefully see their supervisors advocating for the needs of their patients, but senior psychiatrists may have their own personal views about justice-involved patients that may or may not reflect an advocate's stance. As such, it is important to expose residents to a variety of attending physicians to cross-pollinate ideas and help the residents settle into their own views. Also, basic education on the very significant challenges patients face when involved with the criminal justice system is important to limit the formation of bias and stereotypes within trainees and early-career psychiatrists.

In addition to having exposure to mentors, it is important for psychiatrists to tour facilities to gain a greater understanding of their patients' experiences with conditions of confinement. This may include tours of community settings, jails, prisons, and state forensic hospitals. Training should also include some formal exposure to advocacy, advocacy theory, and advocacy in practice. Examples of how advocacy training could be developed are given in the American Psychiatric Association's resource document on this topic (Kennedy and Vance 2018). (See also Chapter 8, "Education as Advocacy," for more information on developing advocacy curricula.)

Formal training on advocacy, however, might not include specifics about the mental health–criminal justice interface. For this area of interest, trainees would benefit from understanding the landscape of organizations that participate in advocacy efforts in this space (see section "Examples of Organizations That Work at the Mental Health–Criminal Justice Interface" later in this chapter). This can help a prospective advocate stay abreast of the latest activities on particular topics of interest, as well as identify potential advocacy partners to strengthen the development of advocacy coalitions. The natural affinity groups often align through years of experience working on particular issues, but changes over time create the need to keep following the work of these participating groups and to extend friendly welcomes to promising new advocates who emerge on the scene where established advocates have already identified their "space."

Conclusion

Individuals with mental illness and substance use disorders in the criminal justice system are some of the most disenfranchised and stigmatized of populations. Training on the justice and mental health systems and their intersection can be one way to learn about these complex systems and how to advocate for positive change. Policy frameworks for advocacy are useful when setting an organizing agenda with which to tackle both local smaller issues and larger systemic barriers in order to foster prevention and diversion from the justice system. Advocacy for individuals at the mental health–criminal justice interface is critical and can have profound impacts on the quality of individuals' lives and their basic longevity, health, and well-being. This population has not always received a sympathetic ear and is often among the most stigmatized and disenfranchised of populations. As individuals with mental illness and substance use disorders enter into the justice system, they may navigate between state and county systems and providers, and risks of disrupted episodes of care and poor outcomes are high. Psychiatrists have a crucial role to play in addressing the needs of these individuals, as for any patient in their offices. To advocate effectively, partnerships with a variety of stakeholders are key. Working through whatever prejudice and stigma exist surrounding the justice-involved population is a first step in moving forward.

Examples of Organizations That Work at the Mental Health–Criminal Justice Interface

American Psychiatric Association: www.psychiatry.org/psychiatrists/advocacy

Bureau of Justice Assistance: www.bja.gov/default.aspx

Council of State Governments: www.csg.org
Mental Health America: www.mhanational.org
National Alliance on Mental Illness: www.nami.org
National Association of State Mental Health Program Directors:
www.nasmhpd.org
Policy Resource Associates and SAMHSA GAINS Center:
www.prainc.com and www.samhsa.gov/gains-center
Substance Abuse and Mental Health Services Administration:
www.samhsa.gov

References

Abreu D, Parker TW, Noether CD, et al: Revising the paradigm for jail diversion for people with mental and substance use disorders: intercept 0. Behav Sci Law 35(5–6):380–395, 2017 29034504

Advocates: Worcester Initiative for Supported Reentry (WISR). Framingham, MA, Advocates, 2019. Available at: www.advocates.org/services/worcester-initiative-supported-reentry-wisr. Accessed September 4, 2019.

Anderson T: Female addicts given an alternative to prison. Boston Globe, February 4, 2016. Available at: www.bostonglobe.com/metro/2016/02/04/taunton-unit-will-give-women-addicts-alternative-prison/i4Va3TEE5ARiQLtJYft6iJ/story.html. Accessed September 4, 2019.

Baxstrom v. Herold, 383 U.S. 107 (1966). No. 219. Argued December 9, 1965. Decided February 23, 1966, 383 U.S. 107

Brolin M: WISR: Results Oriented Status Report. Waltham, MA, Brandeis University, 2016

Cuddeback GS, Wright D, Bisig NG: Characteristics of participants in jail diversion and prison reentry programs: implications for forensic ACT. Psychiatr Serv 64(10):1043–1046, 2013 24081403

Fisher WH, Roy-Bujnowski KM, Grudzinskas AJ Jr, et al: Patterns and prevalence of arrest in a statewide cohort of mental health care consumers. Psychiatr Serv 57(11):1623–1628, 2006 17085611

Governor's Press Office: Baker-Polito administration signs contract to boost patient care at Bridgewater State Hospital (press release). Boston, Commonwealth of Massachusetts, February 7, 2017. Available at: www.mass.gov/news/baker-polito-administration-signs-contract-to-boost-patient-care-at-bridgewater-state-hospital. Accessed September 4, 2019.

Hinckley v. Fair, No. C.A. 88-064, Mass. Sup. Ct. (1990)

Kennedy KG, Vance MC: Resource Document: Advocacy Teaching in Psychiatry Residency Training Programs. Washington, DC, American Psychiatric Association, 2018

Lamb HR, Weinberger LE: Understanding and treating offenders with serious mental illness in public sector mental health. Behav Sci Law 35(4):303–318, 2017 28612397

Maruschak LM, Berzofsky M, Unangst J: Medical Problems of State and Federal Prisoners and Jail Inmates, 2011. Washington, DC, Bureau of Justice Statistics, 2016

Munetz MR, Griffin PA: Use of the Sequential Intercept Model as an approach to decriminalization of people with serious mental illness. Psychiatr Serv 57(4):544–549, 2006 16603751

NYC Mayor's Office of Criminal Justice: Mayor's Task Force on Behavioral Health and Criminal Justice. New York, NYC Mayor's Office of Criminal Justice, 2014. https://criminaljustice.cityofnewyork.us/reports/mayors-task-force-on-behavioral-health-and-criminal-justice. Accessed September 4, 2019.

Pinals DA: Forensic services, public mental health policy, and financing: charting the course ahead. J Am Acad Psychiatry Law 42(1):7–19, 2014 24618515

Quantum Units Education: Information sharing between criminal justice and healthcare communities to enhance public safety. San Luis Obispo, CA, Quantum Units Education, 2019. Available at: www.quantumunitsed.com/get-material.php?id=504. Accessed September 4, 2019.

Ragsdale T: Bail reform advocates make push for change in Kentucky. WDRB.com, January 22, 2019. Available at: https://www.wdrb.com/news/bail-reform-advocates-make-push-for-change-in-kentucky/article_e3e62912–1e87–11e9-aa00–6310a27c714c.html. Accessed September 4, 2019.

Ranapurwala SI, Shanahan ME, Alexandridis AA, et al: Opioid overdose mortality among former North Carolina inmates: 2000–2015. Am J Public Health 108(9):1207–1213, 2018 30024795

Rezendes M: Bridgewater State Hospital patients sue care providers. Boston Globe, January 29, 2015. Available at: www.bostonglobe.com/metro/2015/01/29/bridgewater-state-hospital-patients-sue-care-providers-for-civil-rights-violations/GmHSWl3ysRtkU6HxxUjKFN/story.html. Accessed September 4, 2019.

Rezendes M: Humane care given a place at state's harshest hospital. Boston Globe, September 9, 2017. Available at: www.bostonglobe.com/metro/2017/09/09/humane-treatment-comes-last-bridgewater-state-hospital-where-prisoners-have-become-persons-served/YXvoxK2XUpSQub-wV8E4X2L/story.html. Accessed December 16, 2019.

Schwirtz M: Rikers Island struggles with a surge of violence and mental illness. New York Times, March 18, 2014. Available at: https://www.nytimes.com/2014/03/19/nyregion/rise-in-mental-illness-and-violence-at-vast-jail-on-rikers-island.html?_r=1. Accessed September 4, 2019.

Steadman HJ, Osher FC, Robbins PC, et al: Prevalence of serious mental illness among jail inmates. Psychiatr Serv 60(6):761–765, 2009 19487344

Subramanian R, Delaney R, Roberts S, et al: Incarceration's front door: the misuse of jail in America. Vera Institute of Justice, 2015. Available at: www.safety andjusticechallenge.org/wp-content/uploads/2015/01/incarcerations-front-door-report.pdf. Accessed September 4, 2019.

Swanson JW, Frisman LK, Robertson AG, et al: Costs of criminal justice involvement among persons with serious mental illness in Connecticut. Psychiatr Serv 64(7):630–637, 2013 23494058

U.S. Congress: S.264: Excellence in Mental Health Act. February 7, 2013. Available at: https://www.congress.gov/bill/113th-congress/senate-bill/264. Accessed September 4, 2019.

U.S. Food and Drug Administration: 21st Century Cures Act (PL-114-255). March 29, 2018. Available at: https://www.fda.gov/regulatory-information/selected-amendments-fdc-act/21st-century-cures-act. Accessed September 4, 2019.

Wilson AB, Draineb J, Hadley T, et al: Examining the impact of mental illness and substance use on recidivism in a county jail. Int J Law Psychiatry 34(4):264–268, 2011 21839518

Index

Page numbers printed in **boldface** type refer to tables, figures, or boxes.